D0275013

Current Topics in Pathology
86

Managing Editors

C.L. Berry E. Grundmann

C.L. Berry (Ed.)

The Pathology of Devices

Contributors

M.M. Black · I. Bos · C.H. Buckley · A. Coumbe
J.N. Cox · G. Dasbach · P.J. Drury · T.R. Graham
C.M. Hill · W. Konertz · U. Löhrs · K.-M. Müller
M.D. O'Hara · H.H. Scheld

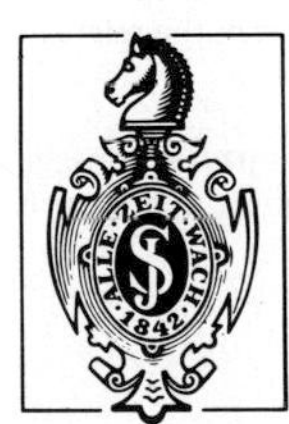

Springer-Verlag
Berlin Heidelberg New York
London Paris Tokyo
Hong Kong Barcelona
Budapest

SIR COLIN BERRY DSC, MD, PhD, FRCPath, FRCP, FFPM
Professor of Morbid Anatomy
The London Hospital Medical College
University of London
London El 1BB
England

With 156 Figures, Some in Colour, and 9 Tables

ISBN 3-540-54393-7 Springer-Verlag Berlin Heidelberg NewYork
ISBN 0-387-54393-7 Springer-Verlag NewYork Berlin Heidelberg

Library of Congress Cataloging-in-Publication Data. The Pathology of devices / C.L. Berry, ed.: contributors, M.M. Black . . . [et al.], p. cm.— (Current topics in pathology: v. 86) Includes bibliographical references and index. ISBN 0-387-54393-7 (New York). —ISBN 3-540-54393-7 (Berlin) 1. Biocompatibility. 2. Medical instruments and apparatus—Toxicology. I. Berry, Colin Leonard, 1937– . II. Black, Martin M. III. Series. RB1. E6 vol. 86 [R857.M3] 616.07 s—dc20 [610'.28] 93-32868

Printed in Germany

Typesetting: Thomson Press (India) Ltd., New Delhi

25/3130/SPS – 5 4 3 2 1 0 — Printed on acid-free paper

List of Contributors

BLACK, M.M., Prof. Dr	Department of Medical Physics and Clinical Technology, University of Sheffield, Royal Hallamshire Hospital, Glossop Road, Sheffield S10 2JF, UK
BOS, I., Dr.	Institute of Pathology, Medical University of Lübeck, Ratzeburger Allee 160, 23562 Lübeck, Germany
BUCKLEY, C.H., Dr.	Department of Gynaecological Pathology, St. Mary's Hospital for Women and Children, Whitworth Park, Manchester M13 0JH, UK
COUMBE, A., Dr.	Department of Morbid Anatomy, The Royal London Hospital, Whitechapel, London E1 1BB, UK
COX, J.N., Dr.	Department of Pathology, CMU, 1 rue Michel-Servet, CH–1211 Geneva 4, Switzerland
DASBACH, G., Dr.	Institute of Pathology, University Hospital, Berufsgenossenschaftliche Krankenanstalten Bergmannsheil, Gilsingstraße 14, 44789 Bochum, Germany
DRURY, P.J., Dr.	Institute of Biomedical Equipment Evaluation and Service, University of Sheffield, Redmires Road, Sheffield S10 4LH, UK
GRAHAM, T.R., Dr.	Department of Cardiothoracic Surgery, The Royal London Hospital, Whitechapel London E1 1BB, UK

HILL, C.M., Dr.
Department of Pathology, Institute of Pathology, The Queen's University, Grosvenor Road, Belfast BT12 6BA, Northern Ireland

KONERTZ, W., Prof. Dr.
Department of Thoracic and Cardiovascular Surgery of the Westphalian Wilhelm's University Münster, Albert-Schweitzer-Str. 33, 48149 Münster, Germany

LÖHRS, U., Prof. Dr.
Institute of Pathology, Medical University of Lübeck, Ratzeburger Allee 160, 23562 Lübeck, Germany

present address:
Director, Institute of Pathology, University Munich, Thalkirchner Str. 36, 80337 München, Germany

MÜLLER, K.-M., Prof. Dr.
Institute of Pathology, University Hospital, Berufsgenossenschaftliche Krankenanstalten Bergmannsheil, Gilsingstraße 14, 44789 Bochum, Germany

O'HARA, M.D., Dr.
Department of Pathology, Institute of Pathology, The Queen's University, Grosvenor Road, Belfast BT12 6BA, Northern Ireland

SCHELD, H.H., Prof. Dr.
Department of Thoracic and Cardiovascular Surgery of the Westphalian Wilhelm's University Münster, Albert- Schweitzer-Straße 33, 48149 Münster, Germany

Preface

In much of the world, improved living standards and the increasing average age of the population have increased the demands made on the medical profession. These demands relate less to the acute phase of illness than to the desire that diseases accompanying aging – notably chronic disease processes or diseases resulting from wear and tear – do not compromise the quality of life. Consequently there has been progress in the development of replacement vessels, joints, and valves; changes affecting drug delivery systems; and the development of new forms of bone, fascia, or inert materials. Tissue engineering is a real possibility, which can be used to treat tissue defects.

In a recent article in *Science* (1993, 260:920–926), Langer and Vacanti estimated that more than 8 million Americans a year undergo skin reconstructions, joint replacements, valve substitutions, tendon repairs, vascular grafts, or dental prosthetic replacements. In this volume we consider developments in these fields for two reasons: to inform pathologists about their role in evaluating these devices, and to demonstrate that a proper documentation and understanding of the successes and failures of this type of therapy is necessary in order to improve treatment.

London, November 1993 SIR COLIN BERRY

Preface

Contents

The Pathology of Artificial Joints

U. LÖHRS and I. BOS

Current Topics in Pathology
Volume 86. Ed. C. Berry

1 Introduction

The significance of artificial joint pathology has become clear in view of the approximately 600 000 joint prosthesis implantations performed worldwide each year. Today the chief indications for endoprosthetic joint replacement are serious degenerative joint disease and femoral neck fracture in combination with osteoarthrosis and rheumatoid arthritis; the procedures are less liberally applied in younger patients because of their greater life expectancy and the risk of long-term complications.

Charnley's pioneering introduction of polymethyl methacrylate cement for fixation in 1958 enabled successful primary stabilisation of hip joint implants to be achieved regularly, and since 1965 prosthetic joint replacement has been widely practised. Cement-free implants had been developed prior to this. In 1939 Smith-Petersen introduced mould arthroplasty, in which metal plates formed an artificial "discus interarticularis". The Judet prosthesis, designed for femoral head replacement, consisted of a Plexiglas (later metal) head, and was fixed with a post in the femoral neck. Early results seemed to be encouraging, but grave complications developed over time, most notably loosening and fracturing of the prosthesis. Intramedullary fixation of a prosthesis in the femur was introduced by Moore and Thompson in 1952. They employed femoral head prostheses made of metal that are still used in a similar form but with bone cement fixation. The metal total endoprostheses developed in 1959 by McKee and Farrar were widely used at first, but became less popular with the inauguration of Charnley's "low-friction arthroplasty" in 1961.

The older all-metal models produced considerable friction between the articulating surfaces. Charnley attained a notable reduction in friction by combining stainless steel femoral components with sockets originally of Teflon and later of polyethylene. Boutin, in 1972, and Mittelmeier, in 1974, introduced a highly dense alumina ceramic as the material for both head and socket. The friction between two highly polished ceramic counterfaces was markedly less than that produced between metal and polyethylene. Sporadically, however, considerable ceramic wear developed secondary to cup malpositioning or loosening so that later a ceramic–polyethylene design was preferred to ceramic–ceramic combinations. Nevertheless, dimensional changes and abrasive wear from the relatively soft polyethylene gradually proved to be a significant problem in these models threatening the implant life expectancy, especially after long-term implantation.

Even greater material-related problems are associated with the application of bone cement. Whereas good short-term and intermediate results are achieved by cemented prostheses, long-term observation reveals complications in up to about 50% of cases (LING 1981). Late loosening is the most common reason for revision surgery, which is a difficult and tedious operation that has to be performed on patients who are generally elderly and threatened by high complication rates. Because of cement-related problems, attempts at cement-free implantation were subsequently re-instituted and new models designed. Here primary stabilisation, which is not always optimal, constitutes the main problem.

Prostheses for other joints, especially for the knee and hand joints, appeared soon after hip joint prostheses. The first artificial knee joints were all-metal hinge constructions but successive designs with an added gliding function imitated natural knee function more closely.

Evaluation of reactive and pathological reactions in the vicinity of prostheses is becoming increasingly important to the pathologist as the number of implants grows. Tissue specimens derive from two sources. The pseudocapsules and the peri-articular soft tissues taken from loosened prostheses are obtained at the time of revision surgery. Here the greatest diagnostic difficulties lie in the differentiation of the various wear particles, which in some cases are positively identifiable only by physical methods.

In autopsy material it is possible to examine tissue reactions around firmly fixed intact implants. This allows differentiation between adaptive processes and the pathological reactions that lead to loosening. Such pathomorphological investigations are important not only for diagnostic reasons but also for clarifying the pathogenetic mechanism of implant loosening. This also may provide information on how different implant materials and designs influence surrounding tissues, thus enabling comparison of the biological compatibility of the various devices.

2 Systemic and Local Complications in Prosthesis Implantation

2.1 Local Complications

Bone fracture and nerve injury are known intraoperative local complications. Postoperative early infection occurs in a small percentage of cases.

2.2 Systemic Complications

Systemic complications related to joint implantation primarily concern the cardiovascular and respiratory systems. Of particular importance are hypotensive circulatory reactions which can, in some cases, lead to irreversible cardiac arrest (Convery et al. 1975; Patterson et al. 1991; Zichner 1987). Lethality due to such incidents is estimated to be between 0.02% and 1.3% (Rinecker and Höllenriegel 1987).

Toxic methyl methacrylate monomers in the venous blood and fat or bone marrow emboli from prosthetic stem insertion have been considered to be the cause of pathological sequelae. Authors disagree about the relative importance that can be ascribed to these two factors. Despite the fact that monomer infusion produced an impairment in lung function and a fall in arterial blood pressure in animal experiments, Feith (1975) considers that a general pharmacological effect of the monomer is not established. Oedema and pulmonary haemorrhage have been seen as the morphological basis of the reduction in lung function (Holland et al. 1973; Homsy et al. 1972).

In man, abnormal liver enzyme levels have been found following prosthesis insertion, and correlated with the amount of bone cement used (Poble and Philipps 1988). However, there is no correlation between serum monomer concentration and falling blood pressure (Crout et al. 1979).

Pulmonary embolism caused by insertion of the prosthesis can cause longer-lasting alterations in pulmonary function. Fat and bone marrow emboli with or without spongiosa fragments can be found regularly at autopsy and are also seen

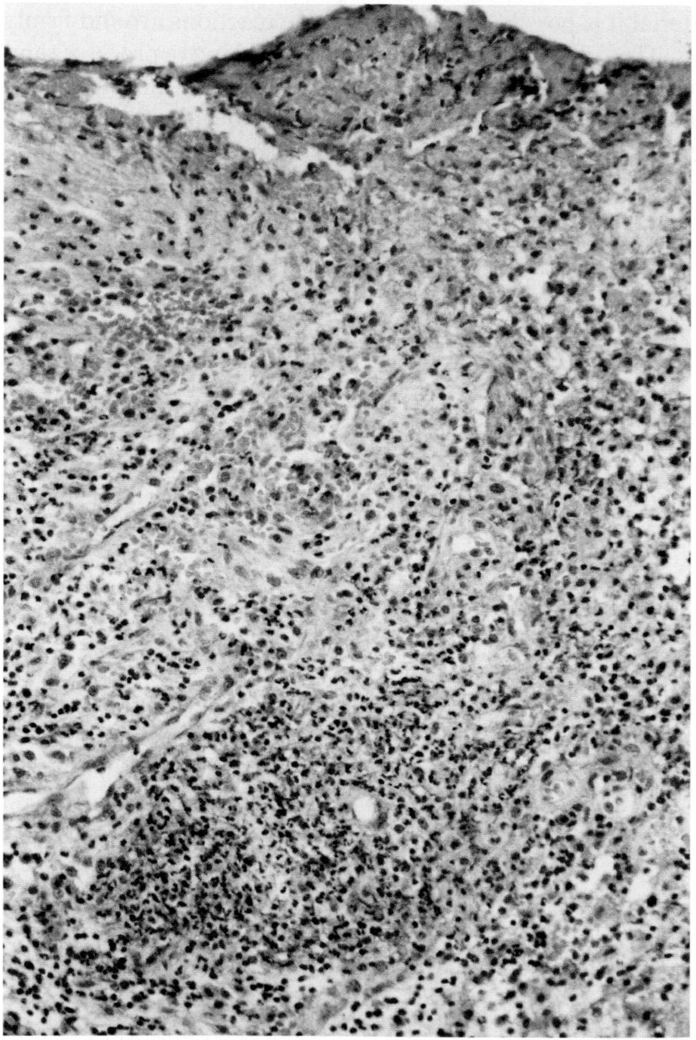

Fig. 1. New synovial tissue with infectious inflammation 2 months after implantation. Loose vascular granulation tissue and granulocytic infiltration with the development of microabscesses. H&E, × 160

after longer periods (Modig et al. 1974; Zichner 1987). The decreasing arterial blood pressure is regarded by some authors as a consequence of impaired pulmonary circulation (Patterson et al. 1991; Schulitz and Dustmann 1976).

2.3 Early Infections

Bacterial infection is one of the most serious complications arising in artificial joint replacement. It is usually accompanied by severe pain and leads inevitably to prosthesis loosening. The incidence of infection is difficult to assess. In the literature figures vary from 0% to 12% (Eftekhar 1973; Konermann 1983). Since the advent of "hypersterile" operating rooms and prophylactic antibiotic therapy, the rate of early infections has been reduced (Gaudillat 1987; Konermann 1983).

Early infection is defined as an infection with acute or subacute inflammation which appears in the first 6 months post-implantation. It can be traced to intraoperative bacterial contamination (Konermann 1983). *Staphylococcus aureus* is most often the causal organism in early infection, followed by *Staphylococcus epidermidis* and *Streptococcus* (for comparison with late infections, see Sect. 8.1). Early infection is characterised histologically by polymorphonuclear granulocytic infiltration (Fig. 1), vascular granulation tissue, fibrinous exudates and microabscesses (Bos and Löhrs 1991; Forest 1987). Differentiation from non-infectious inflammation is achieved primarily by the detection of granulocytes, which appear only infrequently and sparsely in non-infectious inflammation (Bos and Löhrs 1991; Mirra et al. 1976, 1982). The inflammatory infiltrates may extend from the newly formed joint capsule into the surrounding bone as a purulent osteomyelitis.

3 Early Morphological Changes Following Implantation

3.1 Formation of the New Articular Capsule

The articular capsule, which is usually completely removed during prosthesis implantation, restores itself as a pseudocapsule resembling the original within 6 months. However, the structures regenerate in a rather crude fashion with layers that are often less distinctly separated from one another (Bos and Löhrs 1991; Willert and Semlitsch 1976b). Well-vascularised granulation tissue with siderophages fills the postoperative surgical cavity, resorbing necrotic tissue and haemorrhages. After complete resorption of fibrin, necrotic tissue and coagulated blood, a cubic or columnar superficial cell layer forms (Fig. 2), which is later transformed into a flattened synovial cell layer. In subsequent months the granulation tissue is replaced by loose synovial fibrous tissue and dense connective tissue in the periphery. The newly formed synovial tissue, which matches the

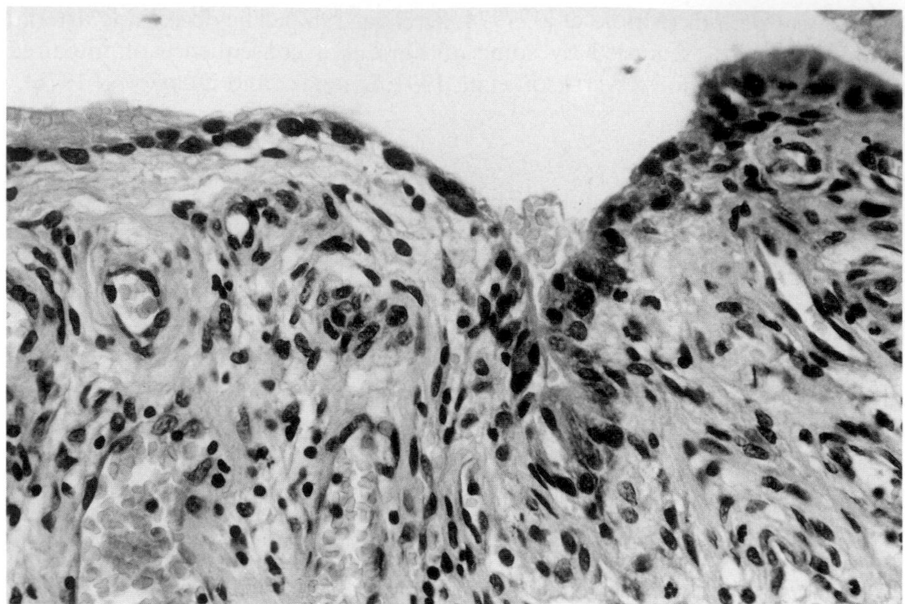

Fig. 2. Newly formed, mainly cubic superficial synovial cell layer in the reparation phase a few weeks post implantation. New synovial tissue consisting of granulation tissue is seen. H&E, $\times$ 400

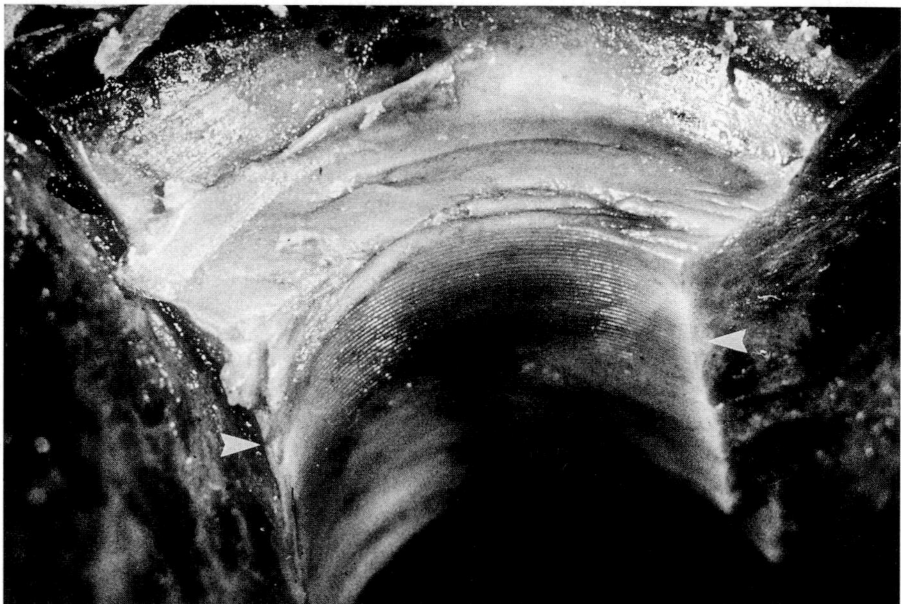

Fig. 3. Sector of a pseudocapsule after 2 years in situ. The capsule presents an exact imprint of the prosthesis surface with corrugation (arrowhead) of the new synovial surface adjacent to the neck of the prosthesis

contour of the prosthetic surface (Fig. 3), demonstrates fibrosis in relatively early stages. Fibrin layers and haemorrhages (frequently found) indicate a state of chronic irritation even before the appearance of wear particles (MAßHOFF and NEUHAUS-VOGEL 1974).

3.2 Early Changes in the Bony Implant Bed

Published data concern cemented prostheses almost exclusively. According to WILLERT and PULS (1972) the transformations take place during an initial phase lasting approximately 3 weeks post implantation and a reparative phase that can extend over several months to a maximum of 2 years.

The initial phase is characterised by a 3- to 5-mm-wide band of necrosis, encompassing the cement mantle, which involves both marrow and cancellous bone (VERNON-ROBERTS and FREEMAN 1976; WILLERT and PULS 1972; WILLERT and SEMLITSCH 1976a; WILLERT et al. 1974). Cortical bone shows a comparatively variable zone of necrosis ranging from 0.5 mm to about one-third of the cortex.

During the reparative phase within the first few weeks to several months, bone marrow, haemorrhages and fibrin exudates are phagocytosed by macrophages, replaced by vascular granulation tissue and finally converted into a cell-rich connective tissue membrane (CHARNLEY 1964; DELLING et al. 1987; REVELL 1982; WILLERT and SEMLITSCH 1976a; WILLERT et al. 1974). The replacement of fractured bone trabeculae and layers of necrotic cortical bone takes more time. Removal of necrotic bone by osteoclasts and new bone formation proceed simultaneously (WILLERT and PULS 1972). Bone and marrow necrosis is attributable to three factors: (a) the mechanical trauma associated with femoral head removal and reaming of the bone marrow, (b) the cytotoxic effects of unpolymerised methyl methacrylate monomers and (c) thermal damage secondary to the heat generated by the exothermic polymerisation of the cement in situ.

Mechanical trauma and monomer toxicity in particular have been verified as causes of extensive necrosis in animal experiments (GOEBEL and OHNSORGE 1973). Pre-implantation reaming of the implant bed leads not only to fractures of the bone trabeculae but also to widespread necrosis of the inner cortex secondary to the destruction of intramedullary arteries, as RHINLANDER et al. (1979) have shown in animals. Numerous investigations on the local tissue toxicity of methyl methacrylate monomer exist (see for example ALBREKTSSON and LINDER 1984; MOHR 1958). These authors document the monomer toxicity as a lipolytic substance capable of eliciting irreversible necrosis in relatively small amounts.

Temperatures from 40° to 120°C were measured on the cement surface as a result of thermal effects during polymerisation (FEITH 1975), and thermal tissue damage may occur since body proteins coagulate from 56°C. However, the heat generated by polymerisation is dependent upon the volume and form of the cement mantle (WILLERT and PULS 1972), and thin layers of bone cement interspersed between bone trabeculae develop less polymerisation heat (Goebel and Ohnsorge 1973). Thus the use of optimal implantation technique does not lead to thermal damage.

4 Wear Particles of Endoprostheses and Their Bone Cement Mantle

The following types of wear particles are released during function of the hip and knee joint prostheses currently used: bone cement debris, consisting primarily of polymethyl methacrylate and x-ray contrast medium, polyethylene particles, alumina ceramic wear particles and metal particles. In small joint prostheses, particularly in those used for hand joints, silicone wear particles from the articulating surfaces have been reported. Smaller wear particles (< 30 μm) are phagocytosed by monocytic histiocytes after their release, while the larger ones are surrounded by multinucleated giant cells.

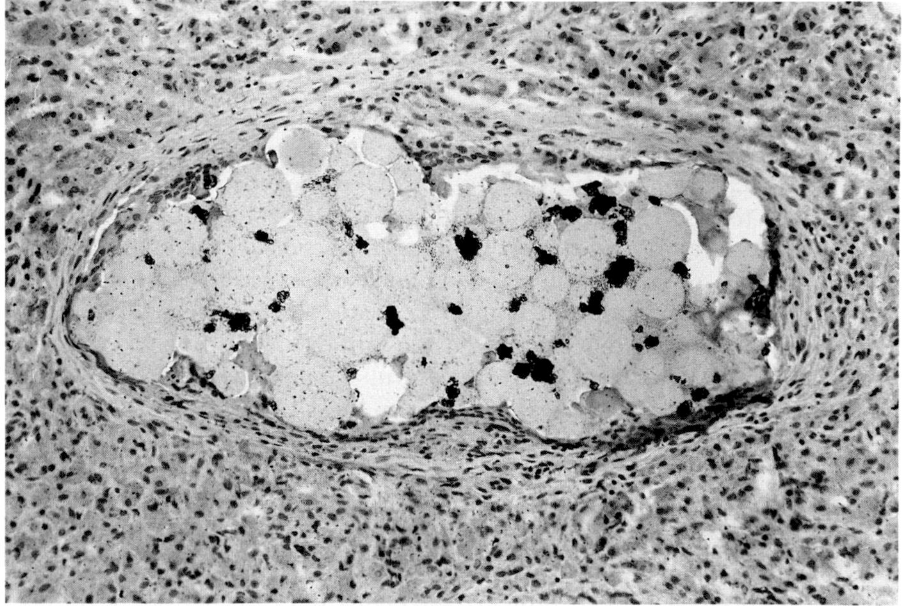

Fig. 4. Larger bone cement inclusion in a histiocytic infiltrate, consisting of polymer spherules of variable size, in between particles of the contrast medium (black). In the periphery, there is a seam of foreign body giant cells. Modified Sudan stain, × 160

4.1 Bone Cement Wear

Bone cement is found in the form of variably sized wear particles in periprosthetic tissue. There are larger extracellular fragments of several millimetres in size and small intracytoplasmic granules.

4.1.1 Extracellular Bone Cement Particles

The larger extracellular bone cement particles have a characteristic mulberry-like configuration (Fig. 4) that results from aggregation of spherical polymethyl methacrylate (PMMA) pearls of variable size during polymerisation.

4.1.2 Polymethyl Methacrylate Wear Particles

The fine granular intracytoplasmic PMMA particles have a different configuration. In light microscopy they appear as oval-, bar- or lancet-shaped fragments with a diameter ranging from 1 to 30 μm (Fig. 5). Electron microscopy of human

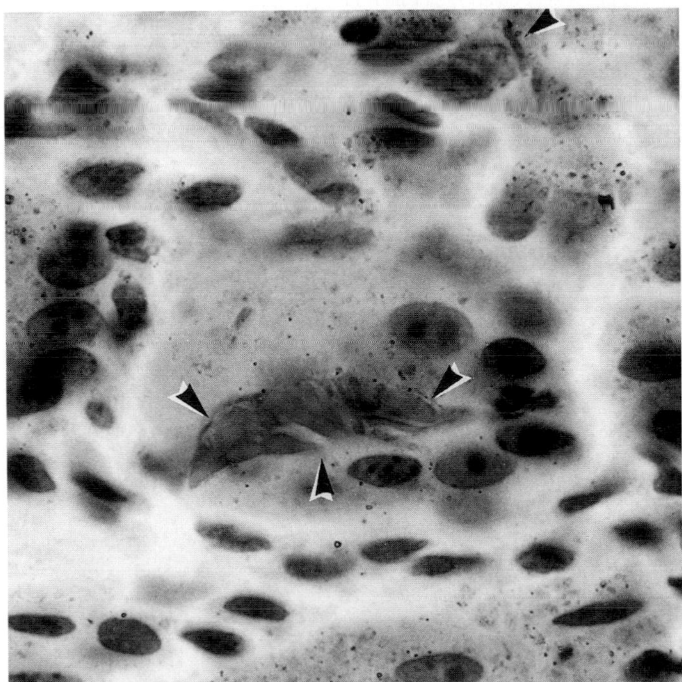

Fig. 5. Intracellular polymethyl methacrylate wear particles (*arrowheads*) of variable size and zirconium oxide particles in histiocytes showing degenerative alterations. Modified Sudan stain, × 750

tissue from implant sites of cemented hip joint prostheses (Bos et al. 1990a) as well as of artificially produced bone cement particles implanted intramuscularly in experimental animals (Pedley et al. 1979) showed identical cytoplasmic inclusions. These exhibited creviced outlines (Fig. 6) which most probably developed during the wear process. Few inclusions were surrounded by a membranous coat.

Large bone cement particles are largely dissolved in the course of ordinary tissue processing for light microscopy due to their PMMA content, but are nevertheless recognisable because of the characteristic configuration of the

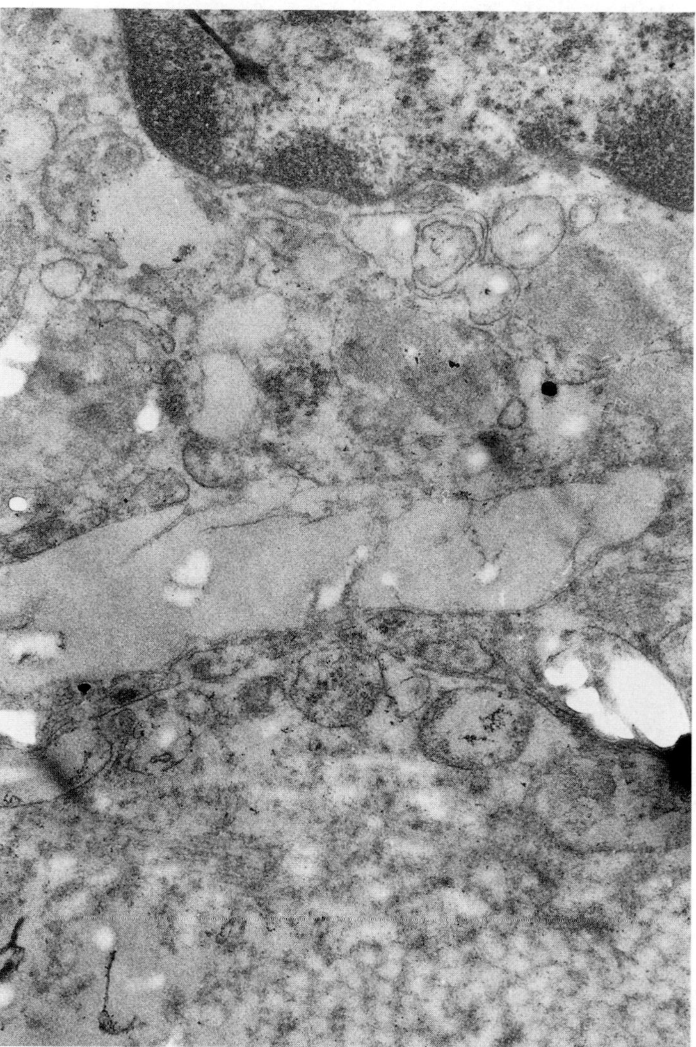

Fig. 6. Cytoplasmic area of a histiocyte centrally containing a polymethyl methacrylate wear particle with marginal tears. × 34 000

resulting gaps. Intracytoplasmic wear particles, however, are identified only in modified Sudan stains of frozen sections or after gelatine embedding.

4.1.3 Radiological Contrast Material

Barium sulphate and zirconium oxide are used as x-ray contrast media in bone cement. Both substances are composed of fine granular particles which can be demonstrated after routine histological processing.

4.1.3.1 Zirconium Oxide. Zirconium oxide particles are readily detectable in the cytoplasm of histiocytes in cases of severe bone cement wear (Fig. 7). As zirconium oxide particles are released simultaneously and in a constant volume ratio with PMMA fragments, the extent of bone cement wear can be estimated by the amount of phagocytosed zirconium oxide when PMMA has been dissolved by routine tissue processing. The particles appear intracellularly as round yellow-brown grains of approximately 0.5 µm in diameter (Bos and Löhrs 1991; Bos et al. 1990a, b; Löer et al. 1987; Szyszkowitz 1973). They are seen solitary or in small clusters in the cytoplasm. Frequently, larger mulberry-shaped con-

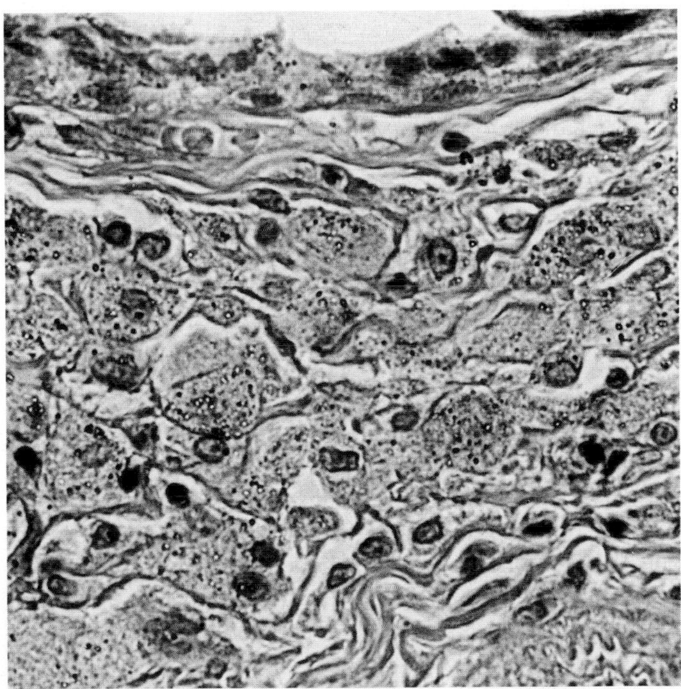

Fig. 7. Histiocytic infiltrate with phagocytosed zirconium oxide particles. H&E, × 470

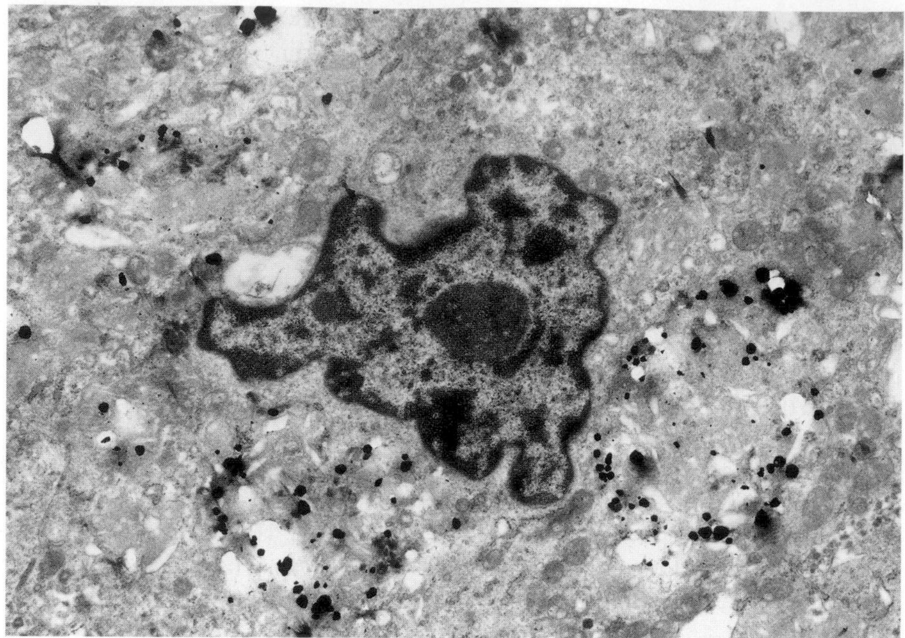

Fig. 8. Electron micrograph of a histiocyte with zirconium oxide particles (black granules) of different size in the cytoplasm. × 10 500

glomerates of up to 20 μm diameter (Willert et al. 1981) are found in the spaces left in the tissues at the sites of dissolved large bone cement fragments. These conglomerates, which presumably develop secondarily due to physical forces, are characteristic for zirconium oxide and facilitate distinction from bone cement wear containing barium sulphate. In electron microscopy, zirconium oxide particles appear to be completely electron dense (Fig. 8), with a diameter between about 0.005 and 0.5 μm (Bos et al. 1990a; Löer et al. 1987). Solitary small grains are therefore not detectable in light microscopy.

4.1.3.2 Barium Sulphate. Barium sulphate granules in the cytoplasm of histiocytes are almost undetectable in the light microscope. After routine tissue processing the cytoplasm appears to be free of foreign particles. However, spaces remaining from dissolved large bone cement fragments have been noted to contain yellow-green round to oval foreign particles, ranging in size from 0.5 to 2 μm (Forest 1987; Mirra et al. 1976; Willert et al. 1981). Electron microscopy reveals intracellular electron-dense particles of variable diameter between 0.003 and 0.3μm. In contrast to zirconium oxide, barium sulphate apparently does not form larger intracellular conglomerates and hence remains for the most part unnoticed under the light microscope. Larger aggregates develop extracellularly and these also fail to reach the size of those formed by zirconium oxide.

4.1.4 *Site of Origin and Distribution of Bone Cement Wear Particles*

Bone cement wear develops apparently chiefly at the bone-cement interface (BEAN et al. 1987; Bos et al. 1990a; JOHANSON et al. 1987; WILLERT 1987; WILLERT et al. 1990b) within the femur shaft as well as in the acetabulum. Micromotions between cement and cancellous bone in the course of stress transmission (ALDINGER 1987; DIENEL et al. 1984; MAGUIRE et al. 1987) lead to the abrasion of small bone cement particles even in firmly fixed implants after longer periods in situ (DELLING et al. 1987; GOLDRING et al. 1986; GROSS et al. 1984). Wear arising from implant and bone cement interaction seems to be of less importance.

How do the wear particles find their way from the bone-cement interface into the pseudocapsule? We found bone cement wear to be evenly distributed in the pseudocapsule and the interface membranes in periprosthetic tissue obtained at revision surgery of loose prostheses. As extensive necrosis often develops in these soft tissue membranes (Bos et al. 1990a; GROSS et al. 1984; JOHANSON et al. 1987; LENNOX et al. 1987), it seems most probable that shear and compressive forces acting on the limb during use promote the migration of wear particles via void spaces in the necrotic tissues into the joint cavity where they are phagocytosed by synovial lining cells (LINDER et al. 1983; WROBLEWSKI et al. 1987). Further, distribution via lymphatic and blood vessels seems possible, as was postulated by WILLERT (1987), in the opposite direction from the articular wear. In an autopsy study of firmly fixed prostheses we were able to demonstrate fine granular bone cement wear appearing after 7 months in situ. As in surgical material from loosened prostheses, the amount of wear increased continuously with the time in situ (up to 20 years). In capsules from loosened prostheses we found moderate to severe bone cement wear in over 60%.

4.1.5 *Toxicity of Bone Cement Wear Particles*

Conflicting reports about the toxicity of bone cement are found in the literature. It is generally thought that systemic toxic effects develop only intraoperatively, through those methyl methacrylate monomers which enter the blood circulation. However, local damage due to toxic effects of one or more bone cement components is discussed, in particular as a possible sequel of phagocytosis leading to a high intracellular concentration of the particles (BENEKE et al. 1973; BÖSCH et al. 1982, 1987; COTTA and SCHULITZ 1970; HOPF et al. 1989; LENNOX et al. 1987; LINTNER and BÖSCH 1987; LINTNER et al. 1984; MOHR 1958; RUDIGIER et al. 1976, 1987; VERNON-ROBERTS and FREEMAN 1976).

Polymerised bone cement in bulk form is viewed by some authors as being biologically inert (CHARNLEY 1970; HULLIGER 1962; KALLENBERGER 1984). Other investigators, however, have observed rounding and reduced phagocytic capacity of macrophages after attachment to PMMA surfaces (LEAKE et al. 1981; NICASTRO et al. 1975), suppression of DNA synthesis by pulverised bone cement (Horowitz et al. 1988), inflammatory changes in the adjacent soft tissue (Hopf et al. 1989; Mohr 1958; Rudigier et al. 1987) and demineralisation of the surrounding bone (Lintner et al. 1982, 1987). These changes are all taken to be signs of toxicity that is attributed to the highly toxic residual monomers (Cotta and Schultiz 1970; Mohr 1958) which, according to Löer et al. (1983), diffuse from the pores of the polymerised cement casts. The concentration of residual monomers is estimated at between 2% and 8% of total cement weight. Beneke et al. (1973) found that monomers are released from the intact bone cement mantle up to 400 days postimplantation. However, by abrasion of fine bone cement debris the release of residual monomers could be amplified due to the opening of new pores in the bone cement (Bos et al. 1990a).

Since bone cement consists of numerous different compounds (PMMA, methyl methacrylate and its monomers, zirconium oxide or barium sulphate and catalyser components, primarily benzoyl peroxide and dimethyl para-toluidine), each of these substances needs to be tested separately for its toxicity.

The x-ray contrast medium zirconium oxide, which, like barium sulphate, is added in a concentration of about 10% of bone cement by weight, is regarded as being generally well tolerated (Hopf et al. 1989). In the literature there is no evidence of toxic effects in either human or animal investigations (Schröder and Balassa 1966; Shelley and Hurley 1958).

Barium sulphate, however, is mostly considered to have toxic effects (Hopf et al. 1989; Rudigier et al. 1976, 1987). Its dissociated form is known to be highly toxic; however, the dissociation rate is very low (Löer et al. 1987). In contrast to Linder (1977), who found no differences in tissue reaction to bone cement plugs with or without barium sulphate, Hopf et al. (1989) and Rudigier et al. (1976, 1987) describe more extensive initial necroses, more intense chronic inflammation after long-lasting implant duration and more serious bone injury with barium sulphate-containing bone cement. With regard to these degenerative changes and necroses in the peri-articular tissue, we were unable to substantiate such differences between cases in which barium sulphate- and zirconium oxide-containing cements had been used.

Catalyser components of the bone cement are also known to have a toxic effect. Benzoyl peroxide combined with dimethyl *para*-toluidine is generally used as an initiator of polymerisation and is non-toxic (Mohr 1958) but dimethyl *para*-toluidine alone is noxious even at the lowest concentrations. Bösch et al. (1982, 1987) found substantial amounts of dimethyl *para*-toluidine in bone cement even after more than 10 years in situ. They believed that adjacent bone lesions had been caused exclusively by this substance.

In conclusion, it seems probable that several toxic substances are released – though in low concentrations – from the bone cement, particularly from the small wear particles. Toxic effects may be responsible in part for the degenerative changes of wear particle-containing histiocytes.

4.2 Polyethylene Wear

Wear fragments from the polyethylene cups and articulating surfaces currently in wide use for hip or knee prostheses have been found in the pseudocapsule and the membranes at the bone–cement interface (Bos et al. 1990b, 1991; Forest 1987; Howie et al. 1990; Maguire et al. 1987; Revell et al. 1978; Willert and Semlitsch (1977). In our own experience these fragments were the second most prevalent form of foreign material, only bone cement particles being more frequent Bos et al. 1991). Polyethylene fragments, which appear translucent or yellowish in routine light microscopy, are easily identified by a bright silver luminescence in polarised light. Typical is a thread-like or lancet-shaped form varying in diameter from 0.5 μm to 1 mm (Fig. 9). The smaller polyethylene particles (less than 30 μm), like the small granular bone cement particles, are found primarily in the cytoplasm of mononuclear histiocytes and in the interstitium. Larger particles, however, are seen mostly in histiocytic giant cells which often contain asteroid bodies in their cytoplasm (Fig. 10). Cases of high-grade polyethylene wear were characterised histologically by the predominance of giant cells (Fig. 9). Polyethylene fragments in our autopsy cases first appeared at 3 months and showed a notable increase with the length of time in situ.

A great number of in vitro and in vivo reports exist addressing the cause and extent of polyethylene wear from articular surfaces in hip endoprostheses. Wear in the relatively soft polyethylene sockets is known to develop through friction as

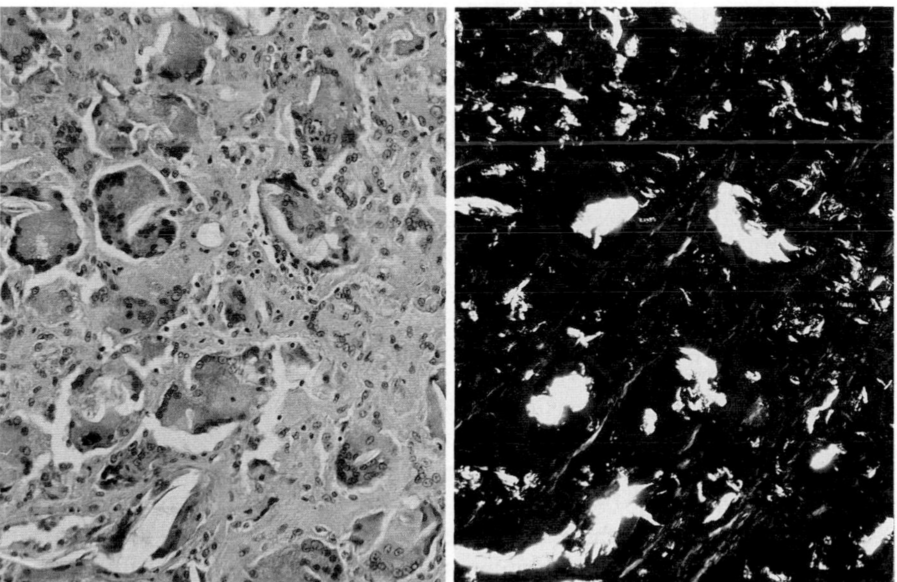

Fig. 9. Synovial tissue with extensive polyethylene wear. Histiocytic infiltration with numerous foreign body giant cells containing polyethylene fibres (right: polyethylene fibres in polarised light) H&E, × 190

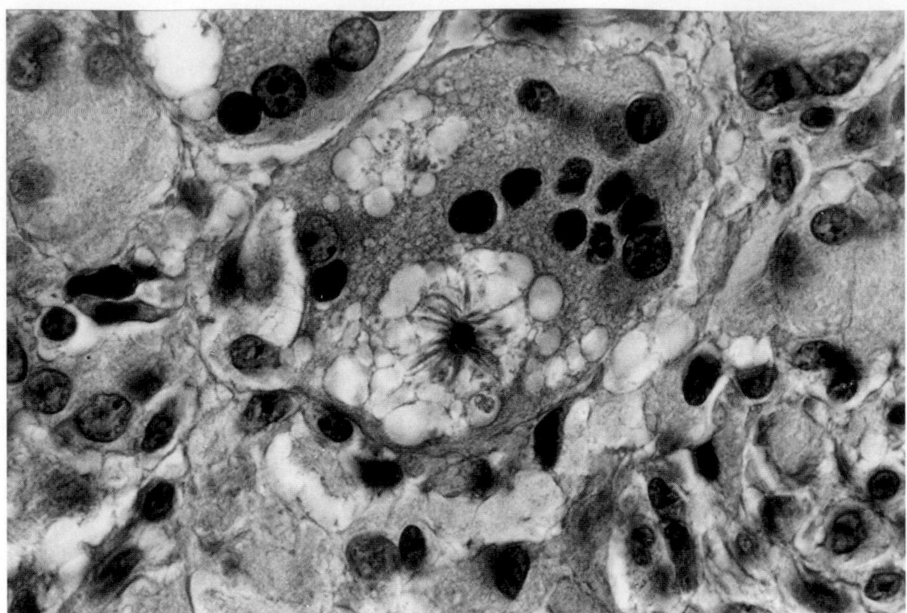

Fig. 10. Multinucleated foreign body giant cell with an asteroid body in the cytoplasm. H&E, × 600

adhesive, abrasive or fatigue wear with characteristic manifestation of defects on the contacting surfaces (ATKINSON 1975; BROWN et al. 1976; CLARKE 1981; CLARKE et al. 1976; DOWLING et al. 1978; GOLD and WALKER 1974; LANCASTER 1969; ROSE et al. 1980; ROSTOKER et al. 1978; UNGETHÜM and WINKLER-GNIEWEK 1983; WALKER and BULLOUGH 1973). Loose particles, moreover, work abrasively as they get between the articular counterfaces (DOWLING et al. 1978; WALKER and BULLOUGH 1973). Of special interest is the interposition of bone cement fragments (CARAVIA et al. 1990; POSTEL and COURPIED 1987; REVELL et al. 1978; ROSE et al. 1979) which get into the joint cavity, even in stable prostheses, after a longer period (BOS et al. 1990a; WILLERT et al. 1978).

The extent of socket wear in vivo is dependent on the materials used for the prosthetic head and socket, the design employed and the mechanical forces imposed on the individual prosthesis (CLARKE 1981; ROSE and RADIN 1982). A finely polished head surface is of particular importance (DAWIHL et al. 1979; SEMLITSCH et al. 1977; WILLERT et al. 1978), as are quality differences in the manufacture of "ultra high molecular weight" (UHMW) polyethylene (ROSE and RADIN 1982; ROSE et al. 1978, 1980).

At present most prosthetic heads are composed of metal or aluminium oxide ceramic. The advantage of aluminium oxide ceramic lies in the smoothness of its polishable surface, its superior wettability and its corrosion resistance, all of which result in improved wear resistance (DAWIHL et al. 1979; DÖRRE and DAWIHL 1978; DÖRRE et al. 1977). Due to the inherent properties of aluminium oxide ceramic, all simulator tests show polyethylene wear from friction against ceramic heads to be less than that from friction against metal heads. However, only the examination of explanted sockets after long-term service and the quantitative evaluation of wear particles in the surrounding tissues can give a true picture of how the polyethylene sockets will behave in patients.

A comparative semiquantitative evaluation of wear particles in pseudocapsules obtained from autopsies showed prostheses of metal-polyethylene combination to release three times as many polyethylene fragments as ceramic-polyethylene implants (Bos et al. 1991).

Considerable deterioration in polyethylene sockets after long-term service suggests that polyethylene sockets, increasingly used as parts of cement-free implants, are becoming the weakest link in the chain of materials employed.

4.3 Silicone Wear

Silicone is used primarily in the replacement of small joints, particularly for articular surfaces in the hand (Gordon and Bullough 1982). Silicone wear particles develop following implant fractures as well as in totally intact joint prostheses (Christie et al. 1977). The prevalence of wear particles in the synovial tissue lies between 1% (Nalbandian et al. 1983) and 25% (Griffiths and Nicolle 1975; Swanson 1972). They are irregularly shaped amorphous fragments that can be translucent to yellowish and, unlike polyethylene particles, are not birefringent in polarised light (Christie et al. 1977; Gordon and Bullough 1982; Kircher 1980; Nalbandian et al. 1983). These particles, which are demonstrable in the joint capsule and medullary cavity of adjacent bone, can lead to chronic histiocytic synovitis with a concomitant decline in joint function.

4.4 Ceramic Wear

Ceramic wear has exclusively been described in artificial hip prostheses with aluminium oxide ceramic heads and sockets (Bos and Löhrs 1991; Mittelmeier and Harms 1979a, b; Trepte et al. 1985).

Ceramic fragments appear histologically as yellow-brown fragments up to 5 µm in diameter (Fig. 11). Electron microscopy reveals particles as small as 0.2 µm. Apparently, the original ceramic grains, whose diameter is reported to be 4.0 µm on average (Dörre et al. 1975), fragment even further in the process of wear generation. In contrast to zirconium oxide particles, which appear very similar in light, ceramic grains show a sharp-edged polygonal configuration in electron microscopic investigations.

Ceramic wear usually originates from the articular surfaces of prosthetic heads and sockets. There is considerable controversy in the literature about its extent. Most simulator tests have demonstrated superior tribological properties

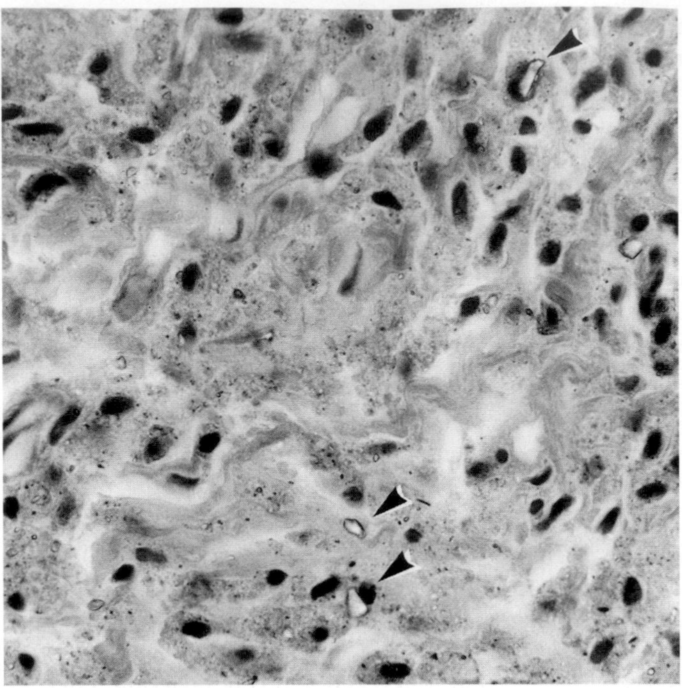

Fig. 11. Histiocytes with ceramic and zirconium oxide wear. Polygonal sharply edged, mainly larger, ceramic particles (arrowheads) besides smaller round zirconium oxide particles. H&E, × 470

of ceramic-ceramic combinations, which exhibit outstanding friction and wear behaviour (DÖRRE et al. 1975; HEIMKE et al. 1973, 1974; HINTERBERGER and UNGETHÜM 1978; SEMLITSCH et al. 1976, 1977; UNGETHÜM and REfiOR 1974).

According to CLARKE et al. (1988) the wear rates are approximately 500 times less than for metal-polyethylene systems. Satisfactory clinical implantation correlates, in most cases, with good clinical performance (GRISS and HEIMKE 1981; HEISEL and SCHMITT 1987; MITTELMEIER and HARMS 1979a,b; SEDEL et al. 1990; STOCK et al. 1980). In a few cases excessive wear has been described in ceramic components retrieved during revision surgery of loosened prostheses (PLITZ et al. 1984).

PLITZ et al. (1984) assumed that excessive wear is initiated when ceramic grains are torn from the high-gloss polished articular surfaces. Other authors have viewed this type of catastrophic wear as a consequence of loosening followed by malpositioning or subluxation of the cup (HEISEL and SCHMITT 1987; MITTELMEIER et al. 1982). Surgical errors leading to cup malorientation can also be responsible for a high wear rate due to dry friction at the socket rim (HEISEL and SCHMITT 1987; MITTELMEIER et al. 1982). So far there are no adequate studies on a sufficient number of autopsy cases with satisfactory and stable ceramic-ceramic implants.

Ceramic components have the disadvantage of possessing little tensile strength, a feature associated with a risk of fracture due to trauma or inadequate head alignment, which occurs in approximately 0.3% of cases (HEISEL and SCHMITT 1987; HINTERBERGER and UNGETHÜM 1978; PLITZ et al. 1984; TREPTE et al. 1985). The corrosion resistance of alumina ceramic, which, in contrast to metal alloys, releases no free ions can be seen as an advantage, as alumina wear particles have no toxic effects (GRISS et al. 1973a,b; HARMS and MÄUSLE 1976; HULBERT and KLAWITTER 1976).

4.5 Metallic Wear

Metallic wear was particularly frequent in the older all-metal prostheses used in hip and knee joint arthroplasty (CHAROSKY et al. 1973; MIRRA et al. 1982; VERNON-ROBERTS and FREEMAN 1976; WILLERT and SEMLITSCH 1976b).

Data collected from the prostheses in present use show disagreement about the incidence and extent of metallic wear, which, however, is regarded as negligible by most authors (HEILMANN et al. 1975; WILLERT and SEMLITSCH 1976b).

In contrast to other prosthetic materials, the cobalt-chrome alloys most frequently used today lead to particulate wear and to corrosion and diffusion of metal ions into body fluids (PRETZSCH and HEIN 1986; SEMLITSCH and WILLERT 1971; VERNON-ROBERTS and FREEMAN 1976; WINTER 1974).

In light microscopy metal particles appear black and granular; they are often needle, bar or lancet shaped (Fig. 12), varying in diameter between 0.5 and 5.0 μm (BOS and LÖHRS 1991; CHAROSKY et al. 1973; WILLERT and SEMLITSCH 1976b; WILLERT et al. 1981; WINTER 1974). Occasionally fragments as large as 100 μm have been observed, surrounded by foreign body giant cells (WILLERT and SEMLITSCH 1976b; WILLERT et al. 1981). Reddish luminous lines along the margins and edges of the particles become evident in polarised light (BOS and LÖHRS 1991; MIRRA et al. 1982; WILLERT and SEMLITSCH 1975, 1976b; WILLERT et al. 1981). Electron microscopy reveals that the particles, which appear solid by light microscopy, are often a conglomerate of metal splinters (Fig. 13) presumably held together by physical forces (WILLERT et al. 1981).

All metal surfaces of joint prostheses can serve as a source of metallic debris. In contrast to the all-metal prostheses no longer used, which regularly released articular wear particles (CHAROSKY et al. 1973; VERNON-ROBERTS and FREEMAN 1976), no significant metal wear is to be expected in the articulation of a cobalt–chrome head against polyethylene (HEILMANN et al. 1975; VERNON-ROBERTS and FREEMAN 1976; WILLERT and SEMLITSCH 1976b). However, in some cases the heads of titanium-based alloys have developed excessive wear leading to osteolysis and aseptic loosening of the implants (AGINS et al. 1988; BLACK et al. 1990; LOMBARDI et al. 1989). In our investigations metallic debris from cemented prostheses occurred in less than 20% of the cases, usually in small amounts. Excessive wear was found only where fractures of the metallic stem had not been immobilised immediately.

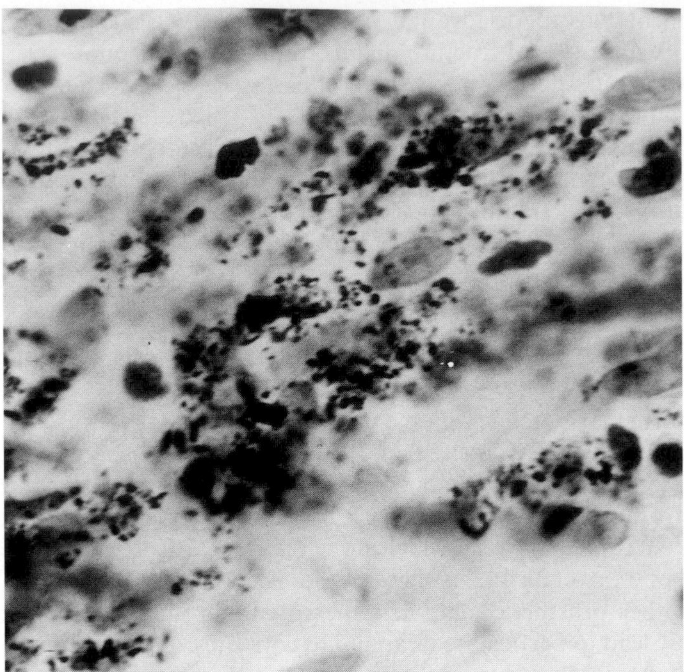

Fig. 12. Predominantly granular or bar-shaped metallic wear particles in the cytoplasm of histiocytes and in the interstitial space. H&E, × 750

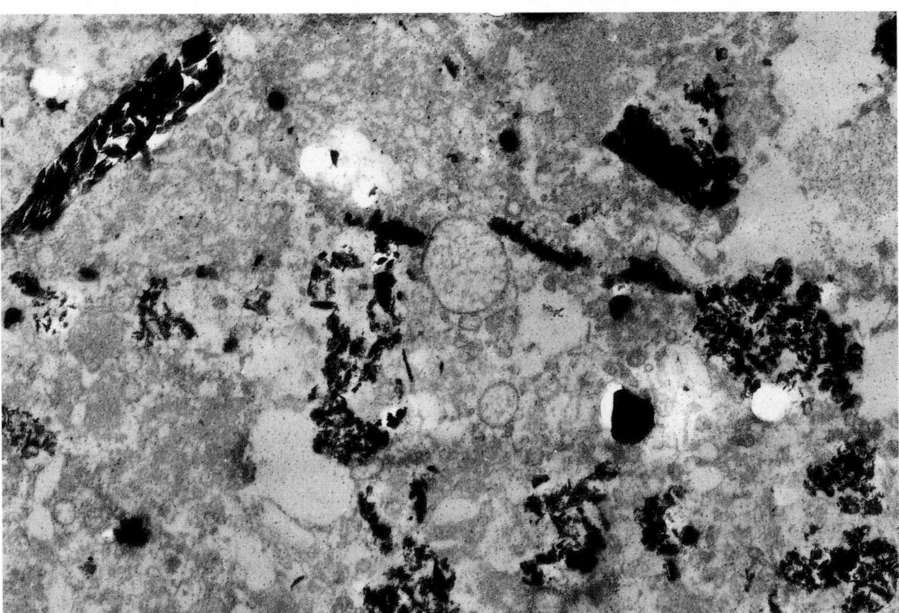

Fig. 13. Electron micrograph of metal wear particles. Needle or bar-shaped electron-dense fragments, some of which form bar-shaped aggregates. × 21 000

Among the non-cemented implants available, numerous variations with enlarged surfaces of the stem and metal-backed acetabular sockets have been developed to achieve tighter interlock between the porous implant and the ingrowing bone trabeculae. Frequently, at the time of implantation, moderate metallic wear results from friction of the rough porous metal surface against the bone of the implant bed (BUCHERT et al. 1986). If tight initial fixation by bony ingrowth is not achieved, excessive metal wear from the rough porous stem surfaces can follow (AGINS et al. 1988; BOBYN et al. 1987; BUCHERT et al. 1986; DORR et al. 1990). With respect to the toxicity of metal debris, systemic effects are considered to be more detrimental than local effects in the peri-articular soft tissue (WILLIAMS 1973). A number of studies have shown that patients with endoprostheses have increased levels of metal ions in internal organs as well as hair, blood and urine (BLACK et al. 1983; COLEMAN et al. 1973; DOBBS and MINSKY 1980; DORR et al. 1990; JONES et al. 1975; JORGENSEN et al. 1983). Numerous investigations have been conducted on cell cultures to assess the extent of toxic effects from different metals. The results indicate that cobalt, nickel and vanadium are likely to lead to cell damage in these systems, as well as the powders of cobalt–chrome alloys (DANIEL et al. 1963; RAE 1975, 1976, 1978, 1981; SCHWIERENGA and BASRUR 1968). The accumulation of metal ion concentrations at a level sufficiently high to cause toxic effects probably can only occur in the vicinity of loose all-metal prostheses. Some authors have pointed out that this may be true for loose cement-free prostheses as well (COLEMAN et al. 1973; DORR et al. 1990; RAE 1979). Even moderately increased body concentrations of the metals used in cobalt-chrome based alloys, functioning physiologically as essential trace elements, are generally considered potentially harmful for the organism (DORR et al. 1990; MICHEL et al. 1980; PRETZSCH and HEIN 1986) and may lead to subsequent changes in the concentrations of other trace elements (DOBBS and MINSKY 1980; MICHEL et al. 1980; PRETZSCH and HEIN 1986).

4.6 Methods of Wear Particle Detection

Whereas polyethylene and PMMA can be visualised by special Sudan staining (for details see BOS et al. 1990a), and polyethylene is easily identified by birefringence in polarised light, small granular wear particles can be detected with certainty only by physical methods. For this purpose and electron beam microprobe combined with a scanning or transmission electron microscopy (SEMLITSCH and WILLERT 1971; WILLERT and SEMLITSCH 1976b; WILLERT et al. 1981), semi-quantitative spectral analysis (SEMLITSCH and WILLERT 1971), instrumental neutron activation analysis (LÖER et al. 1981), atomic absorption spectrometry (SEMLITSCH and WILLERT 1971; WILLERT et al. 1980, 1981) and laser microprobe mass analysis (LAMMA) (BOS et al. 1990a, b; LÖER et al. 1987) have all been used. Some of these methods have the disadvantage of destroying the tissue so that the foreign material cannot be localised. In contrast, the LAMMA technique appears to be particularly

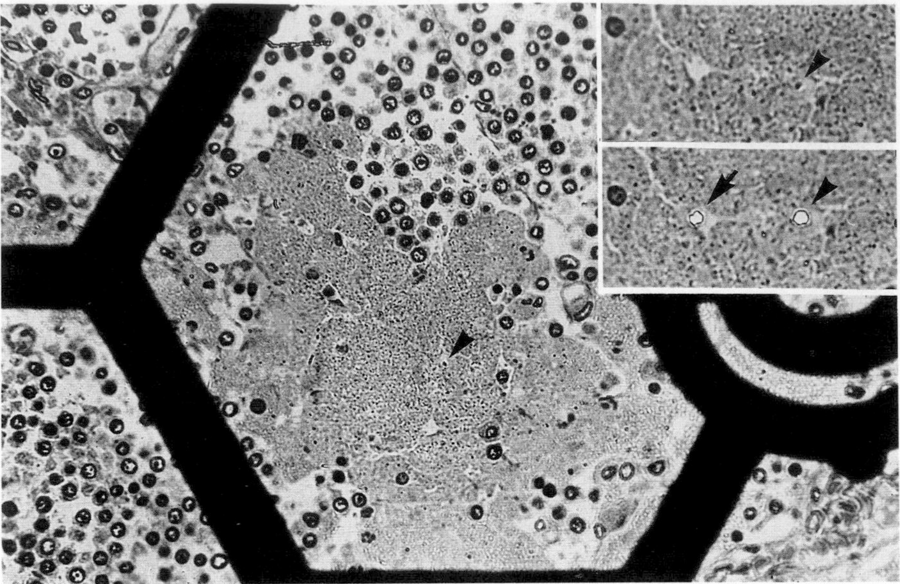

Fig. 14. Semithin section on an electron microscopic grid for LAMMA analysis. Histiocytes with foreign material. *Insets*: Area around the analysed wear particle (*arrowhead*) at higher magnification before LAMMA analysis (*top*). Perforation by laser pulse (*bottom*). Second perforation (*arrow*) for background spectrum. Toluidine blue, × 180; *insets*: × 450

well suited for the analysis of particles which have been detected by light microscopy (Fig. 14) and which subsequently can be focussed and analysed in a sharply defined sample area (Bos et al. 1990a, b).

5 Non-infectious Inflammation in Long-Term Implantations

The non-infectious inflammatory reaction found in peri-articular soft tissues after long-term implantation is characterised predominantly by infiltrates of histiocytes with abundant cytoplasm. These cells engulf wear particles from the prosthesis and its cement mantle (BENEKE et al. 1973; BOS et al. 1990a; FOREST 1987; GOODMAN et al. 1989; HAYASHI and INOUE 1986; LINDER et al. 1983; MIRRA et al. 1976, 1982; PIZZOFERRATO et al. 1981; REINUS et al. 1985; VERNON-ROBERTS and FREEMAN 1976; WILLERT and SEMLITSCH 1976b).

5.1 Origin and Histochemical Characterisation of the Histiocytes

The circulating monocyte is the precursor of tissue macrophages (histiocytes). The factors that control the accumulation of monocytic macrophages at the sites of wear particles are largely unknown. It has not been shown that the wear particles have a genuine chemotactic influence on monocytes. SANTAVIRTA et al. (1990b, 1991) were able to demonstrate that the phagocytes were C3bi receptor- and non-specific esterase-positive monocyte-macrophages. Lysozymes, acid phosphatases (GOLDRING et al. 1983; HAYASHI and INOUE 1986; HEILMANN et al. 1975; LENNOX et al. 1987; LINDER et al. 1983), collagenases (DORR et al. 1990; GOLDRING et al. 1986; SANTAVIRTA el al. 1990 b) and prostaglandin E_2 (DORR et al. 1990; GOLDRING et al. 1983, 1986; HERMAN et al. 1989; SPECTOR et al. 1990) have all been detected in the histiocytes. Some of these factors are mediators of bone resorption, especially prostaglandin E_2, which has been found in larger amounts in interface membranes of loose prostheses (GOODMAN et al. 1989). Thus it seems likely that the macrophages play an important role in the process of loosening of endoprostheses.

The exact mechanism of cytokine involvement or the sort of interaction with other inflammatory cells is still largely unclear. A minimal to moderate degree of lymphocytic infiltration usually appears within accumulations of histiocytes (HAYASHI and INOUE 1986; REVEL 1982; WILLERT and SEMLITSCH 1975, 1976b). According to SANTAVIRTA et al. (1990b, 1991), these lymphocytes belong to resting, interleukin-2 and transferrin receptor-negative T lymphocytes. In contrast, the data of HERMAN et al. (1989) suggest that the T lymphocytes are involved in the activation of monocytes.

Interleukin-1, a macrophage product which is of general importance in inflammatory diseases, was also detected in the inflammatory infiltrate around joint endoprostheses (DORR et al. 1990; HERMAN et al. 1989). HERMAN et al. (1989) found that the in vitro exposure of blood monocytes to PMMA caused release of interleukin-1, tumor necrosis factor and prostaglandin E_2.

5.2 Quantity and Distribution of Histiocytes in Surgical Specimens and Autopsy Material

In the case of a loosened prosthesis, histiocytic infiltrates are not only found in the pseudocapsule but can also be seen as layers of varying thickness around the prosthesis or its cement mantle (BOS et al. 1990a; GOLDRING et al. 1983, 1986; GOODMAN et al. 1989; HEILMAN et al. 1975; JOHANSON et al. 1987; LENNOX et al. 1987). In vertical sections the histiocytic infiltrates appear macroscopically as yellow layers usually a few millimeters thick, and occasionally exceeding 1 cm. A prominent histiocytic reaction frequently is accompanied by marked villous transformation of the newly formed synovial membranes (Figs. 15, 16).

In pseudocapsules of firmly fixed *prostheses* retrieved at autopsy we were able to demonstrate a positive correlation between implant duration and quantity of wear particles, number of phagocytic histiocytes, thickness of the synovial membrane and extent of villous transformation (BOS and LÖHRS 1991; Table 1). In surgical samples from loose *prostheses* a positive correlation between the time

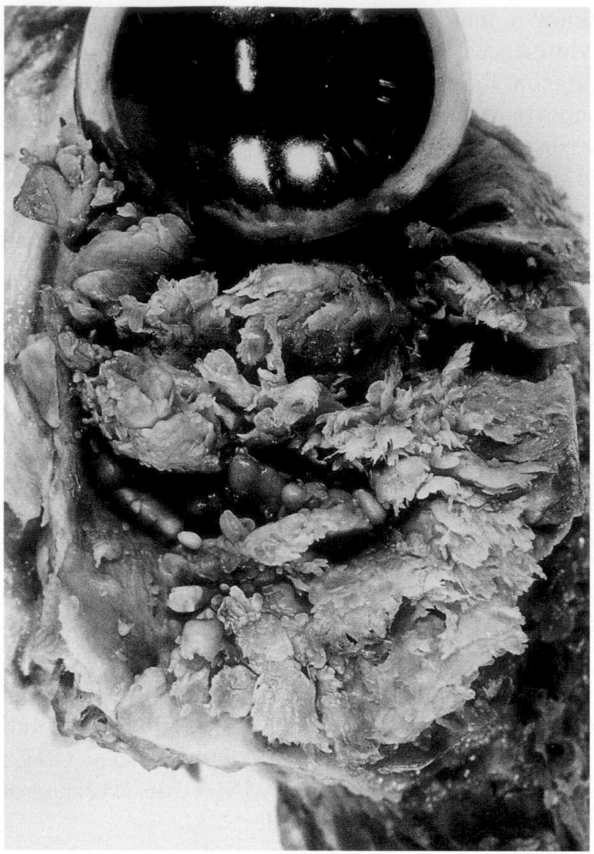

Fig. 15. Marked villous transformation of the synovium from a prosthesis with metal–polyethylene pairing of the contacting surfaces after 12 years in situ (*top*: metal head)

in situ, the extent of wear particles and the histiocytic reaction was also seen. The histology of the inflammatory reaction was primarily dependent on the size and amount of the wear particles rather than on the type of foreign material. A possible exception in this respect is pure ceramic wear, which according to Lennox et al. (1987) does not cause degenerative cell changes.

Even though there were vast differences in the degree of inflammation, we conclude, in agreement with Willert et al. (1978), that the use of the term "aggressive granulomatosis" as a distinct entity (as proposed by Brinkmann and Heilmann 1974; Dannenmaier et al. 1985; Griffiths et al. 1987; Harris et al. 1976; Tallroth et al. 1989; Santavirta et al. 1990a,b, 1991) is not justified. In our investigations of a large number of specimens we were unable to find any clearly defined granulomas. Moreover, the number of giant cells appeared to be dependent exclusively on the size and amount of the wear particles.

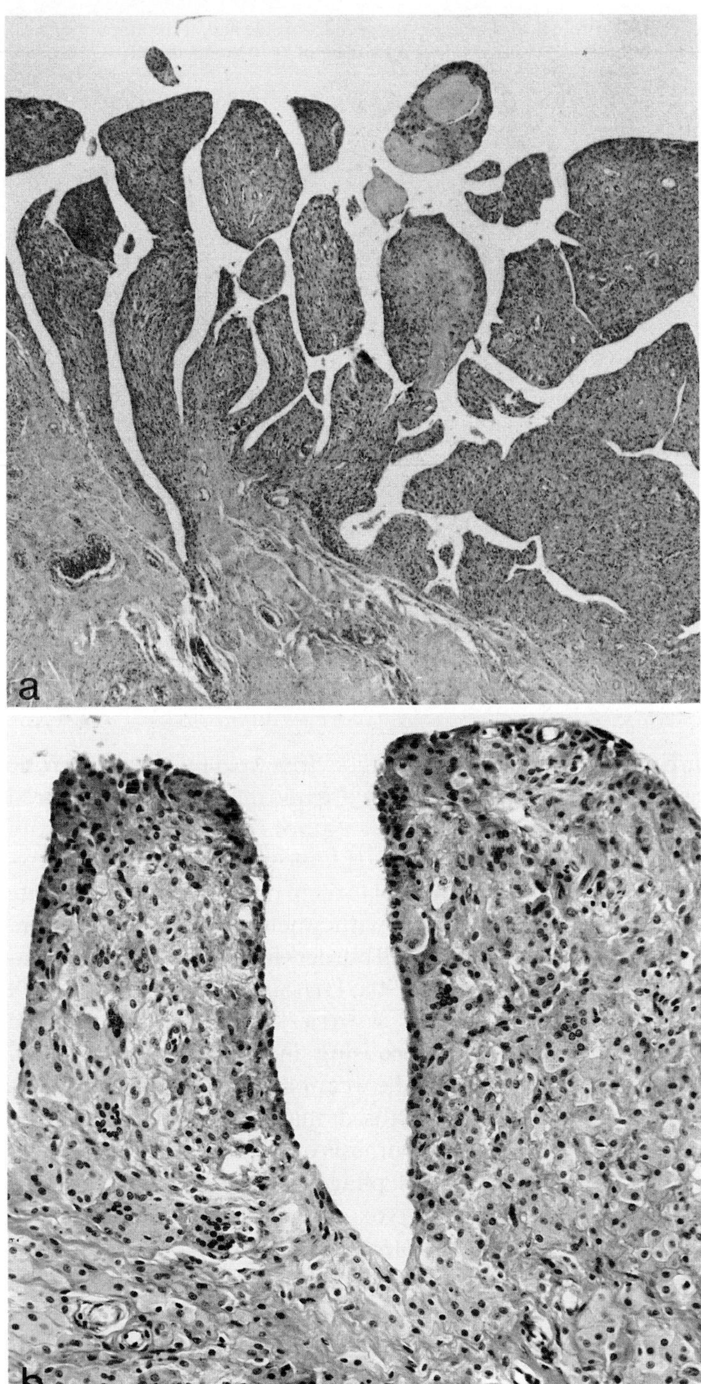

Fig. 16a, b. Pseudocapsule with villous transformation and prominent histiocytic reaction, 5 years after implantation. **a** Overview; H&E, × 40. **b** × 160

Table 1. Grading of the reactive histological changes in the pseudocapsule and of the amount of wear particles: semiquantitative evaluations. Average values on a scale of 1–10 are recorded

Implant duration	<6 mo	6 mo–2 yr	2–4 yr	4–6 yr	6–8 yr	8–10 yr	>10 yr
Average thickness of the synovial membrane (mm)*	2.3	1.8	2.0	2.8	2.3	3.6	3.3
Bone cement wear* (fine granular particles)	0.0	2.0	2.8	3.6	6.7	4.4	5.0
Large bone cement particles**	1.9	6.0	5.5	5.4	6.1	5.8	5.4
Polyethylene wear particles*	0.2	1.6	1.7	3.0	5.2	4.6	4.6
Histiocytic reaction*	2.1	3.2	5.2	5.7	6.7	7.0	7.8
Villous transformation*	0.9	2.6	4.5	3.7	2.6	6.0	5.6
Fibrin	6.9	5.7	3.5	5.9	5.9	4.2	3.6
Granulation tissue	9.1	6.9	6.0	6.0	4.1	5.6	5.4
Necrosis*	2.2	2.7	4.5	7.9	4.8	8.6	7.4
Haemosiderin	6.4	4.2	4.8	3.3	4.4	3.0	5.7
Fibrosis*	6.1	5.9	7.8	7.7	7.9	8.2	8.1
Ectopic ossification	5.0	7.5	5.0	5.4	4.1	6.4	2.8

Asterisks indicate a positive correlation to implant duration: $*P < 0.01$, $P < 0.05$

5.3 Histiocytic Degeneration

Histiocytes from the peri-articular soft tissue phagocytose wear products, necrotic tissue and the debris of haemorrhages. Although organic material can be cleared by lysosomal enzymes, it is accepted by most authors that the debris from endoprostheses cannot be similarly degraded (Lennox et al. 1987; Vernon-Roberts and Freeman 1976). A large amount of foreign material can accumulate in the cytoplasm, which is frequently associated with concurrent cell degeneration. Chromatin agglomeration, disintegration of cell borders followed by cell dissociation and necrosis can all develop (Bos et al. 1990a; Heilmann et al. 1975; Lennox et al. 1987; Willert and Semlitsch 1976b; Winter 1974). The pathogenetic explanation for these degenerative and necrotising changes has not yet been established. Direct toxic effects arising from the wear particles have been considered; in addition the quantity of phagocytosed material may prove to be important. Moreover it is thought that the synthesis of lytic enzymes induced by foreign particles may lead to dissolution of phagosome membranes, enzyme release and, thus, to cell disintegration (Lennox et al. 1987; Riede et al. 1974; Willert et al. 1980; Winter 1974). Our electron microscopic observations, showing that many of the foreign particles lacked surrounding membrane structures, would support this view.

Other tissue changes regularly become manifest after extended implant duration. Areas of necrosis, scar-like fibrosis and haemosiderin deposits can then be found in pseudocapsules and interface membranes between cement mantle and bone. Scattered plasma cell and mast cell infiltrates as well as fibrin exudates and metaplastic ossifications appear somewhat less consistently (Table 1). In contrast to infectious inflammation, granulocytic exudates are sparse.

5.4 Fibrosis

Marked fibrosis frequently develops after longer duration in situ (COTTA and SCHULITZ 1970; LINDER et al. 1983; REVELL 1982; WILLERT and SEMLITSCH 1976b) and is presumably in part the consequence of organisation (COTTA and SCHULITZ 1970; Linder et al. 1983; REVELL 1982; WILLERT and SEMLITSCH 1976b). We observed no material-related differences in the extent of capsular fibrosis and so were unable to substantiate the findings of LINTNER et al. (1984), who reported increased fibrosis with ceramic-ceramic and ceramic-polyethylene combinations.

5.5 Necrosis

Necrosis is also prevalent in the soft tissues surrounding endoprostheses (BENEKE et al. 1973; REVELL 1982; VERNON-ROBERTS and FREEMAN 1976; WILLERT and SEMLITSCH 1976b). LINTNER et al. (1984) report an incidence of 75% for cemented

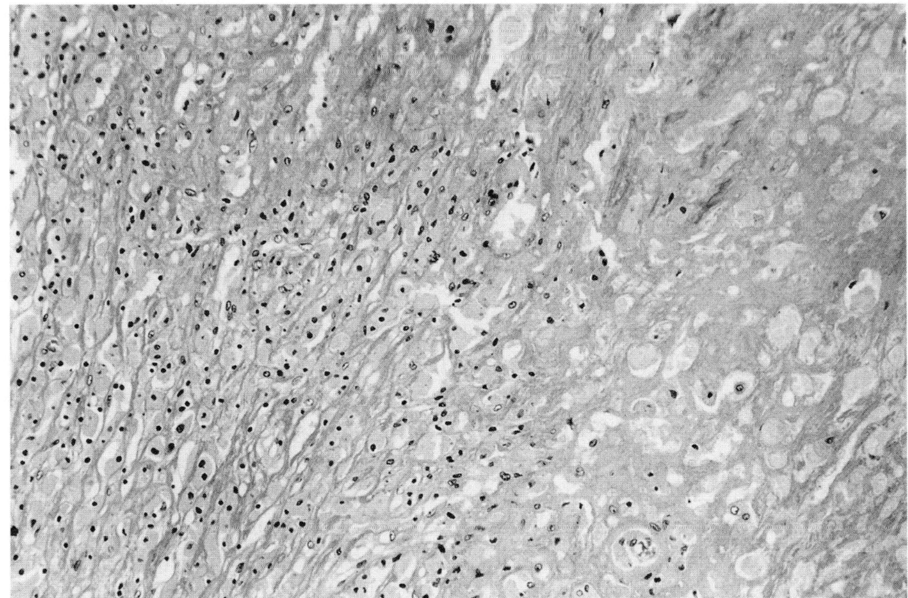

Fig. 17. Extended necrosis of histiocytic infiltrate (right: shadows of necrotic histiocytes with loss of nuclei). Non-decalcified section, Goldner's trichrome, × 160

models. In our study necrosis developed in almost all cases in which cemented prostheses had been implanted for longer than 2 years. In pseudocapsules of firmly fixed prostheses (autopsy material) the amount of necrosis and scar tissue showed a positive correlation with implant duration. After long-term implantation extended, sharply delineated necrotic areas of histiocytic infiltrates (Fig. 17) as well as of fibrotic tissue were seen which sometimes constituted more than one-third of the pseudocapsular sections. This indicates that necrosis is not exclusively the result of degenerative cell changes but also the product of mechanical alterations of the capsule.

5.6 Haemosiderin Deposits

Haemosiderin deposits derived from haemorrhages in the process of resorption were almost always seen in varying degrees (Dielert et al. 1983; Johanson et al. 1987; Vernon-Roberts and Freeman 1976; Willert et al. 1974). The cause was considered to be microtrauma with small blood vessel rupture and possibly vascular necrosis (Dielert et al. 1983; Vernon-Roberts and Freeman 1976).

5.7 Metaplastic Ossifications

The reported incidence of metaplastic ossifications in peri-articular soft tissue varies from 5% to 50% in radiological investigations (Arcq 1973; Brooker et al. 1973; Charnley 1972). We observed that in more than 50% of cases of loosened prostheses the soft tissues contained ectopic ossifications when even the smallest foci were included.

5.8 Comparison Between Cemented and Non-cemented Prostheses

When cemented and non-cemented prostheses were compared, models with cementless fixation showed less inflammatory pseudocapsular changes (Lintner et al. 1984). Minor inflammatory alterations with fibrin exudates, lymphocytic infiltration and fibrosis can also be found in the capsules of stable non-cemented prostheses. Even in the total absence of wear particles enough friction is presumed to exist between capsule and stiff prosthetic components to induce mechanical irritation. Histiocytic infiltration has also been seen in isolated cases with loosened prostheses without release of wear particles, obviously as a consequence of fibrin resorption, necrosis and bleeding. If marked metal wear of a porous stem surface takes place, the histological appearance can be similar to that of cemented prostheses (Bobyn et al. 1987; Dorr et al. 1990; Lennox et al. 1987). A final comparison between cemented and non-cemented prostheses will be possible only after longer implant duration. Results of preliminary studies indicate that markedly less pronounced inflammatory changes are to be expected with the non-cemented designs.

5.9 Histology of the Bone–Cement Interface Membranes in Loosened Prostheses

In comparison with pseudocapsule tissue, interface membranes between bone and cement mantle have several special characteristics (Fig. 18). Some authors have described the membranes as having three distinct histological zones: a synovial-like lining on the cement side, a middle layer containing histiocytes and giant cells and peripheral fibrosis on the membrane's bone side (GOLDRING et al. 1983; JOHANSON et al. 1987; MAGUIRE et al. 1987). In a study which included material from implants as long as 19 years in situ, we were unable to verify such a regular arrangement (BOS et al. 1990a). LENNOX et al. (1987) and GOODMAN et al. (1989) also found that a synovial-like lining at the bone–cement interface was only inconsistently present. More often necroses, fibrin sheaths, fibrocytes or collagen

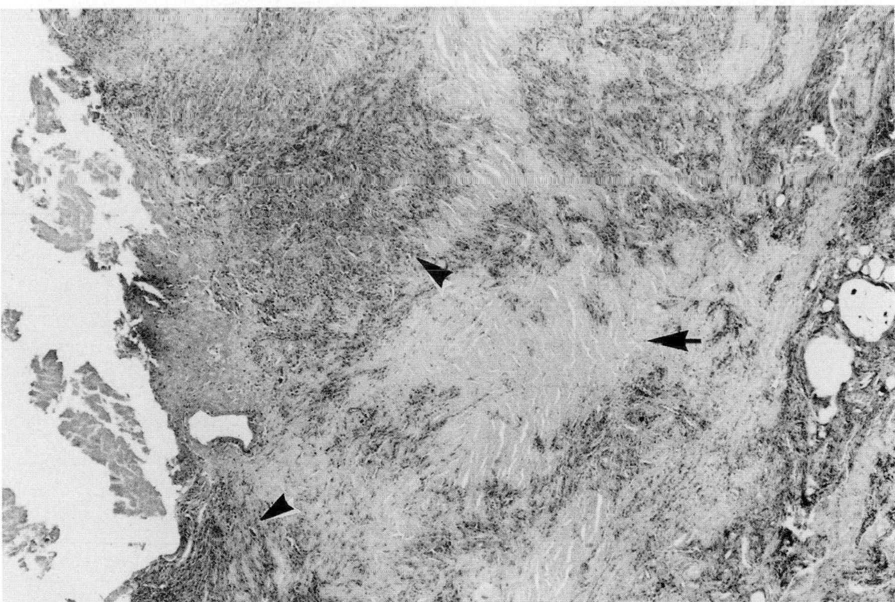

Fig. 18. Soft tissue membrane in the femur bone marrow surrounding a loose hip prosthesis. Inner layer (*left*): necrotic histiocytic infiltrates (*arrowheads*) and fibrosis. Middle layer: degenerative changes and partial necrosis of connective tissue (*arrow*). Outer layer: histiocytes and connective tissue with numerous large bone cement inclusions. H&E, × 40

fibres were found to border on the cement mantle (Bos et al. 1990a, Lennox et al. 1987). In cancellous bone histiocytic infiltrates were frequently observed to be in direct contact with the surface of the bone trabeculae. These exhibited the signs of remodelling predominantly; occasionally resorption lacunae with osteoclasts were seen (Bos et al. 1990a, Linder et al. 1983; Willert et al. 1990b). According to Lennox et al. (1987), interface membranes from loose non-cemented prostheses are composed of poorly vascularised dense fibrous tissue with rare macrophages and other inflammatory cells. Wear particles of mainly metal debris were only sporadically present.

6 Bone Changes in Stable Endoprostheses After Extended Implant Duration

The majority of publications have been concerned with changes in the femur in cemented implants. According to Willert (1973) reparative process in bone traumatised during hip prosthesis implantation takes 1–2 years. Delling et al.

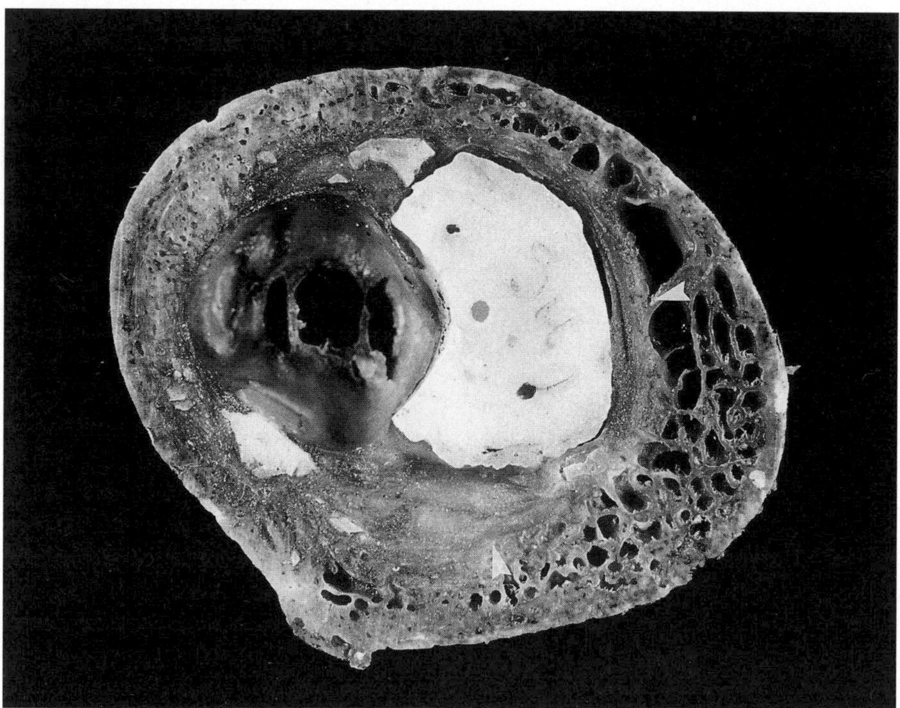

Fig. 19. Femoral cross-section in the area of the lower end of the prosthesis after 7 years in situ. Segmental broad soft tissue membrane between cement and bone (*arrowheads*) with eccentrically lying prosthesis stem

(1987) found that the stabilisation phase begins as soon as a few months after implantation. It is generally accepted that after this period, no further time-dependent alterations take place. Studies on non-weight-bearing cement implants in animals demonstrate a complete encircling of the bone cement plug by newly formed bone which is in direct contact with the cement (DRAENERT et al. 1976). Weight-bearing prostheses, in contrast, are usually separated from bone by a connective tissue membrane of varying width (Fig. 19) in the stabilisation phase (CHARNLEY 1964; DELLING et al. 1987; FREEMAN et al. 1982; GROSS et al. 1984; LINTNER et al. 1982; MALCOLM 1988; REVELL 1982; VERNON-ROBERTS and FREEMAN 1976; WILLERT and PULS 1972). Only JASTY et al. (1990) describe a predominantly direct bone–cement contact, even after an extended implant time. DELLING et al. (1987) found that prostheses of short implant duration showed direct bone–cement contact over as much as 20% of the circumferential surface. Data concerning the width of the connective tissue membrane vary from 5 μm after 6 months in situ (CHARNLEY 1964) to 1.5 mm (VERNON-ROBERTS and FREEMAN 1976; WILLERT and PULS 1972). CHARNLEY (1964) documents a progressive reduction in membrane thickness from 1.0 mm in the proximal part of 0.25 mm in the distal part for prostheses of up to 3.5 years in situ. This interface membrane consists of relatively acellular collagen fibres (REVELL 1982), with an incomplete layer of foreign body giant cells facing the cement surface (LINTNER et al. 1982). Other authors describe a cell composition comparable to the soft tissue membranes found around loose prostheses with marked histiocytic reaction (Figs. 20, 21), fibrin exudates, haemorrhages, necroses and granulation tissue (MALCOLM 1988;

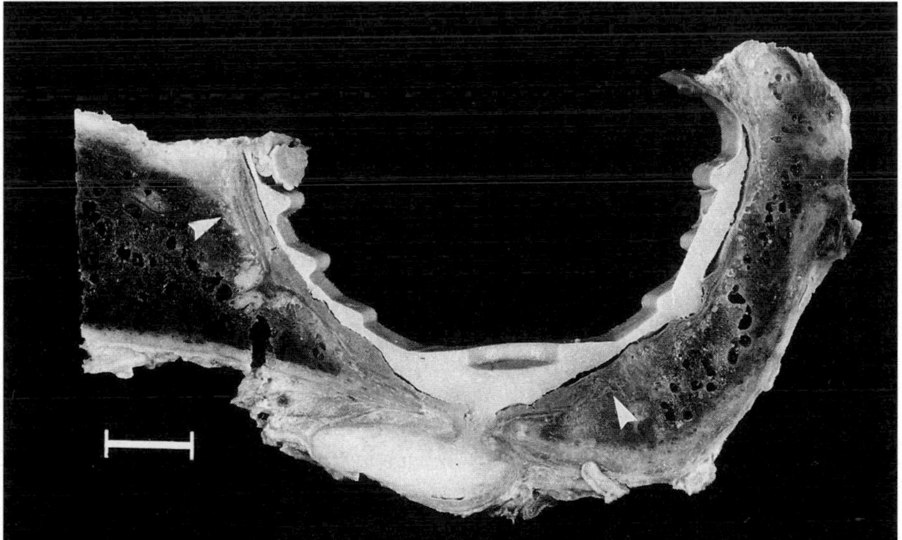

Fig. 20. Section through the acetabular region after 8 years in situ. Broad continuous soft tissue membrane (*arrowheads*) between cement and bone. At the bottom, there is a defect of compact bone bordering the minor pelvis with fibrous encapsulated herniation of bone cement (*bar* = 1 cm)

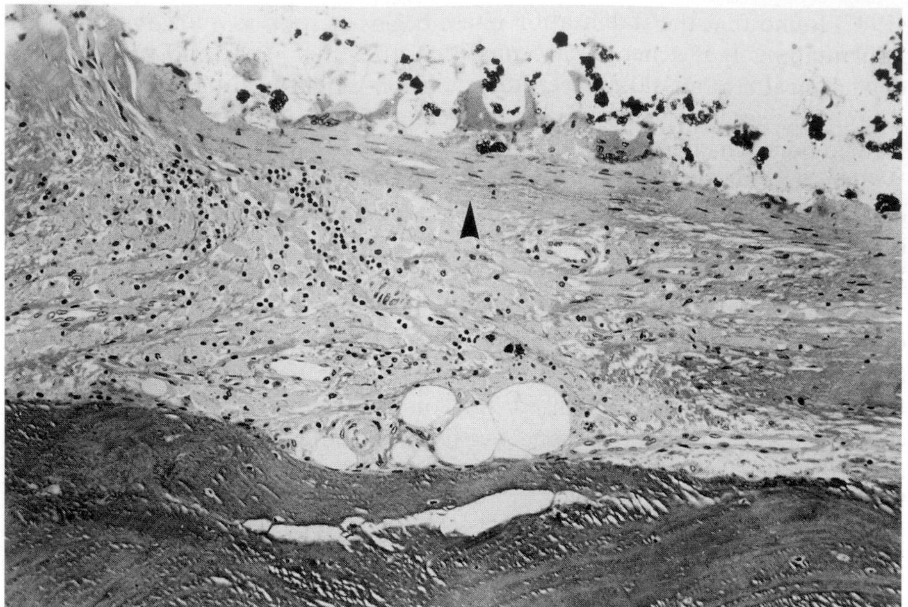

Fig. 21. Interface membrane of the acetabular region of a firmly fixed prosthesis with zonal arrangement in layers. *Top*: bone cement with PMMA spherules, bordered by giant cells, adjacent to a thin connective tissue membrane (*arrowhead*). *Middle*: mainly histiocytic infiltration with scattered lymphocytes. *Bottom*: newly formed compact bone. Non-decalcified section, Goldner's trichrome, × 160

Szyskowitz 1973; Willert 1973; Willert and Puls 1972). Spherical polymethyl methacrylate inclusions were frequently found (Vernon-Roberts and Freeman 1976) as well as small wear particles of bone cement, metal and polyethylene (Malcolm 1988). According to Delling et al. (1983) non-cemented prostheses show extended connective tissue membranes between the prosthetic stem and bone, too. However, macrophages are present only when these membranes also contain metal or ceramic wear particles (Lennox et al. 1987).

In the literature various opinions about the significance of this connective tissue membrane can be found. Willert and Puls (1972) believed it to have a biomechanically beneficial function in dampening physical stresses. Other authors have considered it to be the product of mechanical irritation at the bone–cement interface leading to a reactive fibroblastic proliferation (Draenert und Rudigier 1978; Szyskowitz 1973). Willert (1973) thought the haemorrhages and fibrin exudates in the membrane were the result of microtrauma exceeding the membrane's elastic capacity. Delling et al. (1987) considered the accumulation of histiocytes and giant cells to be due to minimal bone cement wear.

As the changes in the femur are not progressive with increased implant duration, it can be assumed that moderate histiocytic infiltration of the membrane is not a sign of incipient prosthetic loosening.

Our own investigations on the acetabulum around cemented polyethylene sockets revealed different findings. Even in short-term implants we found, in accordance with DELLING et al. (1987), practically no direct bone–cement contact. The thickness of the interface membrane (Figs. 20–22), which varied markedly, nevertheless correlated significantly with implant duration. Most of the soft tissue membranes contained aggregates of histiocytes which had phagocytosed predominantly bone cement wear, and polyethylene fibres to a lesser degree. Histiocytic infiltration was also frequently found in the adjacent cancellous bone (Figs. 22,23).

Numerous studies have also been done on bone remodelling in the femur with a hip endoprosthesis. It has generally been observed that after extended time in situ, cemented prostheses show resorption of the stump of the femoral neck next

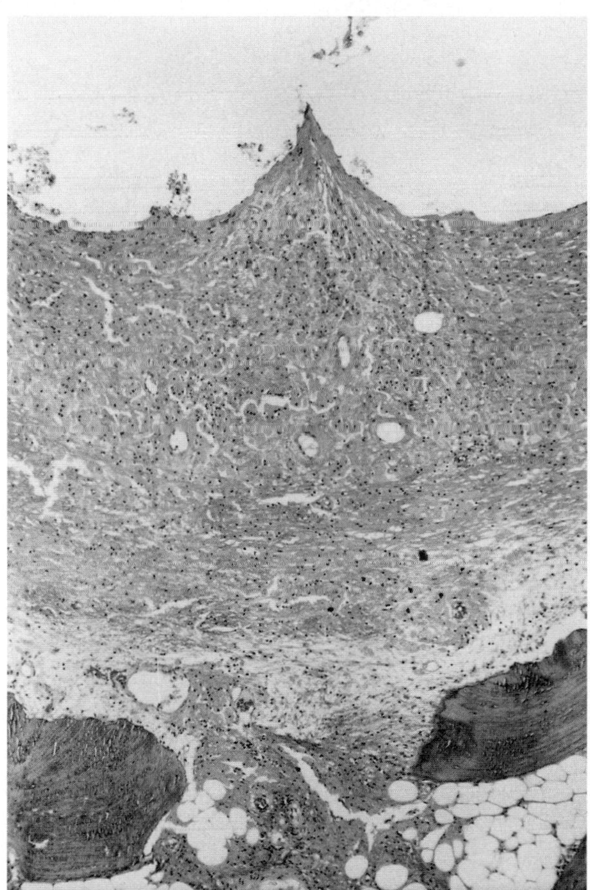

Fig. 22. Soft tissue membrane between bone and cement (*top*) adjacent to a firmly fixed polyethylene socket with broad seams of histiocytes. *Below*: beginning histiocytic infiltration of the bone marrow invading through a gap of the neocortical bone. Non-decalcified section, Goldner's trichrome, × 60

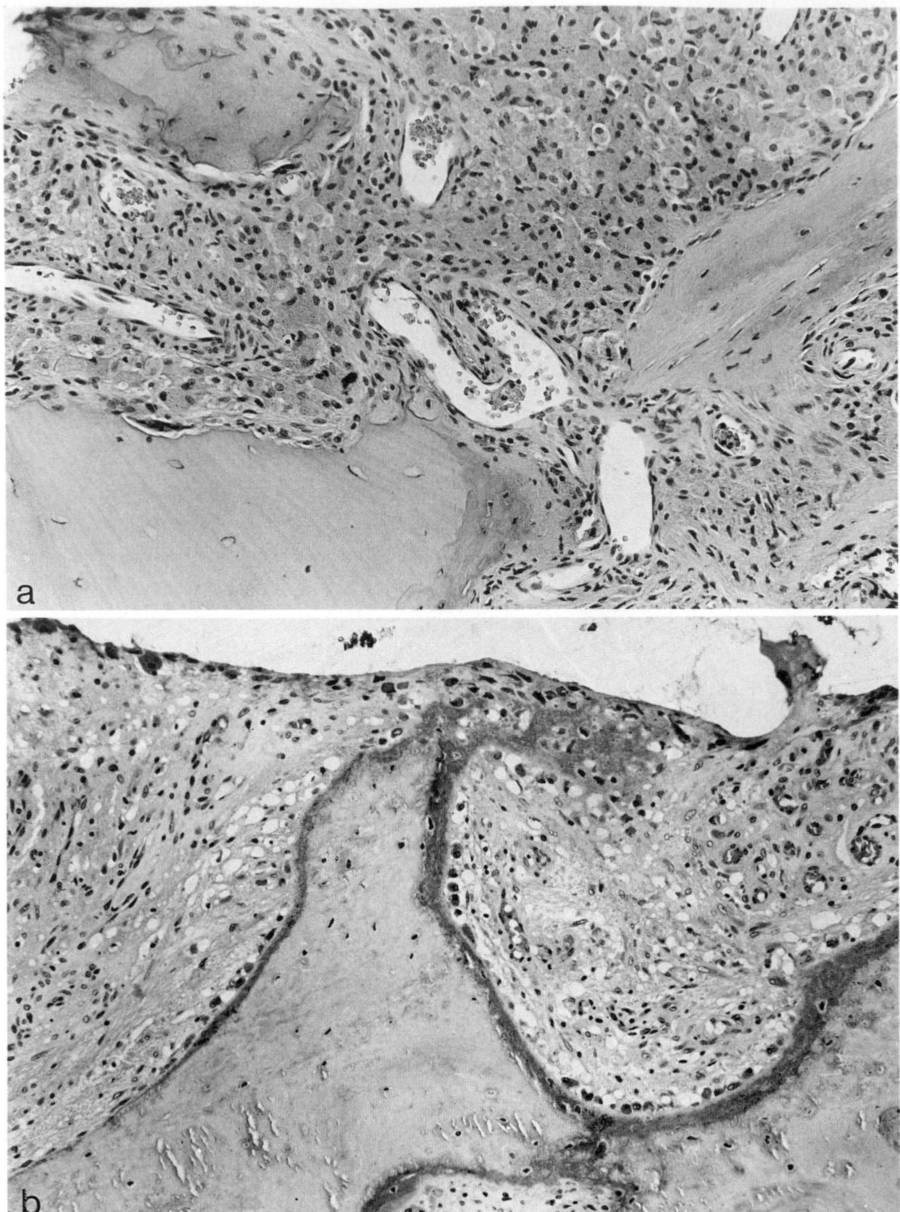

Fig. 23 a, b. Cancellous bone with histiocytic infiltration around a loose (**a**) and a stable (**b**) socket. Bone trabeculae showing signs of remodelling with osteoclastic resorption lacunae (**a**) and seams of osteoid and osteoblasts (**b**). **a** H&E, **b** non-decalcified section, Goldner's trichrome, × 160

to the collar, i.e. the calcar femorale (CHARNLEY 1964; EYB 1987; FAGAN and LEE 1986; JASTY et al. 1990; KÖLLER et al. 1990). The cause of this progressive bone resorption is considered to be disuse osteoporosis since post-transplantation load transfer is no longer transmitted via the cortical bone of the femoral neck, but rather via the bone cement to the distal two-thirds of the stem (CHARNLEY 1964; GROSS et al. 1984; WILLERT and SEMLITSCH 1976 a). Destruction of the blood supply during removal of the femoral head is seen as another possible cause (CHARNLEY 1964). Other factors responsible for the bone resorption at the calcar femorale may be increased micromotion between bone and cement (FAGAN and LEE 1986) and inflammatory changes caused by a higher concentration of wear particles (BOCCO et al. 1977; EYB 1987; GRISS et al. 1978). There is some controversy about the trabecular and cortical bone volume in the other areas of the femur. KÖLLER et al. (1990) did not find reductions in femur bone density of cortical bone or spongiosa in their morphometric studies. Other histological investigations revealed a decrease in cortical bone density or less frequently an increase in the thickness of the cortex (CHARNLEY et al. 1968; COMADOLL et al. 1988; GROSS et al. 1984; JASTY et al. 1990). REVELL (1982) and VERNON-ROBERTS and FREEMAN (1986) observed atrophy of the cancellous bone.

Marked changes in cancellous bone generally occur after longer implant duration. The architecture and the density of the trabecular bone basically reflect the alteration of the mechanical stresses (FAGAN and LEE 1986). A circumferential arrangement of newly formed lamellar bone around the cement cast or prosthesis stem, termed "neocorticalis" by some authors, has been noted in numerous investigations (DRAENERT 1981; DRAENERT and RUDIGIER 1978; GROSS et al. 1984; JASTY et al. 1990; MITTELMEIER and HARMS 1979a). We were able to observe the same phenomenon in the acetabular bone (Figs. 21, 22, 24). New bone formation occurs both as appositional bone on viable as well as necrotic trabeculae and as woven bone in the fibrous tissue, which is later reorganised into a lamellar structure. New bone formation is associated with simultaneous osteoclastic resorption of parts of the original trabeculae. After completion of the remodelling process the inner concentrically aligned layers of bone adjacent to the prosthesis are connected with the cortical bone through radially orientated trabeculae with cross-connections parallel to the cement surface (REVELL 1982; VERNON-ROBERTS and FREEMAN 1976; WILLERT and PULS 1972). Femora with endoprostheses demonstrate a continuous remodelling of bone that is independent of implant duration and considerably more extensive than that found in the femur under normal circumstances (DELLING et al. 1987; GROSS et al. 1984; Jasty et al. 1990; REVELL 1982). In particular, osteoid layers and osteoblast rims (Fig. 23b) have been described as evidence of this transformation (GROSS et al. 1984; WILLERT and PULS 1972; WILLERT et al. 1974). Osteoid layers have been viewed both as a sign of bone apposition by some authors and as a result of secondary demineralisation due to bone cement toxicity by others (DELLING et al. 1987; LINTNER et al. 1982, 1987). We also observed resorption lacunae with osteoclasts (Fig. 23a), though they are present only infrequently (KÖLLER et al. 1990; LINTNER et al. 1982; WILLERT and PULS 1972). Several investigations on cement-free femur implants

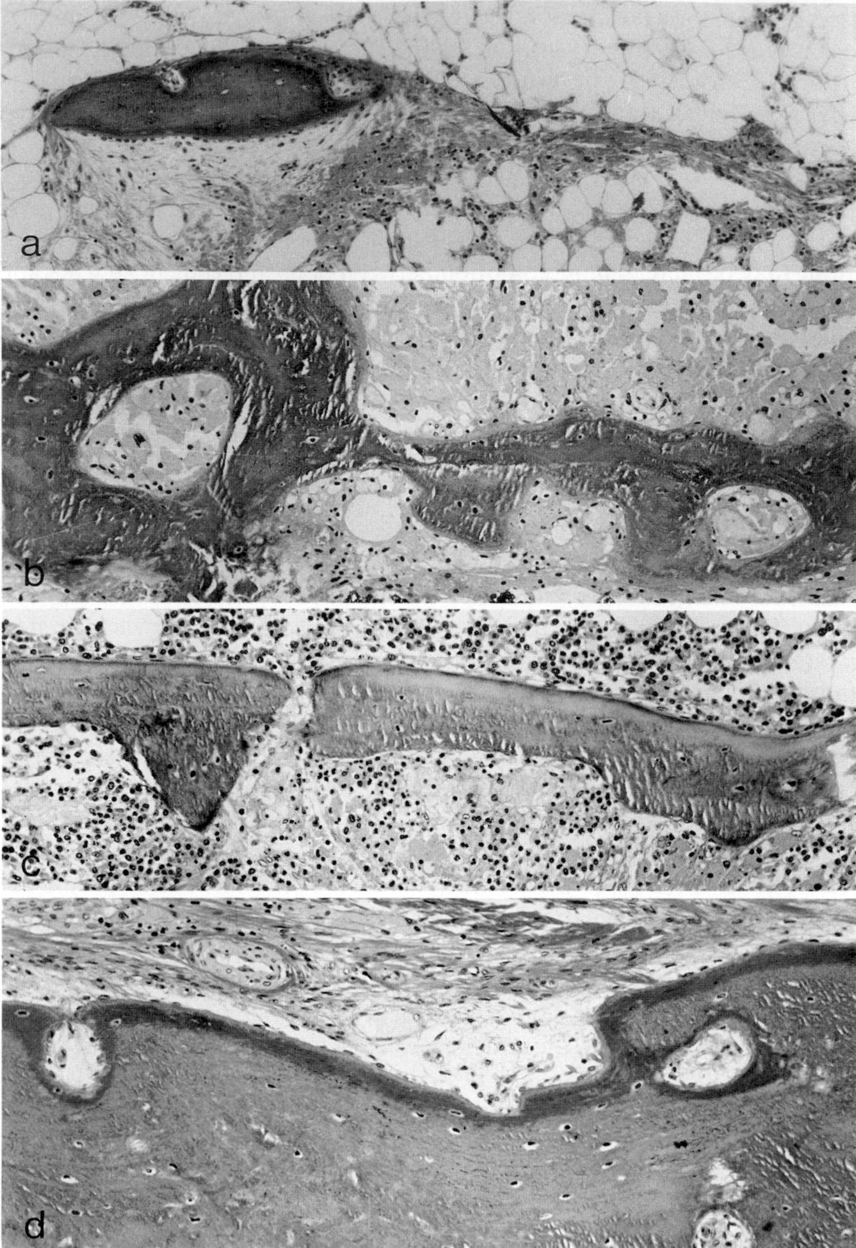

Fig. 24 a–d. Progressive development of neocortical bone in the acetabular region in firmly fixed hip joint prostheses. **a** Initial development of a thin bone trabecula showing osteoid and osteoblast seams. **b** Broad continuous layer of newly formed bone with abundant osteoid and poor mineralisation. **c** Regularly structured, minimally broadened trabecular bone layers without signs of remodelling. **d** Broad continuous layer of neocortical bone with a structure that appears almost identical to cortical bone. Non-decalcified sections, Goldner's trichrome, × 160

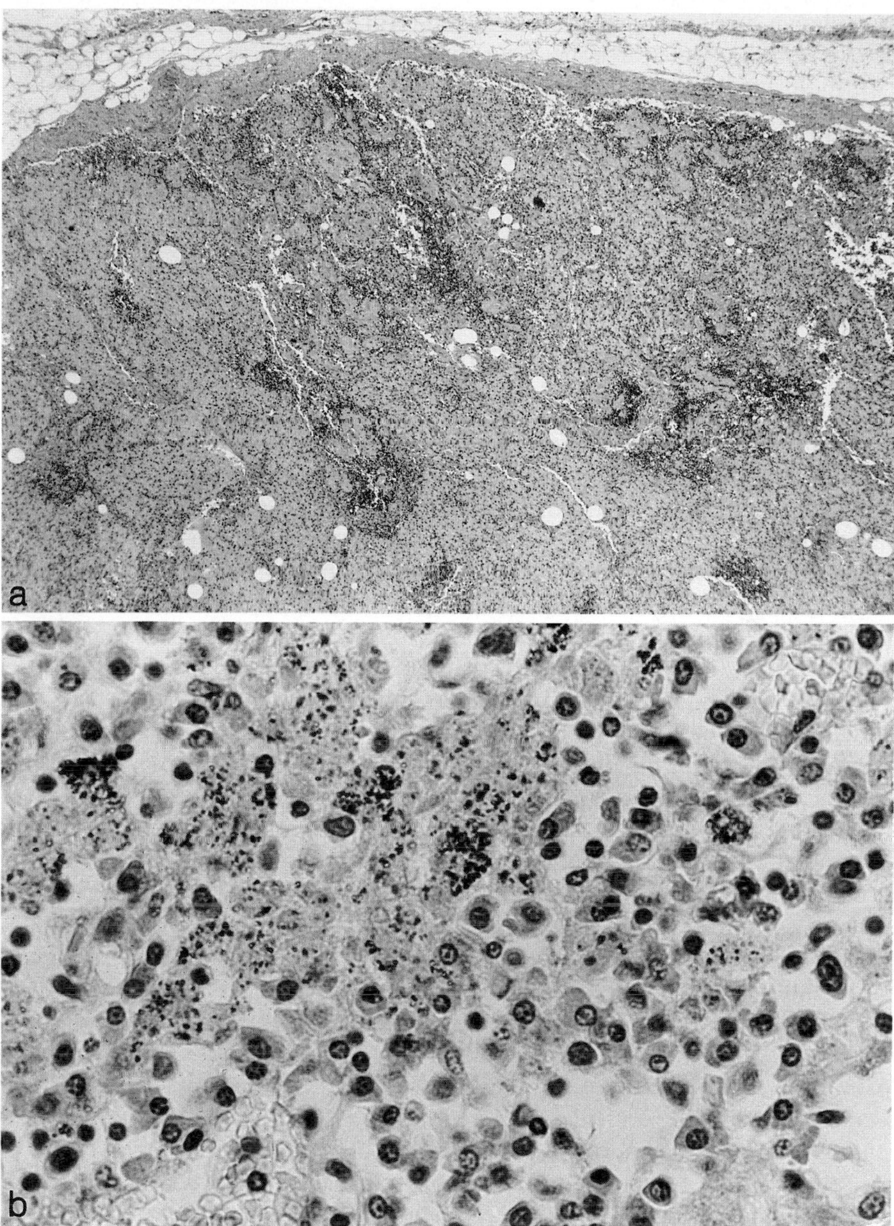

Fig. 25 a, b. Lymph node with marked histiocytosis and partial effacement of the nodal architecture. **a** Overview; H&E, $\times 40$. **b** Histiocytes with degenerative changes and abundant, predominantly metal wear particles; H&E, $\times 400$

have shown similar evidence of remodelling (Biehl et al. 1975; Mittelmeier and Harms 1979b). Cortical bone resorption on the femoral calcar presents an exception which, according to Eyb (1987), is less prominent in cement-free prostheses.

7 Spread of Wear Particles Through the Lymphatic System

In the literature sporadic descriptions of wear particles in lymph nodes with a histiocytic reaction are found (Gray et al. 1989; Heilmann et al. 1975; Jozsa and Reffy 1980; Mendes et al. 1974; Vernon-Roberts and Freeman 1976; Walker and Bullough 1973). Mostly, metal and polyethylene wear fragments have been described (Josza and Reffy 1980; Walker and Bullough 1973). Silicone lymphadenopathy has been found to be among the most frequently described foreign body reactions in lymph nodes (Christie et al. 1977; Kircher 1980; Nalbandian et al. 1983; Travis et al. 1985), Nalbandian et al. reporting it to be encountered in 0.01% of cases with small joint silicone prostheses.

In a systematic autopsy study of subdiaphragmatic lymph nodes we were able to demonstrate bone cement and polyethylene wear particles in all groups of lymph nodes from 32 patients with hip prostheses (Bos et al. 1990b). The amount of wear particles, which appeared as soon as 1.5 years after insertion, correlated positively with the time in situ. In cases with small quantities of wear particles the foreign material was found in a few scattered macrophages or small groups of histiocytes in the nodal sinuses. Larger quantities, however, were found in cohesive histiocytic infiltrates with partial effacement of the nodal architecture (Fig. 25). Wear particles appeared in varying numbers but were seen simultaneously in all lymph node groups. Most were found in the ipsilateral para-iliac nodes and the para-aortic nodes bilaterally. Minor amounts had reached the contralateral para-iliac nodes, probably via lymphatic anastomoses or retrograde spread, and the ipsilateral inguinal and obturator nodes were also involved. As in the pseudocapsules, bone cement debris predominated. Further, the amount of bone cement debris in lymph nodes correlated well with findings in the pseudocapsules. For polyethylene fragments no analogous correlation was demonstrable. In contrast to the pseudocapsules, the lymph nodes contained only small polyethylene fibres. The lymphatic system draining the pseudocapsule appears to have a filtering function, allowing only small polyethylene fibres to pass through to the lymph nodes. Like the histiocytes in the pseudocapsule, histiocytes in the lymph nodes containing wear particles demonstrated degenerative changes and necrosis as well. However, coherent well-demarcated areas of necrosis were not found in the lymph nodes.

8 Late Complications

Among the late complications non-infectious loosening of the prosthesis is of special interest (FOREST et al. 1991). In addition, prosthesis fracture and late infection may occur.

8.1 Late Infection

Infection in artificial joints appearing after 6 months post implantation is defined as late infection. It usually develops by haematogenous spread of bacteria from a distant focus. A distinction is made between acute and chronic infection. In acute infections of late onset the same spectrum of pathogenic organisms is seen as in early infections, with *Staphylococcus* aureus predominating (see Sect. 2.2) The chronic forms, however, are mostly due to infection with *Staphylococcus epidermidis* (GAUDILLAT and DEPLUS 1987).

Histologically acute late infections are characterised by granulocytic infiltration (FOREST 1987), while chronic inflammations are recognised by infiltrates of lymphocytes and plasma cells which appear in considerably greater numbers than in non-infectious inflammation.

8.2 Pathogenesis of Non-infectious Loosening

Most research has been done concerning loosening of the femoral components in cemented hip prostheses. In the literature very different figures with respect to the loosening rate are found, varying from 5.2% (COURPIED and POSTEL 1987) to 57% (LING 1981) after 10 years. Increased activity, obesity, suboptimal implant design, insufficient initial fixation due to poor cementation technique or malpositioning of the prosthesis (varus or eccentric stem position) and a defective implant bed as in osteoporosis or after revision surgery are all considered to be predisposing factors (ALDINGER 1987; EYB 1987; HARRIS et al. 1982; JOHANSON et al. 1987; KÖLLER et al. 1990; KRAUSE and MATHIS 1988; WILLERT et al. 1974). The incidences recorded for socket loosening are similarly divergent, with figures from 1.4% after 8 years (EFTEKHAR 1971) to over 50% after less than 10 years (CHANDLER et al. 1981). Poor cement distribution in the acetabulum and malpositioning (especially with the cup in vertical position) have been associated with premature loosening (COURPIED and POSTEL 1987; KÖLBEL and BOENICK 1972).

A multifactorial process evidently underlies prosthesis loosening (BOS et al. 1990a; KRAUSE and MATHIS 1988, LENNOX et al. 1987), which, according to JOHANSON et al. (1987), can be divided into a mechanical and a biological phase

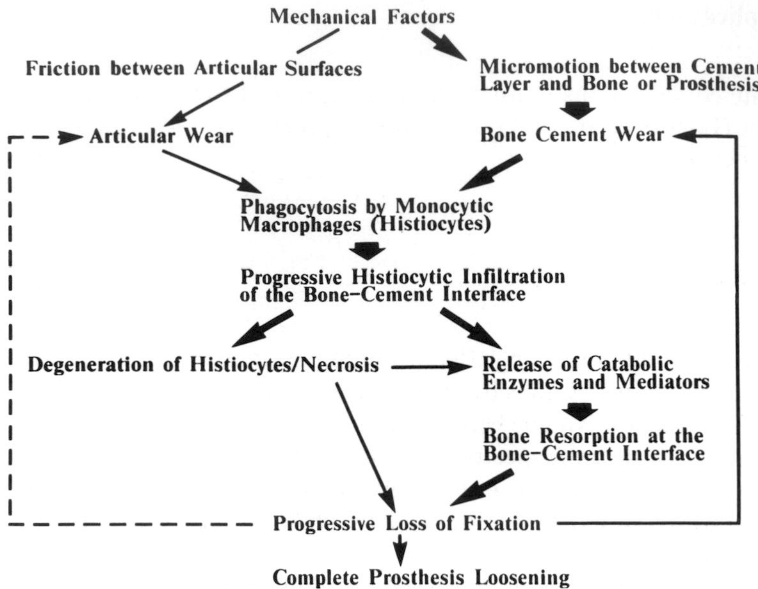

Fig. 26. Pathogenetic concept of non-infectious loosening in cemented joint prostheses

(Fig. 26). Some authors believe that mechanical factors are predominantly or exclusively responsible. Thus SCHNEIDER (1976) suggested loosening to be the consequence of alternating pressure and traction forces with consecutive bone resorption. Loosening mostly takes place at the bone–cement interface, which is regarded as the weakest link in the chain of bone–cement implant systems (BEAN et al. 1987). Because of differences in the mechanical properties of cement and bone, shear stresses result during load transmission which cause minimal relative motion at the bone–cement interface (DIENEL et al. 1984; GEBAUER et al. 1983; JASTY et al. 1990; MAGUIRE et al. 1987).

Uneven stress transfer into the femur, which occurs in malpositioning of the prosthesis or in non-homogeneous bone cement distribution in the medullary cavity (ALDINGER 1987; HUGGLER et al. 1978; KÖLLER et al. 1990), can result in significantly intensified punctual load transmission. This leads to fractures of trabeculae and bone cement intrusions at the bone–cement interface, thus causing mechanical instability (BEAN et al. 1987).

The development of fine particulate bone cement debris by fatigue failure of the bone cement, which demonstrates increased brittleness after many years of service, seems to be of major importance in initiating the process of loosening (BOS et al. 1990a; GROSS et al. 1984; JOHANSON et al. 1987; KRAUSE and MATHIS 1988; WILLERT 1987; WILLERT et al. 1990b). Small amounts of granular foreign material cause an accumulation of histiocytes, which are considered to have a cellular effector function in the biological phase of loosening (BOS et al. 1990a; FREEMAN et al. 1982; JOHANSON et al. 1987; MAGUIRE et al. 1987; SPECTOR et al. 1990). Even though bone cement debris, histiocytes, foreign body giant cells, fibrin exudates and haemorrhages are also seen regularly in stable cemented prostheses (MALCOLM 1988; SZYSKOWITZ 1973; VERNON-ROBERTS and FREEMAN 1976; WILLERT and PULS 1972), there is an apparently long period of equilibrium during which small particles of foreign material are continuously evacuated via lymphatic vessels and necroses and haemorrhages are resorbed. The loosening process is initiated when additional factors such as increased abrasion of bone cement, fractures of bone trabeculae or local bone remodelling lead to decompensation of this equilibrium WILLERT et al. 1990b). Subsequently increased relative motion between bone and cement leads not only to accelerated bone cement wear but also to further necrosis and microhaemorrhage caused by shear and tensile deformation of the soft tissue membranes and thereby to the attraction of histiocytes. The increase in thickness of the interface membrane is associated with resorption of the adjacent bone, causing progressive mechanical instability. Thus, a vicious circle develops that

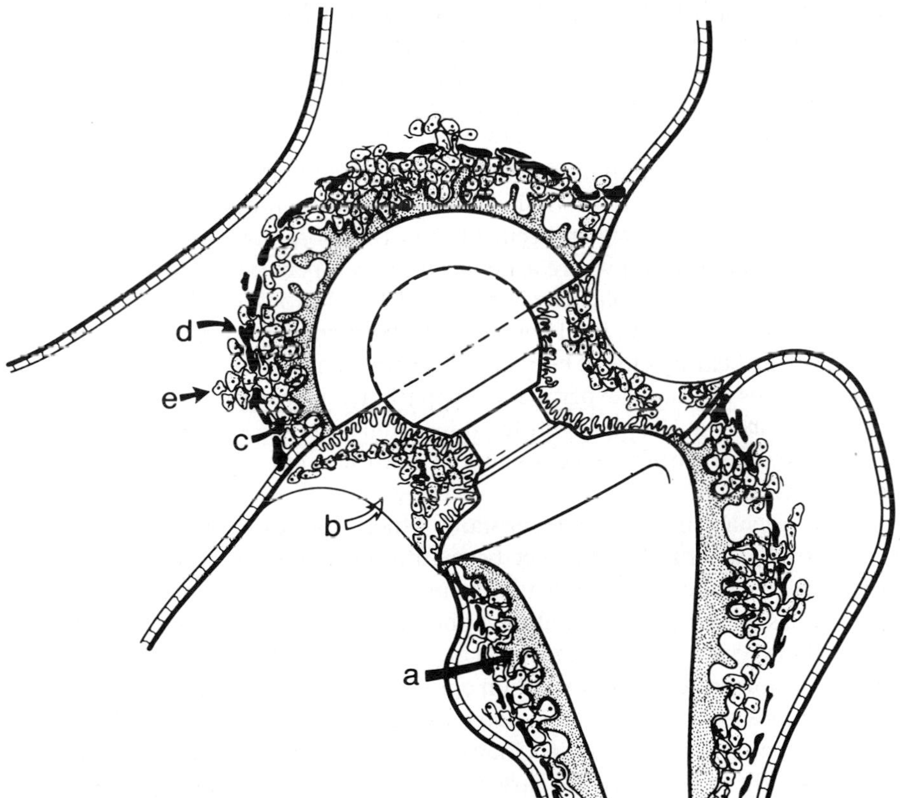

Fig. 27. Diagram of the tissue reaction around a cemented prosthesis after long-term implantation. **a**, Cement mantle; **b**, pseudocapsule with villous transformation and histiocytic reaction containing large extracellular (multispherical) and small granular intracelluar bone cement wear and rod-shaped polyethylene wear; **c**, interface membrane with histiocytic infiltration; **d**, neocortical bone; **e**, histiocytic infiltration of the adjacent bone marrow. (Areas of fibrosis and necrosis are not shown)

leads to complete implant loosening (Fig. 26) when the prosthesis is entirely surrounded by a broad margin of histiocytic infiltration (Bos et al. 1990; Johanson et al. 1987; Lennox et al. 1987; Lintner et al. 1982; Maguire et al. 1987; Spector et al. 1990; Fig. 27). In contrast to the conditions in the femur, the interface membranes around cemented sockets of hip endoprostheses thicken continuously. The process correlates well with a linear increase in the rate of loosening with advancing time in situ (Mattingly et al. 1985; Salvati et al. 1981). The discrepancy between femur and acetabular bone is probably due to the fact that the cement mantle of the socket is entirely surrounded by cancellous bone which is more quickly and more completely resorbable than femoral cortical bone. Investigations to date indicate that the loosening of cemented implants, particularly cemented acetabular sockets, is pre-programmed. It is only the length of time taken by the process of loosening that seems to vary.

It has often been discussed to what extent articular wear, and in particular polyethylene wear, contributes to the loosening process (Bos et al. 1991; Brinkmann and Heilmann 1974; Howie et al. 1990; Linder et al. 1983; Willert et al. 1990a). In our own investigations bone cement wear predominated. Loosening often developed in the absence of articular surface wear. In early investigations Willert and colleagues assumed the wear of the bearing surfaces to be the main cause of prosthesis loosening (Willert 1977; Willert and Semlitsch 1973), probably since the implant materials used at that time, e.g. Teflon, produced excessive wear of the articulating surfaces. At the beginning of the loosening cycle in the proximal femur clefts between bone and cement are often observed (Linder et al. 1983; Wroblewski et al. 1987) where articular wear can penetrate and accelerate the accumulation of macrophages (Bos et al. 1991; Linder et al. 1983; Vernon-Roberts and Freeman 1976). Howie et al. (1988) produced osteolysis adjacent to a non-weight-bearing plug of bone cement by intra-articular injection of polyethylene particles in animal experiments. Apparently, any substance that elicits the accumulation of macrophages at the bone–cement interface leads to loosening, regardless of the type of prosthetic material used (Willert et al. 1990a; Santavirta et al. 1991).

The mechanism of bone resorption, which is an essential prerequisite for prosthesis loosening, has not yet been fully explained. A key role has been attributed to histiocytes. They synthesize and secrete numerous mediators of bone resorption such as acid phosphatase, non-specific esterase, lysozyme and proteinases (Heilmann et al. 1975; Linder et al. 1983; Santavirta et al. 1990b). In vitro studies demonstrated that in addition collagenases and especially prostaglandin E_2, which possesses an osteoclast-activating activity, are produced (Dorr et al. 1990; Goldring et al. 1983, 1986; Goodman et al. 1989; Murray et al. 1989). These products seem to be released in larger quantities after the phagocytosis of wear particles (Lennox et al. 1987), especially when severe degeneration or necrosis of the histiocytes is present (Freeman et al. 1982). The general importance and the relative contribution of these mediator substances to the course of loosening has not yet been clarified. These mechanisms apply to the loosening process as observed in cemented prostheses.

The major problem in non-cemented prostheses is not late loosening but achieving tight initial fixation. Unlike with cemented prostheses, this is not always attainable (ENGH and MASSIN 1989; ROTHMAN and COHN 1990). The prosthetic design has to be well adapted anatomically, with as much direct contact between bone and implant as possible to achieve optimal conditions (SPECTOR et al. 1990). In contrast to cemented prostheses, a reduction in the rate of loosening can be expected with increasing time in situ (HARRIS and SLEDGE 1990). Loosening is quite unlikely, at least in biological ingrowth prostheses, after sufficient trabecular ingrowth into the pores of the metallic implant has been established.

9 Conclusions

Nowadays a wide selection of prostheses for various joints is available. These are mostly capable of providing satisfactory function for many years. However, problems such as infection and most especially non-infectious late loosening have not been completely solved. In non-cemented prostheses, the life expectancy of which is still unknown, achieving initial tight fixation constitutes the major problem to date. Late loosening of cemented implants is seen as a multifactorial process in which bone cement wear seems to play an important role. The macrophages/histiocytes phagocytosing wear particles are considered to be the principal effector cells in late loosening which induce bone resorption by the production of cytokines and enzymes. The resultant mechanical instability starts a vicious cycle of increasing bone-cement wear and consecutive macrophage recruitment finally leading to complete loosening of the prosthesis. The cell biological mechanisms inducing histiocytic inflammation and bone resorption are not yet fully characterised and require further investigations. If it proves possible to retard or prevent bone resorption, for example through cytokine or receptor blocking substances, new therapeutic options would arise for avoiding late loosening in endoprosthetics.

References

Agins HJ, Alcock NW, Bansal M et al. 1988) Metallic wear in failed titanium-alloy total hip replacements. J Bone Joint Surg [Am] 70:347–356

Albrektsson T, Linder L (1984) Bone injury caused by curing bone cement. A vital microscopic study in the rabbit tibia. Clin Orthop 183:280–287

Aldinger G (1987) Der Lockerungsvorgang der Hüfttotalendoprothese unter besonderer Berücksichtigung des Zements. Aktuel Probl Chir Orthop 31:337–341

Arcq M (1973) Die paraartikulären Ossifikationen – eine Komplikation der Totalendoprothese des Hüftgelenks. Arch Orthop Unfallchir 77:108–131

Atkinson JR (1975) Mechanical properties and wear behaviour of plastics in relation to their use in prostheses. Br Polym J 7:93–107

Bean DJ, Convery FR, Woo SL-Y, Lieber RL (1987) Regional variation in shear strength of the bone–polymethylmethacrylate interface. J Arthroplasty 2:293–298

Beneke G, Kuprasch R, Mohr W, Paulini K, Mohing W (1973) Die Reaktion der Gelenkkapsel nach Totalarthroplastik des Hüftgelenkes. Arch Orthop Unfallchir 75:289–301
Biehl G, Harms J, Mäusle E (1975) Tierexperimentelle und histopathologische Untersuchungen über die Anpassungsvorgänge des Knochens nach der Implantation von "Tragrippen-Endoprothesen". Arch Orthop Unfallchir 81: 105–118
Black J, Maitin EC, Gelman H, Morris DM (1983) Serum concentrations of chromium, cobalt and nickel after total hip replacement: a six month study. Biomaterials 4: 160–164
Black J, Sherk H, Bonini J, Rostoker WR, Schajowicz F, Galante JO (1990) Metallosis associated with a stable titanium–alloy femoral component in total hip replacement. A case report. J Bone Joint Surg [Am] 72:126–130
Bobyn JD, Engh CA, Glassman AH (1987) Histologic analysis of a retrieved microporous-coated femoral prosthesis. A seven-year case report. Clin Orthop 224: 303–310
Bocco F, Langan P, Charnley J (1977) Changes in the calcar femoris in relation to cement technology in total hip replacement. Clin Orthop 128: 287–295
Bos I, Löhrs U (1991) Morphologie der Sekundärkapsel bei Hüftgelenkendoprothesen und Bedeutung des Materialabriebs. Eine Untersuchung an Autopsien. Pathologe 12: 82–88
Bos I, Lindner B, Seydel U, Johannisson R, Dörre E, Henβge EJ, Löhrs U (1990a) Untersuchungen über die Lockerungsursache bei zementierten Hüftgelenkendoprothesen. Licht- und elektronenmikroskopische Untersuchung und Laser-Mikrosonden-Massenanalyse. Z Orthop 128: 73–82
Bos I, Johannisson R, Löhrs U, Lindner B, Seydel U (1990b) Comparative investigations of regional lymph nodes and pseudocapsules after implantation of joint endoprostheses. Pathol Res Pract 186: 707–716
Bos I, Meeuwssen E, Henßge EJ, Löhrs U (1991) Unterschiede des Polyäthylenabriebs bei Hüftgelenkendoprothesen mit Keramik- und Metall-Polyäthylenpaarung der Gleitflächen. Eine Untersuchung an Operations- und Autopsiematerial. Z Orthop 129:507–515
Bösch CP, Harms H, Lintner F (1982) Nachweis des Katalysatorbestandteiles Dimethylparatoluidin im Knochenzement, auch nach mehrjähriger Implantation. Arch Toxicol 51: 157–166
Bösch CP, Harms H, Lintner F (1987) Zur Toxizität der Knochenzementbestandteile. Aktuel Probl Chir Orthop 31: 87–89
Brinkmann KE, Heilmann K (1974) Klinische, röntgenologische und feingewebliche Untersuchungen an ausgelockerten Hüftgelenkendoprothesen. Arch Orthop Unfallchir 80: 333–342
Brooker AF, Bowerman JW, Robinson RA, Riley LH (1973) Ectopic ossification following total hip replacement. Incidence and a method of classification. J Bone Joint Surg [Am] 55: 1629–1632
Brown KJ, Atkinson JR, Dowson D, Wright V (1976) The wear of ultrahigh molecular weight polyethylene and a preliminary study of its relation to the in vivo behaviour of replacement hip joints. Wear 40: 255–264
Buchert PK, Vaughn BK, Mallory TH, Engh CA, Bobyn JD (1986) Excessive metal release due to loosening and fretting of sintered particles on porous–coated hip prostheses. J Bone Joint Surg [Am] 68: 606–609
Caravia L, Dowson D, Fisher J, Jobbins B (1990) The influence of bone and bone cement debris on counterface roughness in sliding wear tests of ultra-high molecular weight polyethylene on stainless steel. Proc Inst Mech Eng 204: 65–70
Chandler HP, Reineck FT, Wixson RL, McCarthy JC (1981) Total hip replacement in patients younger than thirty years old. J Bone Joint Surg [Am] 63: 1426–1434
Charnley J (1961) Arthroplasty of the hip: a new operation. Lancet I: 1129–1132
Charnley J (1964) The bonding of prostheses to bone by cement. J Bone Joint Surg [Br] 46: 518–529
Charnley J (1970) The reaction of bone to self-curing acrylic cement. A long-term histological study in man. J Bone Joint Surg [Br] 52: 340–353
Charnley J (1972) The long-term result of low-friction arthroplasty of the hip performed as a primary intervention. J Bone Joint Surg [Br] 54: 61–76
Charnley J, Follaci FM, Hammond BT (1968) The long-term reaction of bone to self-curing acrylic cement. J Bone Joint Surg [Br] 50: 822–829
Charosky CB, Bullough PG, Wilson PD (1973) Total hip replacement failures. A histological evaluation. J Bone Joint Surg [Am] 55: 49–58
Christie AJ, Weinberger KA, Dietrich M (1977) Silicone lymphadenopathy and synovitis. Complications of silicone elastomer finger joint prostheses. JAMA 237: 1463–1464
Clarke IC (1981) Wear of artificial joint materials. Friction and wear studies: validity of wear-screening protocols. Eng Med 10: 115–112

Clarke IC, Black K, Rennie C, Amstutz HC (1976) Can wear in total hip arthroplasties be assessed from radiographs? Clin Orthop 121: 126–142

Clarke IC, Dorlot JM, Graham J, et al. (1988) Biomechanical stability and design. Ann NY Acad Sci 523: 292–296

Coleman RF, Herrington J, Scales JT (1973) Concentration of wear products in hair, blood, and urine after total hip replacement. Br Med J 3: 527–529

Comadoll JL, Sherman RE, Gustilo RB, Bechthold JE (1988) Radiographic changes in bone dimensions in asymptomatic cemented total hip arthroplasties. Results of nine to thirteen-year follow-up. J Bone Joint Surg [Am] 70: 433–438

Convery FR, Gunn DR, Hughes JD, Martin WE (1975) The relative safety of polymethylmethacrylate: a controlled clinical study of randomly selected patients treated with Charnley and Ring total hip replacements. J Bone Joint Surg [Am] 57: 57–64

Cotta H, Schulitz KP (1970) Komplikationen der Hüftalloarthro-plastik durch periartikuläre Gewebereaktion. Arch Orthop Unfallchir 69: 39–59

Courpied J, Postel M (1987) Aseptic loosening among Charnley-type prostheses. In: Postel M, Kerboul M, Evrard J, Courpied JP (eds) Total hip replacement. Springer, Berlin Heidelberg New York, pp 79–83

Crout DHG, Corkill JA, James ML, Ling RSM (1979) Methylmethacrylate metabolism in man. The hydrolysis of methylmethacrylate to methacrylic acid during total hip replacement. Clin Orthop 141: 90–95

Daniel M, Dingle JT, Webb M, Heath JC (1963) The biological action of cobalt and other metals. I. The effect of cobalt on the morphology and metabolism of rat fibroblasts in vitro. Br J Exp Pathol 44: 163–176

Dannenmaier WC, Haynes DW, Nelson CL (1985) Granulomatous reaction and cystic bony destruction associated with high wear rate in a total knee prosthesis. Clin Orthop 198:224–230

Dawihl W, Mittelmeier H, Dörre E, Altmeyer G, Hanser U (1979) Zur Tribologie von Hüftgelenk-Endoprothesen aus Aluminiumoxid-Keramik. Med Orthop Tech 99:114–118

Delling G, Krumme H, Engelbrecht E, Heise K, Kutz R (1983) Reaction of bone tissue after longterm implantation of total joint arthroplasty. A morphological study. In: Kutz R (ed) Proceedings, 2nd international workshop of the design and application of tumor prostheses for bone and joint reconstruction. Egermann, Vienna pp 37–39

Delling G, Kofeldt C, Engelbrecht E (1987) Knochen- und Grenzschichtveränderungen nach Anwendung von Knochenzement—Langzeituntersuchungen an humanem Biopsie-, Operations- und Autopsiematerial. Aktuel Probl Chir Orthop 31: 163–171

Dielert E, Milachowski K, Schramel P (1983) Die Bedeutung der legierungsspezifischen Elemente Eisen, Kobalt, Chrom und Nickel für die aseptische Lockerung von Hüftgelenkstotalendoprothesen. Z Orthop 121: 58–63

Dienel RB, Jungnickel I, Holzweissig F, Manitz L, Hellinger J (1984) Mikrobewegungen von zementfixierten Hüftendoprothesenschäften in Leichenfemora. Beitr Orthop Traumatol 31: 151–158

Dobbs HS, Minsky MJ (1980) Metal ion release after total hip replacement. Biomaterials 1: 193–198

Dorr LD, Bloebaum R, Emmanual J, Meldrum R (1990) Histologic, biochemical and ion analysis of tissue and fluids retrieved during total hip arthroplasty. Clin Orthop 261: 82–95

Dörre E, Dawihl W (1978) Mechanische und tribologische Eigenschaften keramischer Endoprothesen. Biomed Tech 23: 305–310

Dörre E, Beutler H, Geduldig D (1975) Anforderungen an oxidkeramische Werkstoffe als Biomaterial für künstliche Gelenke. Arch Orthop Unfallchir 83: 269–278

Dörre E, Dawihl W, Altmeyer G (1977) Dauerfestigkeit keramischer Hüftendoprothesen. Biomed Tech 22: 3–7

Dowling JM, Atkinson JR, Dowson D, Charnley J (1978) The characteristics of acetabular cups worn in the human body. J Bone Joint Surg [Br] 60: 375–382

Draenert K (1981) The John Charnley award paper. Histomorphology of the bone-to-cement interface remodelling of the cortex and revascularization of the medullary canal in animal experiments. In: Salvati EA (ed) The hip. Proceedings of the ninth open scientific meeting of The Hip Society. Mosby, St. Louis, pp 71–110

Draenert K, Rudigier J (1978) Histomorphologie des Knochen-Zement-Kontaktes. Eine tierexperimentelle Phänomenologie der knöchernen Umbauvorgänge. Chirurg 49: 276–285

Draenert K, Rudigier J, Herrmann W, Willenegger H (1976) Tierexperimentelle Studie zur Histomorphologie des Knochen-Zement-Kontaktes. Helv Chir Acta 43: 769–773

Eftekhar NS (1971) Charnley "Low friction torque" arthroplasty. A study of long-term results. Clin Orthop 81: 93–104
Eftekhar NS (1973) The surgeon and clean air in the operating room. Clin Orthop 96:188–194
Engh CA, Massin P (1989) Cementless total hip arthroplasty using the anatomic medullary locking stem. Clin Orthop 249: 141–158
Eyb R (1987) Die unterschiedlichen Veränderungen am Calcar femoris bei zementierten und zementfreien Hüft-Endoprothesen. Aktuel Probl Chir Orthop 31: 196–200
Fagan MJ, Lee AJC (1986) Role of the collar on the femoral stem of cemented total hip replacements. J Biomed Eng 8: 295–304
Feith R (1975) Side effects of acrylic cement implanted into bone: a histological, (micro)angiographic, fluorescence-microscopic and autoradiographic study in the rabbit femur. Acta Orthop Scand Suppl 161: 1–136
Forest M (1987) Histopathology and the diagnosis of infection. In: Postel M, Kerboul M, Evrard J, Courpied JP (eds). Total hip replacement. Springer, Berlin Heidelberg New York, pp 115–117
Forest M, Carlioz A, Vacher Lavenu MC, Postel M, Kerboull M, Tomeno B, Courpied JP (1991) Histological patterns of bone and articular tissues after orthopaedic reconstructive surgery (artifical joint implants). Pathol Res Pract 187: 963–977
Freeman MAR, Bradley GW, Revell PA (1982) Observations upon the interface between bone and Polymethylacrylate cement. J Bone Joint Surg [Br] 64: 489–493
Gaudillat C (1987) Infective complications of total hip replacement. In: Postel M, Kerboul M, Evrard J, Courpied JP (eds) Total hip replacement. Springer, Berlin Heidelberg New York, pp 105–106
Gaudillat C, Deplus P (1987) Infective complications of total hip replacement. Diagnosis of chronic infection. In: Postel M, Kerboul M, Evrard J, Courpied JP (eds) Total hip replacement. Springer, Berlin Heidelberg New York, pp 110–115
Gebauer D, Blümel G, Rupp G (1983) Der Stellenwert der Reibung beim Lockerungsprozeß von Totalendoprothesen der Hüfte. Z Orthop 121: 634–639
Goebel G, Ohnsorge J (1973) Stand der experimentellen Untersuchungen zur Wechselwirkung zwischen Knochenzement und Lagergewebe: thermische oder toxische Schädigung? In: Cotta H, Schulitz KP (eds) Der totale Hüftgelenkersatz. Grundlagenforschung, Indikation, Komplikationen, Ergebnisse und Begutachtung. Thieme, Stuttgart, pp 164–171
Gold BL, Walker PS (1974) Variables affecting the friction and wear of metal-on-plastic total hip joints. Clin Orthop 100: 270–278
Goldring SR, Schiller AL, Roelke M, Rourke CM, O'Neill DA, Harris WH (1983) The synovial-like membrane at the bone-cement interface in loose total hip replacements and its proposed role in bone lysis. J Bone Joint Surg [Am] 65: 575–584
Goldring SR, Jasty M, Roelke MS, Rourke CM, Bringhurst FR, Harris WH (1986) Formation of a synovial-like membrane at the bone-cement interface. Its role in bone resorption and implant loosening after total hip replacement. Arthritis Rheum 29: 836–842
Goodman SB, Chin RC, Chiou SS, Schurmann DJ, Woalson ST, Masada MP (1989) A clinical-pathological-biochemical study of the membrane surrounding loosened and non-loosened total hip arthroplastics. Clin Orthop 244: 182–187
Griffiths HJ, Burke J, Bonfiglio TA (1987) Granulomatous pseudotumors in total joint replacement. Skeletal Radiol 16: 145–152
Griss P, Heimke G (1981) Five years experience with ceramic-metal-composite hip endoprostheses. I. Clinical evaluation. Arch Orthop Trauma Surg 98: 157–164
Griss P, von Andrian-Werburg H, Krempien B, Heimke G (1973a) Biological activity and histocompatibility of dense A1203/MgO ceramic implants in rats. J Biomed Mater Res (Symp) 4: 453–462
Griss P, Krempien B, von Andrian-Werburg H, Heimke G, Fleiner R (1973b) Experimentelle Untersuchung zur Gewebeverträglichkeit oxidkeramischer (A1203) Abriebteilchen. Arch Orthop Unfallchir 76: 270–279
Griss P, Heimke G, Werner E, Bleicher J, Jentschura G (1978) Was bedeutet die Resorption des Calcar femoris nach der Totalendoprothesenoperation der Hüfte? Eine vergleichende Studie an Charnley-Müller- und Oxidkeramikendoprothesen (Typ Lindenhof). Arch Orthop Trauma Surg 92: 225–232
Gross U, Hahn F, Strunz V (1984) Das Interface von Knochenzement in Autopsie und Experiment. In: Rahmanzadeh R, Faensen M (eds) Hüftgelenksendoprothetik. Aktueller Stand - Perspektiven. Springer, Berlin Heidelberg New York, pp 99–112
Harms J, Mäusle E (1976) Biologishe Verträglichkeitsuntersuchungen von Implantatwerkstoffen im Tierversuch. Med Orthop Tech 96: 103–104
Harris WH, Sledge CB (1990) Total hip and total knee replacement. N Engl J Med 323: 725–731

Harris WH, Schiller AL, Scholler J-M, Freiberg RA, Scott R (1976) Extensive localized bone resorption in the femur following total hip replacement. J Bone Joint Surg [Am] 58: 612–618
Harris WH, McCarthy JC, O'Neill DA (1982) Femoral component loosening using contemporary techniques of femoral cement fixation. J Bone Joint Surg [Am] 64: 1063–1067
Hayashi T, Inoue H (1986) Tissue reaction around loosened prostheses: a histological, x-ray, microanalytic and immunological study. Act Med Okayama 40: 229–241
Heilmann K, Diezel PB, Rossner JA, Brinkmann KA (1975) Morphological studies in tissues surrounding alloarthroplastic joints. Virchows Arch [A] 366: 93–106
Heimke G, Beisler W, von Andrian-Werburg H, Griss P, Krempien B (1973) Untersuchungen an Implantaten aus AL203-Keramik. Ber Dtsch Keram Ges 50: 4–8
Heimke G, Griss P, von Andrian-Werburg H, Krempien B (1974) Aluminiumoxidkeramik, ein neues Biomaterial. Materialeigenschaften und mögliche klinische Anwendungsbereiche. Arch Orthop Unfallchir 78: 216–226
Heisel J, Schmitt E (1987) Implantatbrüche bei Keramik-Hüftendoprothesen. Z Orthop 125: 480–490
Herman JH, Sowder WG, Anderson D, Appel AM, Hopson CN (1989) Polymethylmethacrylate-induced release of bone-resorbing factors. J Bone Joint Surg [Am] 77: 1530–1541
Hinterberger J,Ungethüm M (1978) Untersuchungen zur Tribologie und Festigkeit von Aluminiumoxidkeramik-Huftendoprothesen. Z Orthrop 116: 294–303
Holland CJ, Kim KC, Malik MI, Ritter MA (1973) A histologic and hemodynamic study of the toxic effects of monomeric methylmethacrylate. Clin Orthop 90: 262–270
Homsy CA, Tullos HS, Anderson MS, Differrante NM, King JW (1972) Some physiological aspects of prosthesis stabilization with acrylic polymer. Clin Orthop 83: 317–328
Hopf TH, Scherr O, Glöbel B, Hopf C (1989) Vergleichende tierexperimentelle Untersuchung zur Gewebeverträglichkeit und Messungen der Radioaktivität verschiedener Röntgenkontrastmittel. Z Orthop 127: 620–624
Horowitz SM, Frondoza CG, Lennox DW (1988) Effects of polymethylmethacrylate exposure upon macrophages. J Orthop Res 6: 827–832
Howie DW, Vernon-Roberts B, Oakeshott R, Manthey B (1988) A rat model of resorption of bone at the cement—bone interface in the presence of polyethylene wear particles. J Bone Joint Surg [Am] 70:257–263
Howie DW, Cornish BL, Vernon-Roberts B (1990) Resurfacing hip arthroplasty. Classification of loosening and the role of prosthesis wear particles. Clin Orthop 255: 144–159
Huggler AH, Jacob HA, Schreiber A (1978) Biomechanische Analyse der Lockerung von Femurprothesen. Arch Orthop Trauma Surg 92: 261–272
Hulbert SF, Klawitter JJ (1976) Ceramics as a new approach to the improvement of artificial joints. In: Schaldach M, Hohmann D (eds) Advances in artificial hip and knee joint technology. Springer, Berlin Heidelberg New York, pp 287–293
Hulliger L (1962) Untersuchungen über die Wirkung von Kunstharzen (Palacos und Ostamer) in Gewebekulturen. Arch Orthop Unfallchir 54: 581–588
Jasty M, Maloney WJ, Bragdon CR, Haire T, Harris WH (1990) Histomorphological studies of the long-term skeletal responses to well fixed cemented femoral components. J Bone Joint Surg [Am] 72: 1220–1229
Johanson NA, Bullough PG, Wilson PD, Salvati EA, Ranawat CS (1987) The microscopic anatomy of the bone-cement interface in failed total hip arthroplasties. Clin Orthop 218: 123–135
Jones DA, Lucas HK, O'Driscoll M, Price CHG, Wibberley B (1975) Cobalt toxicity after McKee hip arthroplasty. J Bone Joint Surg [Br] 57: 289–296
Jorgensen TJ, Munno F, Mitchell TG, Hungerford D (1983) Urinary cobalt levels in patients with porous Austin-Moore prostheses. Clin Orthop 176: 124–126
Jozsa L, Reffy A (1980) Histochemical and histophysical detection of wear products resulting from prostheses. Folia Histochem Cytochem (Krakow) 18: 195–200
Kallenberger A (1984) Untersuchungen zur Zellkompatibilität von Knochenzementen. In: Rahmanzadeh R, Faensen M (eds) Hüftgelenksendoprothetik. Aktueller Stand – Perspektiven. Springer, Berlin Heidelberg New York, pp 95–98
Kircher T (1980) Silicone lymphadenopathy. A complication of silicone elastomer finger joint prostheses. Hum Pathol 11: 240–244
Kölbel R, Boenick U (1972) Mechanische Eigenschaften der Verbindung zwischen spongiösem Knochen mit Polymethylmethacrylat bei statischer Belastung. Arch Orthop Unfallchir 73: 89–97
Köller W, Müller U, Henßge EJ (1990) Reaktion des knöchernen Lagers nach Implantation von zementierten Endoprothesen am Femur. Z Orthop 128: 67–72

Konermann H (1983) Endoprothetic des Hüftgelenkes: Reoperation und deren Ergebnisse. Therapiewoche 33: 475–482
Krause W, Mathis RS (1988) Fatigue properties of acrylic bone cements: review of the literature. J Biomed Mater Res 22: 37–53
Lancaster JK (1969) Abrasive wear of polymers. Wear 14: 223–239
Leake ES, Wright MJ, Gristina AG (1981) Comparative study of the adherence of alveolar and peritoneal macrophages, and of blood monocytes to methyl methacrylate, polyethylene, stainless steel, and vitallium. J Retic Soc 30: 403–414
Lennox DW, Schofield BH, McDonald DF, Riley LH (1987) A histologic comparison of aseptic loosening of cemented, press-fit, and biologic ingrowth prostheses. Clin Orthop 225: 171–191
Linder L (1977) Reaction of bone to the acute chemical trauma of bone cement. J Bone Joint Surg [Am] 59: 82–87
Linder L, Lindberg L, Carlsson A (1983) Aseptic loosening of hip prostheses. A histologic and enzyme histochemical study. Clin Orthop 175: 93–104
Ling RSM (1981) Loosening experiences at Exeter. Orthop Trans 5: 351
Lintner F, Bösch P (1987) Das Tierexperiment zur Beurteilung der Verträglichkeit von Knochenzement. Aktuel Probl Chir Orthop 31: 188–191
Lintner F, Bösch P, Brand G (1982) Histologische Untersuchungen über Umbauvorgänge an der Zement-Knochengrenze bei Endoprothesen nach 3- bis 10-jähriger Implantation. Pathol Res Pract 173: 376–389
Lintner F, Bösch P, Brand G, Knahr K (1984) Vergleichende Untersuchungen zur Nekrosebereitschaft des Kapselgewebes bei Arthrose und endoprothetischem Gelenkersatz. Z Orthop 122: 686–691
Lintner F, Bösch P, Brand G (1987) Gewebeschäden durch PMMA-Knochenzement. Aktuel Probl Chir Orthop 31: 172–176
Löer F, Zilkens J, Hofmann J, Michel R (1981) Zum Nachweis körperfremder Spurenelemente nach Langzeitimplantation von Totalendoprothesen aus Kobaltbasislegierungen. Z Orthop 119: 763–766
Löer F, Zilkens J, Michel R, Freisem-Broda G, Bigalke KH (1983) Gewebebelastung mit körperfremden Spurenelementen durch Röntgenkontrastmittel der Knochenzemente. Z Orthop 121: 255–259
Löer F, Zilkens J, Michel R, Bigalke KH (1987) Wechselwirkungen zwischen Röntgenkontrastmitteln der Knochenzemente und den Lagergeweben und Körperflüssigkeiten. Aktuel Probl Chir Orthop 31: 177–183
Lombardi AV, Mallory TH, Vaughn BK, Drouillard P (1989) Aseptic loosening in total hip arthroplasty secondary to osteolysis induced by wear debris from titanium-alloy modular femoral heads. J Bone Joint Surg [Am] 71: 1337–1342
Maguire JK, Coscia MF, Lynch MH (1987) Foreign body reaction to polymeric debris following total hip arthroplasty. Clin Orthop 216: 213–223
Malcolm AJ (1988) Pathology of longstanding cemented total hip replacements in Charnley's cases. J Bone Joint Surg [Br] 70: 153
Maßhoff W, Neuhaus-Vogel A (1974) Die Gelenkkapsel nach Alloplastik. Arch Orthop Unfallchir 78: 175–198
Mattingly DA, Hopson CN, Kahn A, Giannestras NJ (1985) Aseptic loosening in metal-backed acetabular components for total hip replacement. J Bone Joint Surg [Am] 67: 387–391
Mendes DG, Walker PS, Figarola F, Bullough PG (1974) Total surface hip replacement in the dog. A preliminary study of local tissue reaction. Clin Orthop 100: 256–264
Michel R, Hofmann J, Holm R, Zilkens J (1980) Zum Übertritt von Korrosionsprodukten aus Stahlimplantaten in das Kontaktgewebe. Untersuchungen der Implantatoberfläche mit ESCA und instrumentelle Neutronenaktivierungsanalyse des Kontaktgewebes. Z Orthop 118: 793–803
Mirra JM, Amstutz HC, Matos M, Gold R (1976) The pathology of the joint tissues and its clinical relevance in prosthesis failure. Clin Orthop 117: 221–240
Mirra JM, Marder RA, Amstutz HC (1982) The pathology of failed total joint arthroplasty. Clin Orthop 170: 175–183
Mittelmeier H, Harms G (1979a) Derzeitiger Stand der zementfreien Verankerung von Keramik-Metall-Verbundprothesen. Z Orthop 117: 478–481
Mittelmeier H, Harms J (1979b) Hüftalloplastic mit Keramik-Endoprothesesn bei traumatischen Hüftschäden. Unter besonderer Berücksichtigung zementfrei implantierbarer "Autophor"-Tragrippen-Endoprothesen. Unfallheilkunde 83: 67–75
Mittelmeier H, Sitz W, Hanser U (1982) Abriebmessungen bei explantierten Keramik-Hüftendoprothesen. Z Orthop 120: 487
Modig J, Busch C, Olerud S, Salderen T (1974) Pulmonary microembolism during intramedullary orthopaedic trauma. Acta Anaesthesiol Scand 18: 133–143

Mohr HJ (1958) Pathologische Anatomie und kausale Genese der durch selbstpolymerisierendes Methacrylat hervorgerufenen Gewebsveränderungen. Z Exp Med 130: 41–69

Murray DW, Rae T, Rae T, Rushton N (1989) The influence of the surface energy and roughness of implants on bone resorption. J Bone Joint Surg [Br] 71: 632–637

Nalbandian RM, Swanson AB, Maupin BK (1983) Longterm silicone implant arthroplasty. Implications of animal and human autopsy findings. JAMA-250: 1195–1198

Nicastro JF, Shoj H, Rovere GD, Gristina AG (1975) Effects of methylmethacrylate in *S. aureus* growth and rabbit alveolar macrophage phagocytosis and glucose metabolism. Surg Forum 26: 501–503

Patterson BM, Healey JH, Cornell CN, Sharrock NE (1991) Cardiac arrest during hip arthroplasty with a cemented long-stem component. J Bone Joint Surg [Am] 73: 271–277

Pedley RB, Meachim G, Gray T (1979) Identification of acrylic cement particles in tissues. Ann Biomed Eng 7: 319–328

Pizzoferrato A, Savarino L, Lambertini V (1981) Histopathological grading suggestion for the evaluation of the intolerance in hip joint endo- and arthroprostheses. Chir Organi Mov 66: 147–171

Plitz W, Walter A, Jäger M (1984) Materialspezifische Verschleißerscheinungen der Gleitpaarung Keramik/Keramik bei revidierten Hüftendoprothesen. Z Orthop 122: 299–303

Pople IK, Phillips H (1988) Bone cement and the liver. A dose-related effect? J Bone Joint Surg [Br] 70: 364–366

Postel M, Courpied JP (1987) The future of the polyethylene cup. In: Postel M, Kerboul M, Evrard J, Courpied JP (eds) Total hip replacement. Springer, Berlin Heidelberg New York, pp 131–135

Pretzsch J, Hein W (1986) Quantitative Analyse des Chrom-, Nickel-, Molybdän-und Mangangehaltes der Neokapsel nach Totalendoprothesenplastiken der Hüftgelenke. Beitr Orthop Traumatol 33: 120–124

Rae T (1975) A study on the effects of particulate metals of orthopaedic interest on murine macrophages in vitro. J Bone Joint Surg [Br] 57: 44–50

Rae T (1976) Action of wear particles from total joint replacement prostheses on tissues. In: William D, David F (eds) Biocompatibility of implant materials. Sector, London, pp 55–59

Rae T (1978) The haemolytic action of particulate metals (Cd, Cr, Co, Fe, Mo, Ni, Ta, Ti, Zn, Co-Cr alloy). J Pathol 125: 81–89

Rae T (1979) Comparative laboratory studies on the production of soluble and particulate metal by total joint prostheses. Arch Orthop Trauma Surg 95: 71–79

Rae T (1981) The toxicity of metals used in orthopaedic prostheses. An experimental study using cultured human synovial fibroblasts. J Bone Joint Surg [Br] 63: 435–440

Reinus WR, Gilula LA, Kyriakos M, Kuhlman RE (1985) Histiocytic reaction to hip arthroplasty. Radiology 155: 315 318

Revell PA (1982) Tissue reactions to joint prostheses and the products of wear and corrosion. Curr Top Pathol 73–101

Revell PA, Weightman B, Freeman MAR, Vernon-Roberts B (1978) The production and biology of polyethylene wear debris. Arch Orthop Trauma Surg 91: 167–181

Rhinelander FW, Nelson CL, Stewart RD, Stewart CL (1979) Experimental reaming of the proximal femur and acrylic cement implantation. Clin Orthop 141: 74–89

Riede UN, Ruedi T, Rohner YLE, Perren S, Guggenheim R (1974) Quantitative und morphologische Erfassung der Gewebereaktion auf Metallimplantate (Osteosynthesematerial). I. Eine morphometrische, histologische, mikroanalytische und rastereletronenmikroskopische Studie am Schafsknochen. Arch Orthop Unfallchir 78: 199–215

Rinecker H, Höllenriegel K (1987) MMA-Toxizität versus Implantationsembolie: Klinische Untersuchungen. Aktuel Probl Chir Orthop 31: 206–209

Rose RM, Radin EL (1982) Wear of polyethylene in the total hip prosthesis. Clin Orthop 170: 107–115

Rose RM, Schneider H, Ries M, Paul I, Crugnola A, Simon SR, Radin EL (1978) A method for the quantitative recovery of polyethylene wear debris from the simulated service of total joint prostheses. Wear 51: 77–84

Rose RM, Crugnola A, Ries M, Cimino WR, Paul I, Radin EL (1979) On the origins of high in vivo wear rates in polyethylene components of total joint prostheses. Clin Orthop 145: 277–286

Rose RM, Nusbaum HJ, Schneider H, et al. (1980) On the true wear rate of ultra-high-molecular-weight polyethylene in the total hip prosthesis. J Bone Joint Surg [Am] 62: 537–549

Rostoker W, Chao EYS, Galante JO (1978) The appearances of wear on polyethylene – a comparison of in vivo and in vitro wear surfaces. J Biomed Mater Res 12: 317–335

Rothman RH, Cohn JC (1990) Cemented versus cementless total hip arthroplasty. A critical review. Clin Orthop 254: 153–169

Rudigier J, Draenert K, Grünert A, Ritter G, Krieg H (1976) Biologische Effekte von Bariumsulfat als Röntgenkontrastmittelbeimengung in Knochenzementen. Eine tierexperimentelle Studie am Kaninchenfemur. Arch Orthop Unfallchir 86: 279–290

Rudigier J, Rech R, Walde HJ, Degreif J (1987) Der Einfluß von Röntgenkontrastmitteln in Knochenzementen auf Bindegewebe und Knochenstruktur. In: Willert HG, Buchhorn G (eds) Knochenzement. Huber, Bern, pp 181–183

Salvati EA, Wilson PD, Jolley MN, Vakili F, Aglietti P, Brown GC (1981) A ten-year follow-up study of our first one hundred consecutive Charnley total hip replacements. J Bone Joint Surg [Am] 63: 753–767

Santavirta S, Hoikka V, Eskola A, Konttinen YT, Paavilainen T, Tallroth K (1990a) Aggressive granulomatous lesion in cementless total hip arthroplasty. J Bone Joint Surg [Br] 72: 980–984

Santavirta S, Konttinen YT, Bergroth V, Eskola A, Tallroth K, Lindholm TS (1990b) Aggressive granulomatous lesions associated with hip arthroplasy. J Bone Joint surg [Am] 72: 252–258

Santavirta S, Konttinen YT, Hoikka V, Eskola A (1991) Immunopathological response to loose cementless acetabular components. J Bone Joint Surg [Br] 73: 38–42

Schneider R (1976) Der Mechanismus der Protheseninstabilität an der Hüfte. Helv Chir Acta 43: 731–734

Schröder HA, Balassa JJ (1966) Abnormal trace metals in man: zirconium. J Chronic Dis 19: 573–586

Schulitz KP, Dustmann HO (1976) Komplikationen der Totalendoprothese. Arch Orthop Unfallchir 85: 33–50

Schwierenga SHH, Basrur PK (1968) Effect of nickel on cultured rat embryo muscle cells. Lab Invest 19: 663–674

Sedel L, Kerboull L, Christel P, Meunier A, Witvoet J (1990) Alumina-on-alumina hip replacement. Results and survivorship in young patients. J Bone Joint Surg [Br] 72: 658–663

Semlitsch M, Willert HG (1971) Gewebsveränderungen im Bereiche metallischer Hüftgelenke; mikroanalytische Untersuchungen mittels Spektralphotometrie, Elektronenstrahlmikroskopie und der Elektronenstrahl-Mikrosonde. Mikrochim Acta 1:21–37

Semlitsch M, Lehmann M, Weber H, Dörre E, Willert HG (1976) Neue Perspektiven zu verlängerter Funktionsdauer künstlicher Hüftgelenke durch Werkstoffkombination Polyäthylen-Aluminiumoxidkeramik-Metall. Med Orthop Tech 5: 152–157

Semlitsch M, Lehmann M, Weber H, Dörre E, Willert HG (1977) New prospects for a prolonged functional life-span of artificial hip joints by using the material combination polyethylene/aluminum oxide ceramic/metal. J Biomed Mater Res 11: 537–552

Shelley WB, Hurley HJ (1958) The allergie origin of zirconium deodorant granulomas. Br J Dermatol 70: 75–101

Spector M, Shortkroff S, Hsu HP, Lane N, Sledge CB, Thornhill TS (1990) Tissue changes around loose prostheses. A canine model to investigate the effects of an antiinflammatory agent. Clin Orthop 261: 140–152

Stock D, Diezemann ED, Gottstein J (1980) Results of endoprosthetic hip joint replacement with the aluminium ceramic-metal composite prosthesis "Lindenhof". Arch Orthop Trauma Surg 97: 7–12

Swanson AB (1972) Flexible implant arthroplasty for arthritic finger joints. J Bone Joint Surg [Am] 54: 435–454

Szyskowitz R (1973) Zur Problematik der Knochenzementimplantation. In: Cotta H, Schulitz KP (eds) Der totale Hüftgelenkersatz. Thieme, Stuttgart, pp 171–182

Tallroth K, Eskola A, Santavirta S, Konttinen YT, Lindholm TS (1989) Aggressive granulomatous lesions after hip arthroplasty. J Bone Joint Surg [Br] 71: 571–575

Travis WD, Balogh K, Abraham JL (1985) Silicone granulomas: report of three cases and review of the literature. Hum Pathol 16: 19–27

Trepte CT, Gauer EF, Gärtner BM (1985) Erfahrungen mit Endoprothesen mit Keramik/Keramik-Gleitpaarung ganz oder teilweise zementlos fixiert. Z Orthop 123: 239–244

Ungethüm M, Refior HJ (1974) Ist Aluminiumoxidkeramik als Gleitlagerwerkstoff für Totalendoprothesen geeignet? Arch Orthop Unfallchir 79: 97–106

Ungethüm M, Winkler-Gniewek W (1983) Untersuchung des Verschleißes an Polyäthylenkomponenten von Endoprothesen nach klinischem Einsatz. Z Orthop 121: 683–692

Vernon-Roberts B, Freeman MAR (1976) Morphological and analytical studies of the tissues adjacent to joint prostheses: investigations into the causes of loosening of prostheses. In: Schaldach M, Hohmann D (eds) Advances in artificial hip and knee joint technology. Springer, Berlin Heidelberg New York, pp 148–186

Walker PS, Bullough PG (1973) The effects of friction and wear in artificial joints. Orthop Clin North Am 4: 275–293

Willert HG (1973) Die Reaktion des knöchernen Implantatlagers auf Methylmethacrylatknochenzement. In: Cotta H, Schulitz KP (eds) Der totale Hüftgelenkersatz, Thieme, Stuttgart, pp 182–192

Willert HG (1977) Reactions of the articular capsule to wear products of artificial joint prostheses. J Biomed Mater Res 11: 157–164

Willert HG (1987) Die Zerrüttung des Zementköchers. Aktuel Probl Chir Orthop 31: 326–333

Willert HG, Puls P (1972) Die Reaktion des Knochens auf Knochenzement bei der Allo-Arthroplastik der Hüfte. Arch Orthop Unfallchir 72: 33–71

Willert HG, Semlitsch M (1973) Die Reaktion der periartikulären Weichteile auf Verschleißprodukte von Endoprothesenwerkstoffen. In: Cotta H, Schulitz KP (eds) Der totale Hüftgelenkersatz. Thieme, Stuttgart, pp 199–209

Willert HG, Semlitsch M (1975) Kapselreaktionen auf Kunststoff und Metallabrieb bei Gelenkendoprothesen. Tech Rundsch Sulzer 2: 1–15

Willert HG, Semlitsch M (1976a) Problems associated with the cement anchorage of artificial joints. In: Schaldach M, Hohmann D (eds) Advances in artificial hip and knee joint technology. Springer, Berling Heidelberg New York, pp 325–346

Willert HG, Semlitsch M (1976b) Tissue reactions to plastic and metallic wear products of joint endoprostheses. In: Gschwend N, Debrunner HU (eds) Total hip prosthesis. Huber, Bern, pp 205–242

Willert HG, Semlitsch M (1977) Reactions of the articular capsule to wear products of artificial joint prostheses. J Biomed Mater Res 11: 157–164

Willert HG, Ludwig J, Semlitsch M (1974) Reaction of bone to methacrylate after hip arthroplasty. A long-term gross, light microscopic and scanning electron microscopic study. J Bone Joint Surg [Am] 56: 1368–1382

Willert HG, Semlitsch M, Buchhorn G, Kriete U (1978) Materialverschleiß und Gewebereaktion bei künstlichen Gelenken (Histopathologie, Biokompatibilität, biologische und klinische Probleme). Orthopäde 7: 62–83

Willert HG, Buchhorn G, Semlitsch M (1980) Die Reaktion des Gewebes auf Verschleißprodukte von Gelenkendoprothesen der oberen Extremitäten. Orthopäde 9: 94–197

Willert HG, Buchhorn GH, Semlitsch M (1981) Recognition and identification of wear products in the surrounding tissues of artificial joint prostheses. In: Dumbleton JH (ed) Tribology of natural and artificial joints. Elsevier, Amsterdam, pp 381–419

Willert HG, Bertram H, Buchhorn GH (1990a) Osteolysis in alloarthroplasty of the hip. The role of ultra-high molecular weight polyethylene wear particles. Clin Orthop 258: 95–107

Willert HG, Bertram H, Buchhorn GH (1990b) Osteolysis in alloarthroplasty of the hip. The role of bone cement fragmentation. Clin Orthop 258: 108–121

Williams DF (1973) The response of the body environment to implants. In: Williams DF, Roaf R (eds) Implants in surgery. W.B. Saunders, London, pp 203–297

Winter GD (1974) Tissue reactions to metallic wear and corrosion products in human patients. J Biomed Mater Res 5: 11–26

Wroblewski BM, Lynch M, Atkinson JR, Dowson D, Isaac GH (1987) External wear of the polyethylene socket in cemented total hip arthroplasty. J Bone Joint Surg [Br] 61–63

Zichner L (1987) Embolien aus dem Knochenmarkskanal nach Einsetzen von intramedullären Femurkopfendoprothesen mit Polymethylmetacrylat. Aktuel Probl Chir Orthop 31: 201–204

Pathology of Injected Polytetrafluoroethylene

M.D. O'HARA and C.M. HILL

1 Introduction

It is a little over 50 years since the serendipitous discovery of polytetrafluoroethylene (PTFE). As the first fluorocarbon polymer to be commercialised, PTFE is the slipperiest solid in the world, is an excellent electrical insulator, displays remarkable antistick behaviour and is renowned for its chemical inertness, insolubility, weatherability and impermeability to moisture (BANKS 1988). At an early stage it was clear that its properties would be of considerable importance to the study of prosthetic and biomedical devices.

2 History

The discovery of PTFE grew out of the tremendous demand for commercial refrigeration in the early decades of the twentieth century in the United States. By

Current Topics in Pathology
Volume 86. Ed. C. Berry

the 1920s refrigerant gases were based on ethylene, ammonia or sulphur dioxide (PLUNKETT 1986). Leakage resulted in liberation of flammable, noxious and other unpleasant gases into the environment. In the search for alternatives, scientists working for the Frigidaire Division of General Motors postulated, on theoretical and experimental grounds, that organic fluorocarbon compounds might be suitable for the purposes of refrigeration. As a result, the General Motors and Du Pont companies jointly funded the establishment of a new company, Kinetic Chemicals, to undertake research on the identification and development of safer refrigerants. By 1935 five chlorine-containing fluorocarbon gases had been identified (CCl_3F,CCl_2F_2,$CHClF_2$, CCl_2FCClF_2 and $CClF_2CClF_2$). They were non-flammable, possessed a low order of toxicity and came to represent the backbone of the fluorocarbon industry. (Possible effects on the ozone layer were as yet undocumented.) Roy Plunkett, a young research chemist employed by Du Pont and seconded to Kinetic Chemicals, was given the task of developing alternatives to the refrigerant gas $CClF_2CClF_2$, for which the gas tetrafluoroethylene (TFE) stored under pressure in gas cylinders was to be used as a basic chemical building block. One morning in April 1938, Plunkett's assistant noted that a cylinder which had been expected to contain TFE gas appeared to be empty. A check of the cylinder's weight suggested that there was still material inside. More careful examination, ultimately including the cutting open of the cylinder, disclosed the presence of a whitish powder which on subsequent analysis was proven to be polymerised TFE (GARRETT 1962). Initial testing by Du Pont scientists identified remarkable chemical properties including unusual inertness but it was clear that the costs of commercial production of this newly discovered polymer were likely to be of an order of magnitude far greater than for other polymers available at the time, precluding further investment for the time being.

Attitudes were to change when the United States became involved in World War II. Scientists working on the Manhattan Project to develop the atomic bomb suggested adoption of PTFE as an inert material for use as gaskets, packing and linings, in the separation of fissionable uranium-235 from uranium-238, using highly reactive uranium hexafluoride. So began the impetus to produce commercial quantities of the polymer. A veil of secrecy fell over fluorocarbon polymer research at this time but following the end of wartime restrictions, Du Pont had emerged as the only company to develop a significant commercial technology for TFE and PTFE production. In 1950, the company brought on stream the first fully commercial plant at Parkersby, West Virginia.

Polytetrafluoroethylene is now produced widely around the world. As well as the original developer Du Pont, manufacturers include ICI (Fluon), Daikin Kogyo (Polyflon), Hoechst (Hostaflon), Ausimont (Algoflon and Halon) and the USSR (Fluoroplast). In 1945 Du Pont coined the trademark "Teflon" for its PTFE, which word has been incorporated into the English language as synonymous with fluorocarbon PTFE polymer of any origin.

Polytetrafluoroethylene is currently manufactured in three main forms (GANGAL 1989). Granular PTFE is used to produce solid billets or moulds which can be further machined to form accurate shapes. Fine powder, which can be of different grades, is useful in the production of long rods or hollow tubes. Aqueous dispersions can be used for spraying metal substrates to provide chemical resistance, non-stick and low-friction properties. They are also used for spinning PTFE fibres from which woven materials are made. Production of PTFE polymer in the "free" world was of the order of 34 $\times 10^3$ tonnes in 1990.

The history of the events leading up to and immediately following the discovery of PTFE indeed bear testimony to the serendipitous nature of "the right person in the right place at the right time", and have subsequently been well described by BANKS (1988) and PLUNKETT himself (1986).

3 Chemical Properties

The unusual chemical inertness of PTFE is the result of properties conferred on it by its constituent atoms, fluorine and carbon (Fig. 1). The fluorine atom is one of the most reactive known. Following reaction, the chemical compounds formed by fluorine are often of unusual stability. One of the strongest bonds known amongst organic compounds, and incidentally not seen in natural organic compounds, is the carbon–fluorine (C–F) bond. In addition the carbon–carbon bond, which forms the backbone of the polymer chain, is well known to be one of the strongest single bonds capable of forming high-weight polymer molecules [Du Pont (i)].

Another attribute of fluorine atoms is their unique size relative to the carbon atoms which they surround. Their size is such that they form a tight spiral sheath protecting the carbon chain from possible attack by various chemical reagents. Smaller atoms would result in gaps in the cover, larger ones would crowd each other resulting in failure to complete a smooth covering sheath, either case permitting break-up of the carbon–carbon bonds of the polymer chain in adverse circumstances.

Two other factors are of importance in understanding the chemical inertness and temperature resistance of this fluorocarbon polymer. *Firstly*, the molecular weight of the polymer is unusually high. Although difficult to assess in such an unreactive molecule, and varying considerably depending on the production method, it is reported as being between 142×10^3 and 543×10^3 for low-weight polymer, and between 389×10^3 and 8900×10^3 for high-weight polymer (GANGAL 1989). The basic C_2F_4 molecule is repeated between 10 000 and 100 000 times. In other polymers chain lengths do not often exceed 5000 units. In general, chemical reactions which break down polymers commence at the ends of molecules. Fewer "sensitive" ends per unit volume of polymer, which is the case in PTFE, results in considerably enhanced stability (HOMSEY 1973). *Secondly,* secondary valence forces which link the polymer chains are about one-tenth as strong as the primary valence forces and determine to a large extent the physical properties of the molecule.

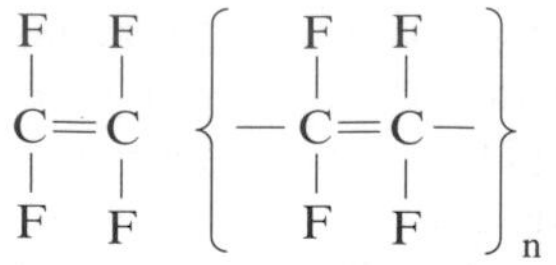

$$\begin{matrix} F & & F \\ | & & | \\ C & = & C \\ | & & | \\ F & & F \end{matrix} \quad \left\{ \begin{matrix} & F & & F & \\ & | & & | & \\ - & C & = & C & - \\ & | & & | & \\ & F & & F & \end{matrix} \right\}_n$$

Fig. 1. Conversion of TFE to polymer

Polytetrafluoroethylene is a highly crystalline orientable polymer [Du Pont (ii)]. Its regular structure is thought to imply relative absence of cross-linking, and branching is presumed to be absent since branching mechanisms would involve breaking the ultrastrong C–F bonds (BILLMEYER 1962).

The consequence of this unusual combination of properties is a polymer that is extremely resistant to attack by the most highly corrosive chemicals including strong acids and alkalis, gaseous chlorine, hydrogen peroxide and a wide range of organic materials such as esters, ketones, alcohols, acid chlorides and highly halogenated organic substances [Du Pont (i)]. Its remarkable inertness is maintained at temperatures up to 400 °C. Above this temperature decomposition eventually occurs. Beyond 990 °C breakdown products burn, but do not support combustion. Prolonged exposure to thermal decomposition products, which include carbon dioxide, carbon tetrafluoride and toxic hydrogen fluoride, causes so-called polymer fume fever, a temporary reversible influenza-like condition (GANGAL 1989).

In view of its remarkable resistance to chemical breakdown, it is not surprising that the chemical environments found in biological systems are unlikely to disrupt the molecular structure of the polymer, and no natural enzymes are known which break down the highly stable C–F bonds (GEBELEIN 1982).

4 Clinical Uses of Injectable PTFE

4.1 Composition

The first use of injectable PTFE was described by ARNOLD (1962). The suspension was prepared by the Ethicon company from a 50% mixture of glycerine and PTFE powder, the particle size of which was recorded as being 6–12 µm. In 1964, WARD and WEPMAN, conscious of the migration of PTFE particles to adjacent lymph nodes, obtained paste with 50- to 100-µm particle size from Ethicon, and this particle size has remained in use from that time. The early use of injectable PTFE was on a "named patient" basis, but by 1970 the product was available for general sale from Ethicon under the name of Polytef. The Ethicon product has used PTFE produced by Du Pont sold under the trade name Teflon. The reader should therefore be aware, in view of the origin of these products within the United States, that in the literature the basic polymer PTFE is more often referred to under the name of "Teflon" or "Polytef" than by its strictly correct "polytetrafluorethylene" chemical name. In this review we have preferred to use PTFE when describing the polymer.

4.2 Vocal Cord Paralysis

BRÜNINGS in 1911 reported on the use of liquid paraffin which he injected into the vocal cord(s) of patients suffering from cord paralysis. The paraffin added bulk to the affected cord (or cords) and allowed re-establishment of phonation and improvement of the strength of cough. The technique attracted something of a following but gradually fell into disrepute following the recognition of the potent ability of paraffin to cause disruptive oleogranulomata (paraffinoma) and to disperse and move from the injection site, even causing embolism. The principle was, however, established that injection of "space-occupying material" into paralysed cords results in considerable clinical improvement. A variety of other materials were investigated in a similar manner to establish their efficacy. Materials examined included semi-liquids such as vaseline (RETHI 1954) and a number of powdered solids, often combined with resorbable glycerine to form an injectable paste. These included cartilage dust (ARNOLD 1955), bone dust (GOFF 1960), tantalum (ARNOLD 1961) and plastics, including acrylic (LIBSERSA 1952) and silicone (RUBIN 1965a; HARRIS and CARLETON 1966).

Polytetrafluoroethylene was first reported as being used in this role by ARNOLD (1962). An injectable paste was made by combining 6- to 12-μm particles of powdered PTFE with glycerine. This was injected under local anaesthesia into the vocal cord, usually in two aliquots, the total of which ARNOLD stressed should not exceed 0.5–0.75 ml. Correct anatomical placement of the injection was considered essential. Post-operative reaction was considered to be mild, with airway narrowing being easily remediable by use of sedatives, ephedrine or steam inhalations. Pain was usually mild and normally disappeared after a few days. A "slightly tender" swelling of ipsilateral thyroid lymph nodes was noted which disappeared shortly thereafter. The clinical results were described as showing "encouraging lasting vocal improvement". The technique was considered not to be difficult for those experienced in intralaryngeal surgery. ARNOLD included with the initial clinical investigation a histopathology study of the tissue reaction following injection of 1 ml PTFE paste into the quadriceps muscle of rabbits which were harvested 2 and 4 months later. A sharp demarcation between the implant and normal muscle was noted, with lymphocytes, macrophages and giant cells being present. Fibrosis was recorded as being minimal.

There have been a number of reports on the use of intracordal PTFE injection following ARNOLD's initial communication. Clinical series reported to date include those of LEWY (1964:32 cases), SIEGLER (1967:20 cases), DEDO et al. (1973:135 cases) and NASSAR (1977:34 cases). The largest clinical series reported to date is that of LEWY (1976), which describes details on 144 of 218 personal cases and presents further data obtained by questionnaire from 38 accredited investigators (within the United States) who had performed a total of 1139 procedures. The commonest cause of cord dysfunction was either planned or accidental injury to the nerve during surgery, malignant disease (especially carcinoma of lung), or idiopathic, which is in accord with most other series. In 67% of patients, voice improvement was reported as well as improvement of other physiological functions of the laryngeal valve including straining, swallowing, coughing and avoidance of aspiration. Whilst few short-term complications were reported, two patients required tracheotomy because of acute laryngeal oedema. In one patient laryngeal carcinoma was recorded as a complication but there was substantial doubt as to whether the tumour was related to the PTFE since the tumour was not adjacent to the implant and the patient was a heavy smoker who, contrary to advice at the time of the implant, had continued to smoke.

It is now accepted by most authors that the technique is likely to be beneficial in those conditions causing unilateral cord paralysis. A poor outcome is probable in bilateral cord paralysis, severe traumatic scarring of the cord region or paralyses which are the result of complex neurological deficit (Dedo et al. 1973).

Ward et al. (1985) have reported on a novel approach in which flexible instrument laryngoscopy is used to monitor the transcutaneous injection of PTFE paste. The basic principle, however, remains the same, i.e. that of medial displacement of the paralysed cord by accurate placement of PTFE paste injection.

Migration of injected semifluid of finely particulate materials, for example paraffin and tantalum, had already been identified as a problem in cordal injection (Arnold 1962). Arnold had stressed the need for anatomical accuracy and the avoidance of injection of excessive quantities of PTFE paste during the procedure. He drew attention to the need to bear in mind anthropomorphic differences and suggested that a total injection quantity of 0.5 ml was sufficient for females, and 0.75 ml for males. Rubin (1965b) further emphasised the need for careful technique, accuracy of injection and avoidance of excessive quantity of injected PTFE paste. He particularly stressed that paste should be precisely injected just lateral to the thyroarytenoid muscle. Using whole larynx histological sections, he elegantly demonstrated the risks of proximal, distal, lateral and intramuscular injection, all of which were associated with poor clinical result and potential risk of migration of PTFE. In a clinical review of 32 cases, Lewy (1964) looked for, but on the basis of clinical examination noted no evidence of, "drift". Kirchner et al. (1966) and Toomey and Brown (1967), using dogs as an experimental model for intracordal injection, found no evidence of migration of PTFE particles to adjacent tissue. Boedts et al. (1967) drew attention to particles of PTFE in small peri-arterial lymphatics in this material but also commented on the risk of intravascular injection of PTFE paste during implantation.

It was clear, however, from a number of reports that PTFE could pass inferiorly and laterally through the cricothyroid membrane into the soft tissues around the thyroid and form a discrete palpable lesion (Lewy 1966; Stone and Arnold 1967; Stone et al. 1970; Stephens et al. 1976). Such migration had on occasion given rise to clinical suspicion of thyroid neoplasia (Walsh and Castelli 1975).

To date, in man there are histopathological descriptions of just less than 30 cases of vocal cord PTFE implantation, chiefly from postmortem material (Table 1). The statement in the majority of such reported cases that migration has not been seen, has, in almost every instance, to be judged against relatively sparse evidence of how the laryngeal specimen was obtained, how carefully the local anatomical area of the larynx was examined and which internal organs, e.g. lung, liver, spleen, kidney and brain, were examined and in what detail (LEWY 1966; STONE and ARNOLD 1967; BOEDTS et al. 1967; GOFF 1969,1973; HARRIS and HAWK 1969; STONE et al. 1970; WALSH and CASTELLI 1975; LEWY and MILLET 1978; DEDO and CARLSÖÖ 1982; CARLSÖÖ et al. 1983).

Reports from Oppenheimer and his group from the early days of investigation of the behaviour of plastics in laboratory animals indicated a significant risk of development of sarcoma in rats and mice following long-term exposure to a wide range of plastics (OPPENHEIMER et al. 1955). This resulted in justifiable anxiety in many investigations concerning the risk of neoplasia following long-term exposure to injected PTFE. The longest human exposure so far reported is 16 years (DEDO and CARLSÖÖ 1982). None of the clinical reports or the reports of animal or human pathological material has shown evidence of dysplasia or neoplastic change directly associated with PTFE injection of the vocal cord. Most authors recognise that it will take 20–30 years at least before a firm reassurance on the risk of possible neoplasia can be given.

POHRIS and KLEINSASSER (1987) reported a case of laryngeal stenosis which had developed 1.5 years following intracordal PTFE injection. The histological pictures provided with this case show quite extensive acute inflammation amongst the PTFE particles which suggests ulceration and/or secondary infection as causative factors.

RUBIN (1975) commented that an intracordal PTFE implant was irretrievable and stressed the need to avoid injection of excessive quantities of paste. He noted the difficulty of removing PTFE from cords in the event of an unsuccessful clinical result and the risk of removal of considerable normal cordal tissue along with the PTFE. He also reported on a case in which an operation to excise a mass of PTFE lying external to the laryngeal cartilage caused a wound discharging PTFE particles through a fistula for 6 weeks which ultimately healed with some induration. HORN and DEDO (1980), using surgical dissection techniques which avoid the free edge of the cord, described how excess PTFE paste could be removed from cords overinjected by paste. KOCH et al. (1987) have described a laser method of removing excess PTFE from the cord, bearing in mind that PTFE burns in oxygen-rich air with the production of gases, some of which are potentially toxic.

4.3 Velopharyngeal Insufficiency

Adequate velopharyngeal closure of the nasal cavity is an essential mechanism in the production of normal speech and in swallowing. Patients with imperfect velopharyngeal closure are chiefly those with unoperated or poorly repaired cleft palate, but other aetiological factors include congenital shortness of palate, neurological and muscular diseases and scarring. In the various operative techniques used to try and ensure phonation and swallowing, an important underlying concept was the creation of a posterior pharyngeal ridge which reduced the gap between palate and pharynx. As in the case of the vocal cord, early investigators used paraffin by injection to move the posterior pharyngeal wall forward (Ekstein 1922). The various problems associated with paraffin injection, i.e. paraffinoma and migration with mediastinitis, caused the use of this substance to fall into disrepute. Implants of fascia and cartilage offered unpredictable and often transitory results because of reabsorption. Blocksma (1963) implanted silicone rubber into the retropharyngeal wall with reasonable success and apparently excellent tissue tolerance.

Following Arnold's (1962) report on the use of PTFE and tantalum in the vocal cord, Ward and Wepman (1964) used these materials in a series of experiments on adult cats. Artificial clefts were created in the cats' palates which were then repaired, simulating the situation commonly found in many human cases of velopharyngeal insufficiency. No comment was made on the quantity of PTFE or tantalum paste injected other than to note the formation of an "adequate ridge" in the posterior pharynx. They noted that tantalum and PTFE were both well tolerated and maintained the ridge in the pharyngeal mucosa. Histologically, however, PTFE and tantalum particles were found in all lymph nodes examined. The particle size of PTFE was therefore increased from 6–12 μm to 50–100 μm. Although greatly reduced in amount, there was still evidence of migration when the larger particle size was used.

Lewy et al. (1965) gave the first report of PTFE injection into the posterior pharyngeal region in a human. They injected 5 ml of 50- to 100-μm particle size paste along Passavant's line in a 15-year-old female who had suffered palatal weakness following acute poliomyelitis at the age of 1 year. Postoperatively a "dramatic" improvement in the quality of her voice was recorded.

Ward et al. (1966) described the injection of five patients under general anaesthesia, with 50- to 100-μm particle size PTFE paste beneath the mucosa of the posterior pharyngeal wall just above the prominence caused by the tubercle of the atlas. From 6 to 12 ml of paste was injected in one session. Injection was confined as far as possible to the submucosa and superior constrictor muscle. Caudal extension was prevented by the pressure of a tongue depressor against the mucosa overlying the first vertebra caudal to the injection site. In some instances where the ridge appeared inadequate, 1–2 ml of PTFE paste was injected into the posterior margins of the palate on each side. Two patients required second injections and their speech was determined to have returned to normal by trained listeners. Two of the remaining three patients with single injections had "good improvement". No clinical evidence of spread was identified although it was noted that up to 24 ml of paste had been used in two procedures.

There have been few reports of use of PTFE paste in velopharyngeal insufficiency since Ward et al.'s original report. Using an identical injection technique, Ward (1968) recorded an excellent or good clinical response in 18 out of 21 patients. The quantity of PTFE paste used by WARD varied between 4 and 30 ml per injection. One patient, following several attempts at surgical correction, received a cumulative total of 98 ml apparently without ill-effect. The technique is now recommended only in selected cases as a treatment of last resort if various plastic and reconstructive surgical techniques and speech therapy have proved unsuccessful. Its use is not thought to be advised in cases with underlying neurological disturbance.

4.4 Other Otorhinolaryngological Uses

Atrophic rhinitis is recorded as being successfully treated by PTFE injection (WARD 1968). One patient is recorded as having a sustained improvement in the condition of his nasal mucous membranes following multiple injections of small quantities of PTFE paste into the floor of the nose under the inferior turbinate and the septum. A total of 19 ml of paste was injected, with good clinical improvement 16 months following the procedure.

Problems of excessive patency of the eustachian tube opening have been helped by PTFE injection of the tubotubarious area (WARD 1968)

The operation of supraglottic hemi-laryngectomy for selected neoplasm has, in some patients been attended by failure of the protective mechanisms of the larynx necessary for normal swallowing. Injection of PTFE paste into the healed scar tissue following operation has allowed a build up of tissue to cause a more complete closure of the glottic chink with good clinical improvement in swallowing and cessation of aspiration (YARINGTON and HARNED 1971).

4.5 Hip Replacement

Polytetrafluoroethylene was introduced to clinical orthopaedic practice when the operation of total hip arthroplasty was developed to deal with severe degenerative articular disease of the hip joint (CHARNLEY 1961). PTFE was initially used (because of its inertness and non-stick properties) to simulate damaged articular cartilage. Later it was formed into a socket articulating with a metal femoral head replacement. In the early stages sockets were not cemented into the acetabular cup. Within a few years it was obvious that PTFE was not ideal because of socket migration, formation of nodular inflammatory masses and extensive bone destruction. CHARNLEY (1963) described how abraded PTFE particles may aggregate to form granulomatous masses, 100–200 ml in volume, with a PTFE content of 13% by dry weight. He described the PTFE aggregates as collections of "sterile pus" which could be called "truly caseous". Numerous giant cells surrounded the PTFE particles. Slowly erosive behaviour was noted when the mass was in contact with bone, which contrasted with the tendency of the masses to become encapsulated in the soft tissues. It became clear that the cause of these destructive masses of particulate PTFE was the combination of continual abrasion of the prosthetic metal femoral head on the PTFE socket and the mechanical pressures of weight bearing and movement. All these factors helped to drive the PTFE particles, and any inflammatory cells in contact, into the musculoskeletal tissues of, and adjacent to, the hip joint. The size of the PTFE particles was described as very large, often up to 300 μm (CHARNLEY 1979). Systematic measurements of wear rates revealed that PTFE could wear at rates of between 2.4 and 3.6 mm per year. In contrast, high molecular weight polyethylene (HMWP) prostheses were shown to have an average mean wear rate of 0.13 mm per year, and HMWP therefore rapidly replaced PTFE as the polymer of choice for use as a prosthetic acetabular socket. (SWANSON and FREEMAN 1977).

Late calcification of the nodular mass of PTFE particles was described by WROBLEWSKI (1988), and this was thought to be indicative of a healing process provided that movement of the granuloma had ceased (EDITORIAL 1990).

Whilst this process is not directly comparable to the external injection of PTFE paste, it represents what might be termed an "endogenous injection" of PTFE debris. The debris is, however, mixed with a variety of whole or fragmented inflammatory cells and highly chemically reactive agents derived from them. That its behaviour may be less than desirable is not surprising.

4.6 Reconstructive Surgical Procedures

The first description of use of PTFE paste to correct a saddle nose deformity was given by WILSON (1964). BARRY (1965) used PTFE paste experimentally in dogs to reconstruct the nasal dorsum. WARD (1968) also recorded the use of PTFE paste injected between the upper and lower lateral cartilages of the nose in a 14-year-old boy to replace intranasal tissues lost following a history of trauma, septal haematoma and abscess formation. A total of 1.5 ml of PTFE paste was required to correct the abnormal nasal contour.

PTFE has also been combined with carbon fibre to form a porous sponge-like material (Proplast) which has a similar modulus of elasticity to that of bone. The material can be easily shaped, and its porous structure allows tissue ingrowth for stabilisation (WILLIAMS 1976). Clearly this material does not equate with injectable PTFE, but the fine dispersion of PTFE in a spongy matrix does allow comparisons to be made. Using rabbits and dogs and experimental animals, HOMSEY and ANDERSON (1976) described extensive interstitial giant cell migration with marked collagenisation within the polymer when used in bone and tendon repair or replacement. Clinical use in a variety of orthopaedic, orofacial and plastic surgical procedures was reported as being successful.

The use of PTFE paste as a substance to alter the shape and profile of the eyelid was reported by DAICKER et al. (1985). About 0.5 ml of paste was used to remodel the upper palpebral furrow in a patient whose lid had been retracted by scars following a road traffic accident. Oedema was very prominent within the first 24 h but proved transient. Large foreign body granulomas occurred which required two excisions at 4 and 7 months. The authors advised against the use of PTFE paste in the well-vascularised loose tissue of the eyelid.

4.7 Urinary Incontinence

Polytetrafluorethylene was introduced into urological practice by POLITANO et al. (1974) who treated post-prostatectomy urinary incontinence by peri-urethral injection of PTFE in the form of Polytef paste. The paste added bulk to the periurethral tissues and increased the resistance to urinary outflow, thus restoring urinary control. The volume of paste injected was 10–14 ml, repeated if necessary. Thirty-two patients received 53 injections and a good to excellent result was achieved in 62%. Complications were minimal. Following his initial success Politano continued to use this method and in 1982 described a larger series of 165 patients with urinary incontinence (POLITANO 1982). A good to excellent result was achieved in 75%. Politano monitored the patients carefully and showed no changes in the main haematological and biochemical parameters in their blood after PTFE injection.

Politano thought that embolisation of the PTFE was a real hazard. However he found no alteration in the chest X-ray appearances before and after PTFE injection and at follow-up. Subsequently MITTLEMAN and MARRACCINI (1983) reported, at autopsy, finding PTFE particles surrounded by foreign body giant cells in the lungs of a patient treated with peri-urethral PTFE injections on two occasions for post-prostatectomy urinary incontinence. The first injection was 2 years prior to death and the second (of 10–15 ml of Polytef paste) was 1 year after the first. Despite the presence of numerous particles in the pulmonary interstitium the reaction to them consisted of foreign body giant cells but only a few lymphocytes (Table 1). This was graded as a mild response without clinical significance. These authors thought that the PTFE particles had reached the pulmonary circulation via the prostatic venous plexuses. They did not regard this finding as a contra-indication to the continued use of PTFE to treat urinary incontinence.

A recent review by POLITANO (1992) described his long clinical experience with PTFE injection for post-prostatectomy urinary incontinence. His series included 720 such patients who had been incontinent for a minimum of 1 year after prostatic surgery. A very high success rate was reported. Among those whose incontinence followed transurethral resection of prostatic tissue 88% were improved by PTFE injection. After radical prostatectomy the success rate was 67%. Particle migration was not a clinicially significant problem and malignancy related to PTFE did not occur in this large series. Politano continued to recommend injection of PTFE for the treatment of urinary incontinence occurring after prostatic surgery.

Table 1. Clinicopathological findings in reports of PTFE implantation in which histopathological details are given

Author(s)	Species	Implant site	Amount injected	Duration	Particle size	Migration	Neoplasia
Arnold 1962	Rabbit	Quadriceps	1 ml	2–4 mo	6–12	NS	NS
Ward and Wepman 1964	Cat	Pharynx	1–3 ml	4–6 mo	6–12	Yes, nodes	NS
					50–100	Yes, nodes	NS
Harris and Carleton 1966	Dog	Vocal cord	NS	3 mo	NS	No. (larynx only)	No
Kirchner et al. 1966	Dog	Vocal cord	0.5–1.0 ml	6–18 mo	NS	No (larynx only)	No
Lewy 1966	Man (1)	Vocal cord	NS	17 mo	NS (E)	No (larynx only)	No
Rubin 1966	Dog	Vocal cord	0.5–1.0 ml	48 h–2 y	50–100	NS	NS
	Man (2)	Vocal cord	NS	10 d, 6 wk	50–100	NS	NS
Stone and Arnold 1967	Man (2)	Vocal cord	1 ml	4, 10 mo &a+72H	50–100	No (larynx only)	No
Toomey and Brown 1967	Dog	Vocal cord	0.2–0.5 ml	2 wk–6 mo	NS	No (larynx only)	No
Boedts et al. 1967	Man (1)	Vocal cord	NS	1 mo	NS	No "various organs" but PTFE noted in lymphatics	NS
Goff 1969	Man (1)	Vocal cord	NS	5 wk	NS (E)	NS	NS
Harris and Hawk 1969	Man (1)	Vocal cord	1.5 ml	25 mo	NS (E)	No (larynx only)	No
Stone et al. 1970	Man (3)	Vocal cord	1 ml	3–16 mo	Polytef	No (larynx only)	No
Goff 1973	Man (2)	Vocal cord	0.5–1.6 ml	4 d, 1.5 yr	Polytef	No	No
Rubin 1975	Man (1)	Vocal cord	NS	NS	Polytef	Cricothyroid	No
Walsh and Castelli 1975	Man (1)	Vocal cord	NS	9 mo	Polytef	Cricothyroid	No
Stephens et al. 1976	Man (2)	Vocal cord	1.5 ml	11, 21 mo	Polytef	Cricothyroid	No
Lewy and Millett 1978	Man (1)	Vocal cord	NS	48 h	NS	–	–

Dedo and Carlsöö 1982	Man (2)	Vocal cord	0.2–0.75 ml	4 wk–16 yr	NS	–	No
Carlsöö et al. 1983	Man (1)	Vocal cord	–	15 yr	NS	–	–
Mittleman and Marraccini 1983	Man (1)	Urethra	10–15 ml	3 yr	NS	Yes, lung	NS
Malizia et al. 1984	Dog Monkey	Urethra	2 ml	50–105 mo	Polytef	Yes, nodes, lungs, spleen kidney, brain	No
Puri and O'Donnell 1984	Piglet	Ureter	0.5–1 ml	1–6 mo	Polytef	NS	NS
Altermatt et al. 1985	Man (1)	Pharynx	NS	6 yr	NS	Yes, small particles	–
Ellis et al. 1987	Dog	Vocal cord	0.5 ml	2 wk–6 mo	Polytef	Yes, regional lymph nodes	–
Pohris and Kleinsasser 1987	Man (1)	Vocal cord	–	1.5 yr	–	–	–
Lacombe 1990	Man (3)	Ureter	NS	3–4 mo	Polytef	NS	NS
Marcellin et al. 1990	Man (4)	Ureter	NS	3–6 mo	NS	NS	NS
Schulman et al. 1990	Man (7)	Ureter	0.2 ml	NS	NS	NS	NS
Wenig et al. 1990	Man (5)	Vocal cord	–	6 mo–15 yr	NS	Cricothyroid	NS

NS, Not stated; NS (E), Ethicon acknowledged as manufacturer.

4.8 Vesico-ureteric Reflux

Another clinical problem for urological surgeons has been the management of vesico-ureteric reflux in children. The need for and the timing of surgical intervention are important questions. Reflux may regress spontaneously in many children. Others may be at risk of progressive renal damage if they have recurrent infections and intrarenal reflux (Report of the International Reflux study Committee 1981; Birmingham Reflux Study Group 1983; WOODARD and RUSHTON 1987). MATOUSCHEK (1981) showed that PTFE injected at the ureteric orifice abolished vesico-ureteric reflux in the one patient whom he treated by this method. The technique of endoscopic subureteric Teflon injection, which became known as STING, was described in animals (PURI and O'DONNELL 1984) and man (O'DONNELL and PURI 1984). Fourteen of their first 18 treated ureters showed complete absence of reflux after one injection of PTFE in the form of Polytef paste, three were successfully treated by a second injection, and the reflux in the remaining case was greatly improved. These early results were encouraging and the technique became more widely used, avoiding the need for ureteric reimplantation in many patients (PURI 1990). It was also a successful form of treatment for reflux into complete duplex systems (DEWAN and O'DONNELL 1991).

Submucosal injection of PTFE in the form of Polytef paste has been used for several years in this centre as an endoscopic treatment for vesico-ureteric reflux in children (DIAMOND and BOSTON 1987a; BROWN 1989). This has included children with neuropathic bladders, some of whom had open neural tube defects (PURI and GUINEY 1986). DIAMOND and BOSTON (1987b) also treated a patient with an orthotopic ureterocoele by subureteric PTFE injection as part of a conservative treatment plan.

The main indications for PTFE treatment were evidence of intrarenal reflux or lower grades of reflux with persistent urinary tract infection. At cystoscopy 0.2–0.6 ml of Polytef paste was injected beneath the mucosa at the vesico-ureteric orifice which in reluxing ureters is abnormally wide. The injection was repeated if reflux did not improve after the first STING treatment, as assessed by micturating cystogram.

Whilst this procedure made anti-reflux surgery unnecessary in many cases, in some patients the reflux was not corrected, and surgical reimplantation of the refluxing ureters was performed later. This operation included excision of injection sites in the distal ureter.

5 Pathological Studies

5.1 Light Microscopy

The initial response noted to PTFE paste injection is a marked neutrophil response with accompanying oedema of the injection site and immediate surrounding tissues (LEWY and MILLET 1978). The oedematous reaction is of relatively minor significance with the exception of the vocal cord, where respiratory obstruction has been described. The oedema fades within 24–48 h. Associated with the oedema is hyperaemia, which causes redness of the skin when PTFE has been injected subcutaneously (CHARNLEY 1963). This is also a transient phenomenon which fades within a week. The neutrophil response may not represent a specific reaction to PTFE and has been described by Rubin (1966) to be identical when glycerine alone is injected. RUBIN also noted that the initial inflammatory response does not necessarily affect the entire sample of PTFE paste, which may be of importance in determining later cellular events within the injected mass. Commencing at about 48 h, there is a mononuclear cell infiltration amongst the PTFE particles. This mononuclear cell response builds up rapidly so that by 5 days well-defined histiocytes and foreign body-type giant cells are easily identified, especially at the margins of the implant. At this stage neutrophils rapidly decline in number and are not a feature of older lesions unless there has been superadded infection or other acute inflammatory irritant. Over the next 3–4 weeks, histiocytes and giant cells become the main cellular component. In young lesions sparse numbers of small lymphocytes are seen, chiefly at the margins of the lesion.

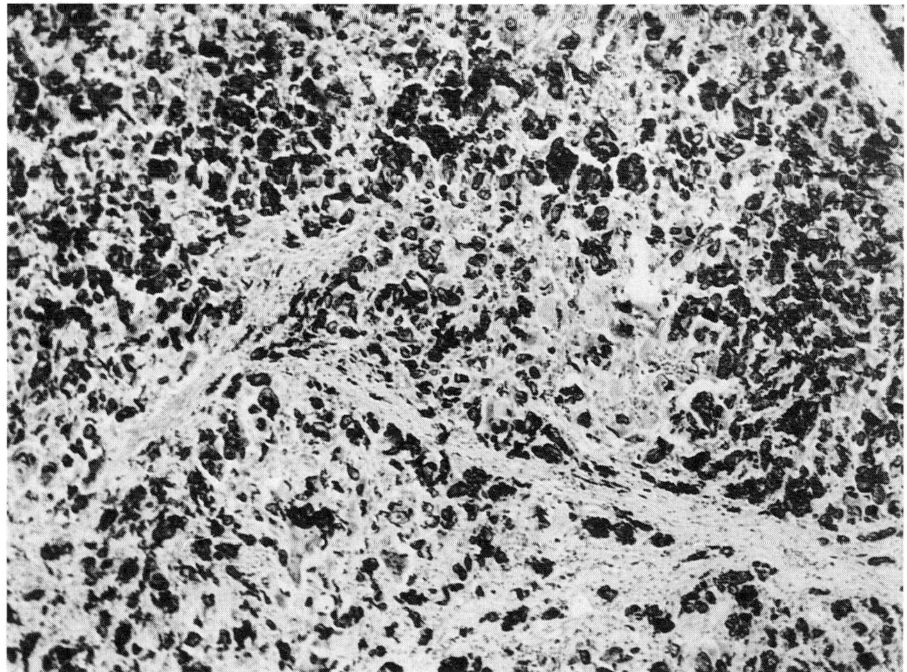

Fig. 2. The PTFE particles, which appear dark at this magnification, are separated by thin fibrous trabeculae. H&E, × 40

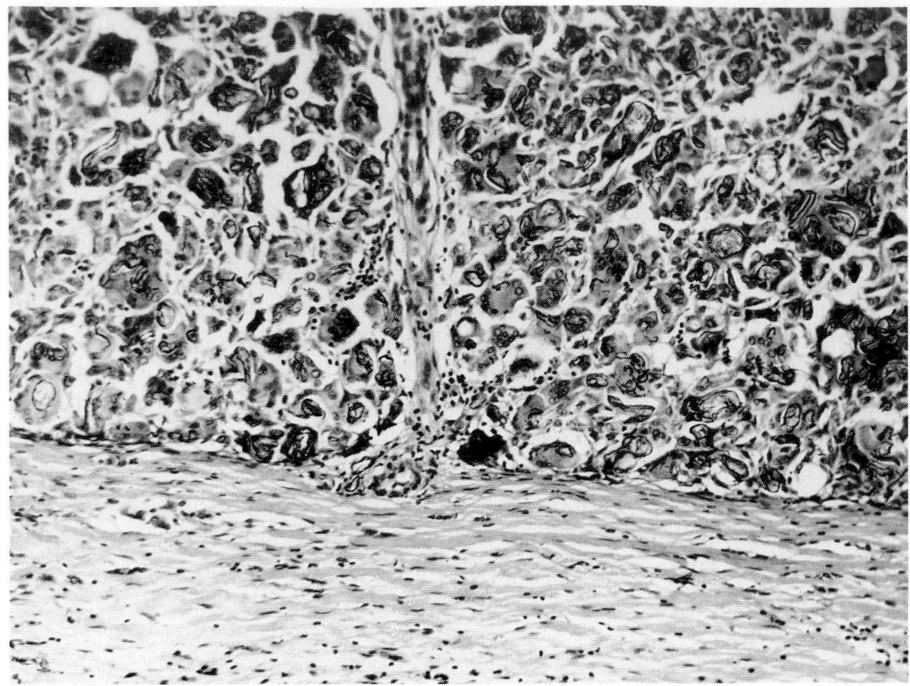

Fig. 3. The PTFE particles form a well-defined edge in the ureteric submucosa. H&E, × 100

Beginning imperceptibly, but described by as early as 2 weeks, there is a delicate collagenisation. The permeation is most marked at the periphery of the lesion but does extend into the centres of the masses, forming what could be described as a "lobular" pattern with septa of denser collagenous tissue dividing the injected mass into discrete areas (Fig. 2). This appearance, however, may be enhanced by the presence of the pre-existing supportive collagen framework of the tissue affected by the injected particles. Amid the confined anatomy of vocal cord or ureter, provided the injected mass is correctly situated, the cleavage of tissue planes which occurs does not result in a nodular lobulated pattern (Fig. 3). On the other hand, if the PTFE is forced through loose fibrovascular and particularly fatty connective tissue, there is an enhanced recruitment of collagenous tissue with much coarser collagen bands being formed in consequence, and less tendency for the injected PTFE to remain as a discrete, continuous mass (Fig. 4). Some investigators have found that the central area of the PTFE mass remains unreactive and comparatively acellular (Fig. 5). This has been noted particularly in the vocal cord (KIRCHNER et al. 1966; STEPHENS et al. 1976) and in the ureter (O'HARA et al. 1989). This central lack of response does not seem to be related to the age or size of the implant.

The giant cell response to PTFE is very characteristic. The cells are almost exclusively of foreign body giant cell type and are noted to partially or completely

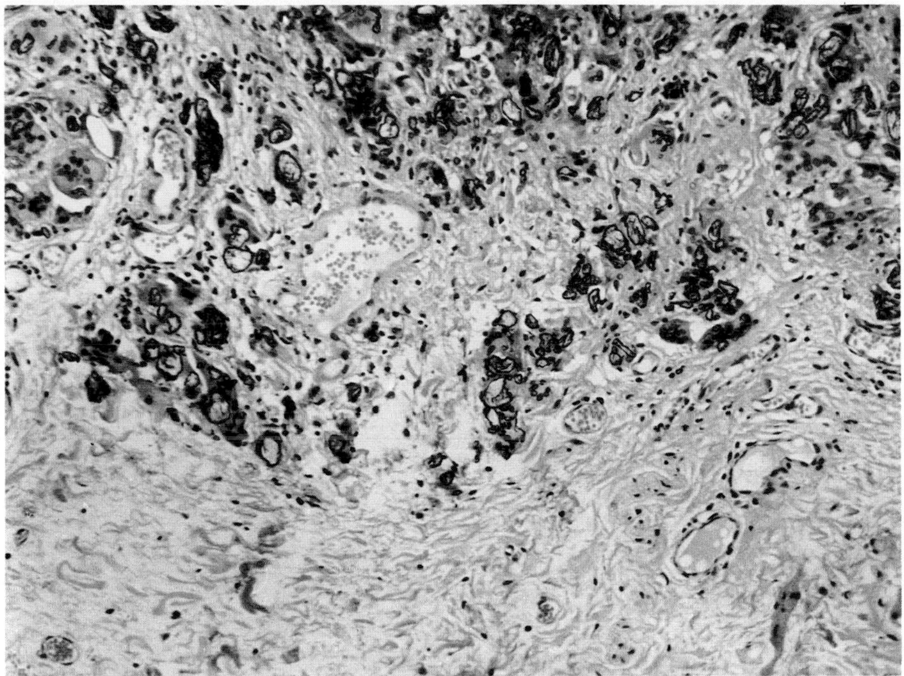

Fig. 4. PTFE particles lie in small separate aggregates, amongst which permeate fibroblasts, small blood vessels and immature collagen. H&E, × 100

envelop PTFE particles, depending on their size (Fig. 6). Langhans-type giant cells are not described. There is little evidence of formation of sheets of epithelioid histiocytes, which would suggest that immune mechanisms are not of importance in the response to PTFE. Asteroid bodies have occasionally been described (Dedo and Carlsöö 1982).

The lymphocytic response in injection sites uncomplicated by infection remains remarkably light throughout the injected mass. There may be a tendency for small aggregates to form at the margins of the masses, especially if the injected material has extended to involve loose areolar fibrofatty connective tissues.

Polytetrafluoroethylene particles are characterised by a variety but yet constancy of appearances. There is a distinct tendency to form nearly rectangular or rhomboid appearances, usually but not invariably with rounding of the angles. Some fragments are virtually semicircular whilst others are highly irregular in outline. Particles occasionally join to form small aggregates. They are thrown into very sharp relief by polarised light, which can be used in diagnostic situations and is of importance in the investigation of migration (Fig. 7). The particle size varies enormously and whilst the upper size limit of the commercial preparation seems to conform well wtih the stated 100 μm size, there are undoubtedly many particles of less than 50 μm size in our material. Particles small enough to be seen in lysomes

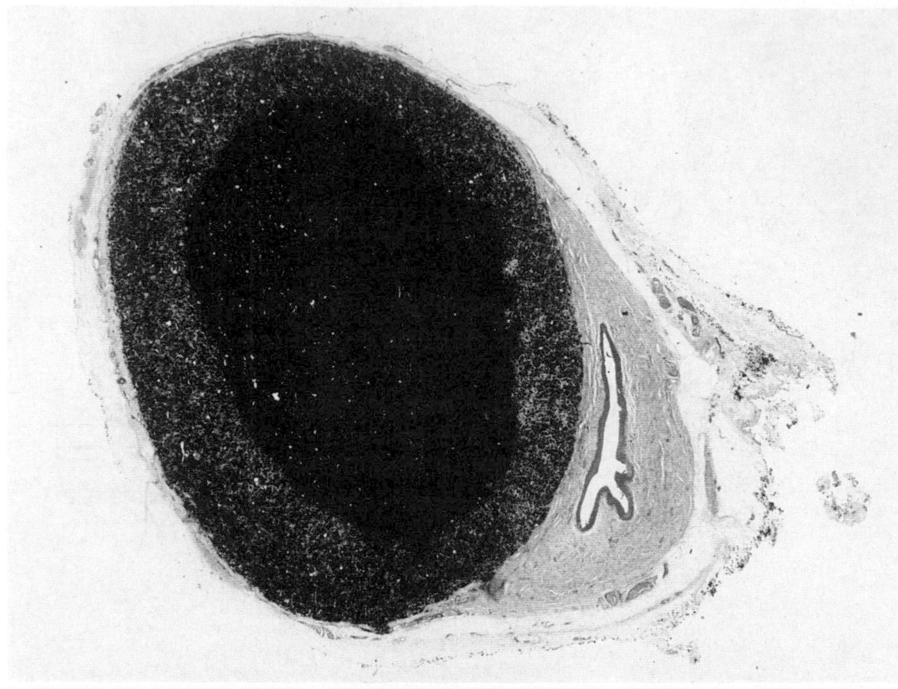

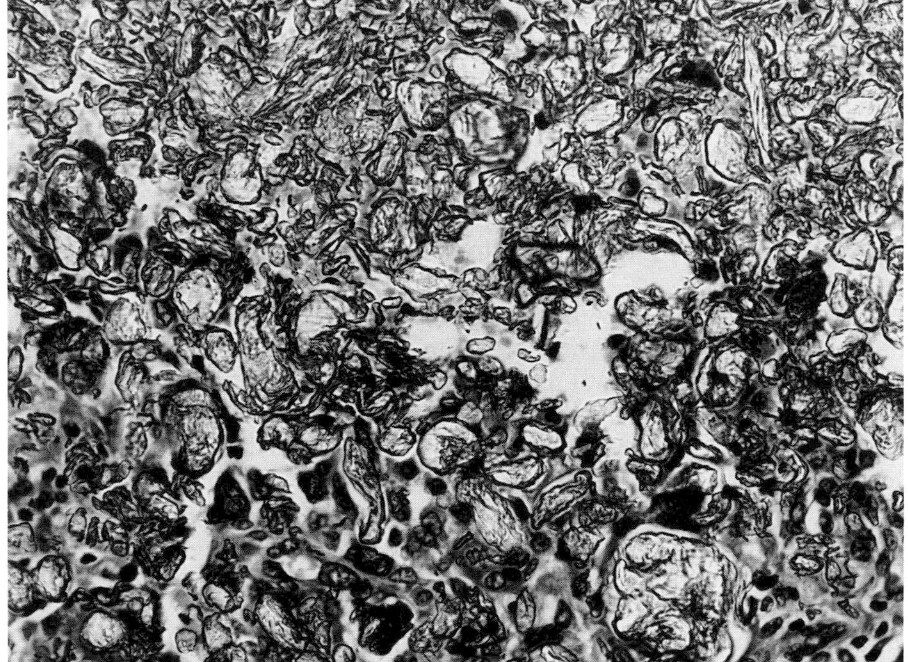

Fig. 5 a. This low-power illustration of ureter clearly demonstrates a central unreactive zone in the PTFE mass. H&E, × 20. **b** In the central zone *(top)* of the PTFE mass, particles are crammed together. The reactive zone *(bottom)* shows separation of particles by histiocytes, lymphocytes and occasional fibroblasts. H&E, × 250

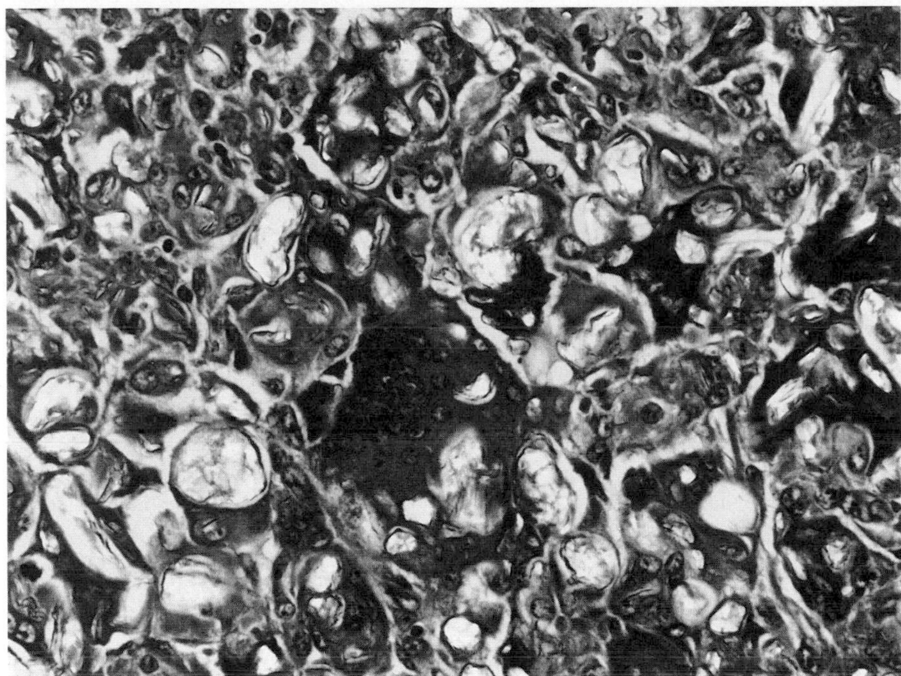

Fig. 6. The PTFE particles are surrounded by mononuclear histiocytes and multinucleated foreign body giant cells, some of which are large enough to engulf several particles. H&E, × 350

using transmission electron microscopy (TEM) suggest that tiny particles must be injected along with the larger 50–100 μm size. MALIZIA et al. (1984) described a particle size of between 4 and 40 μm for 90% of particles within the commercially available product Polytef. Tangential section artefact is not a satisfactory explanation. In view of the chemical inertness of PTFE and the lack of biological systems to break down its chemical bonds, biodegradation is extremely unlikely. It may be that tiny particles, i.e. considerably less than 50 μm, remain adherent to larger particles for a variety of physiochemical reasons during preparation, only to separate in the environment of the body. An alternative explanation may be that some of the 50 to 100-μm particles are already splintered during manufacture but that separation into smaller fragments does not occur until the particles enter the body environment. Some evidence of separation of small fragments is provided by the detection, by means of scanning electron microscopy (SEM), of small "flakes" of PTFE attached to particles (WENIG et al. 1990; see also Sect. 5.3).

One theme which predominates in case reports of PTFE particle histology, with the exception of those particles derived from abraded artificial hip implants, is the remarkable similarity and constancy of the cellular response over many months and years. Our own study of 66 specimens taken from 34 patients three months to six years following STING has shown gross and microscopic

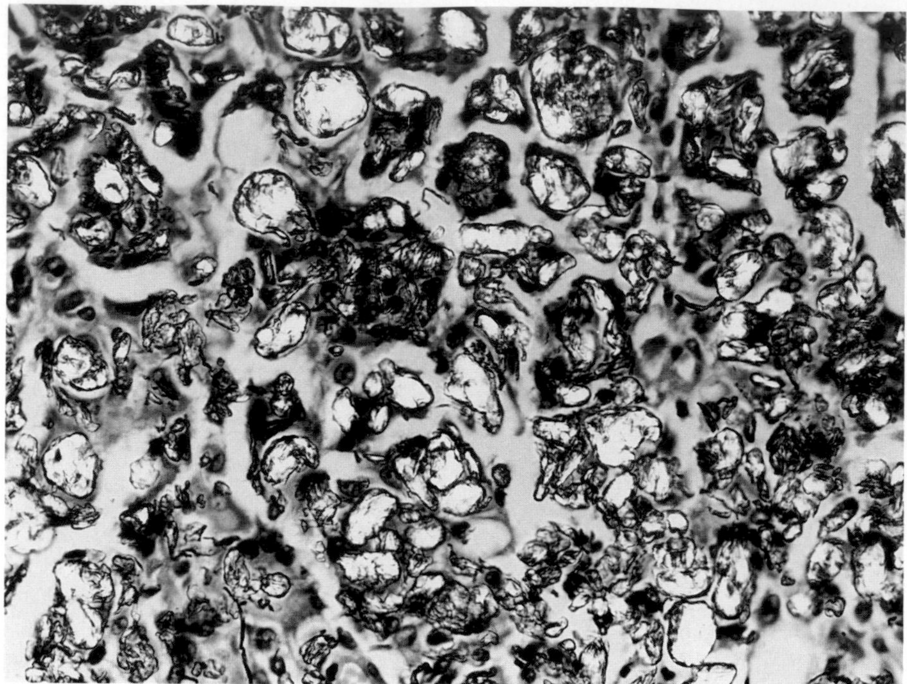

Fig. 7. Polarised light emphasises the rounded-off polyangular, and semicircular shapes of the PTFE particles. Note the relatively large range of particle size present (see text). H&E, ×250

pathological appearances entirely in accord with the description given above. DEDO and CARLSÖÖ (1982), in their description of the longest implant yet described (16 years), stress the similarity of the response to that noted in short-term cases of some 6 months. It appears that once formed, at about 2–3 months following implantation, the histological features of the injected PTFE mass enter a virtual steady state which persists for many years thereafter.

Table 2. Immunostains used in study

Immunostain	Supplier
L26 (CD40)	Dako
UCHL1 (CD45RO)	Dako
MT1 (CD43)	Biotest
KP1 (CD68)	Dako
F. VIII	Ortho
Ulex eur.	Vector

Table 3. Immunohistochemical respone to ureteric PTFE implant

Case no. (range 3 mo–2.5 years)	Central core	Lymphocytes L26 P	L26 C	UCHL1 P	UCHL1 C	MTI P	MTI C	Giant cells/ macrophages CD68	Capillary endothelium F.VIII	Capillary endothelium *Ulex eur.*
1	Y	–	–	++	–	++	+	+	+	++
2	N	–	–	+	–	+	±	+++	+	+
3	N	–	–	+	±	++	+	+++	+	+
4	N	–	–	++	+	++	+	+++	+	+++
5	N	–	–	++	+	++	++	+++	+	+++
6	Y	+	–	++	±	+++	+	+++	+	+++
7	N	–	–	++	+	++	±	+++	±	+
8	Y	–	–	+	±	++	±	+++	++	±
9	Y	–	–	+	±	++	+	+++	+	++
10	N	–	–	+	±	+	+	++	±	+
11	Y	–	–	++	+	++	+	+++	+	±
12	N	–	–	++	+	+++	++	+++	+	+++
13	Y	–	–	++	+	++	+	+++	+	+++
14	Y	–	–	++	+	++	+	+++	+	+++
15	Y	+	–	++	+	++	+	+++	+	+++
16	Y	–	–	++	+	++	+	+++	+	±

Y, yes; N, no; P, periphery; C, central; O, no respones; ± slight; +, mild; ++, moderate; +++, marked

5.2 Immunocytochemistry

There have been very few immunocytochemical studies on the tissue response to injected PTFE particles. ALTERMATT et al. (1985) reported no evidence of positive staining for IgA, IgG, IgM and complement component C3 in the PTFE tissue response. A study was undertaken on 16 examples of ureteric PTFE taken from the files of this Institute. Particular attention was paid to those cases in which there was a central core of PTFE particles virtually devoid of and unaffected by the cellullar response. One-half of the cases were of this type. Sections were immunostained using the P Strept. ABC method to a panel of lymphocyte macrophage and vascular markers (Table 2). Using a simple semi-quantitative method comparison was made of the reaction in the central and peripheral regions of the PTFE particle mass.

The results (Table 3) indicate that in the mature tissue response to PTFE, the lymphocyte response is almost exclusively of T cell type, and that virtually no B cells are present. There is a restrained capillary vascular response amongst the giant cell/macrophage complexes and at the immediate edge of the granulomata. No qualitative or quantitative differences have been identified between the two groups of specimens to account for the lack of cellular response in the central Teflon core. The non-reactive core may reflect the inert nature of the PTFE polymer and features specific to the anatomy of the injection site (O'HARA et al. 1991).

5.3 Electron Microscopy

Although 30 years have elapsed since the initial histopathological observation of the tissue responses to injected PTFE particles, there have been very few reports of either TEM or SEM findings.

Using TEM, DEDO and CARLSÖÖ (1982) examined a vocal cord specimen removed 1.5 years following implantation. They found that the majority of the PTFE particles had been phagocytosed by macrophages and that the phagocytosed material was enclosed in smooth-walled vacuoles. The diameter of the particles varied considerably. Although this was not stated, to judge from the ultrastructural photomicrographs accompanying the papers, particles as small as 1 μm in diameter were present. The cells contained numerous mitochondria, sparse rough endoplasmic reticulum and numerous cytoplasmic lysomes. Free ribosome clusters were observed, as were numerous microvilli and pseudopods on the cellular surfaces. Cell nuclei often contained fibrillogranular intranuclear inclusions up to 0.5 μm in diameter.

In a second TEM report, CARLSÖÖ et al. (1983) detailed a further case of vocal cord PTFE removed 1.5 years following implantation. In this instance many more foreign body giant cells were present. As before, PTFE was desposited as round to oval granules. Although somewhat distorted due to technical artefact, the size of particles ranged from 1 to 15 μm. The majority of the granules were located intracellularly but some were found in the extracellular space. The intracellular granules were separated from the cytoplasm by a dark-staining vesicle membrane. The cytoplasm was crowded with organelles but these were not evenly dispersed. Lysosomes and mitochondria were prominent. No intracellular fibrosis was present and Golgi complexes, microtubules and centrioles were rarely seen.

MALIZIA et al. (1984) submitted the commercially available PTFE paste, Polytef, to SEM. Polytef has been marketed on the basis of a 50–100 μm particle following the observation by WARD and WEPMAN (1964) that the smallar 6–16 μm particle size PTFE paste, originally developed by Ethicon for ARNOLD (1962), migrated easily to the regional lympth nodes of dogs undergoing retropharyngeal PTFE injection. Malizia's group reported that the particles range from 4 to 100 μm, with 90% between 4 and 40 μm. The shapes were angular and irregular. WENIG et al. (1990) used SEM on material removed from the laryngeal region of seven patients with a post-injection interval ranging from 1 month to 15 years. Whilst no comment was made about the size of particles, they drew attention to what they described as a "flaky" appearance of individual PTFE particles. The appearance could be likened to "scales" still loosely attached to the parent particle. These scales or flakes are considerably smaller than the parent particle. If they were to become detached following injection into the body they could account for the often reported presence in pathological material of particles of considerably smaller size than the 50 – 100 μm size said to be the composition of the commercial product.

Energy dispersive X-ray analysis performed on material taken from excised specimens of ureter in this laboratory show strong peaks for carbon and fluorine, the only two atoms in the polymer (Fig. 8). The principal peaks occur at 0.282 keV

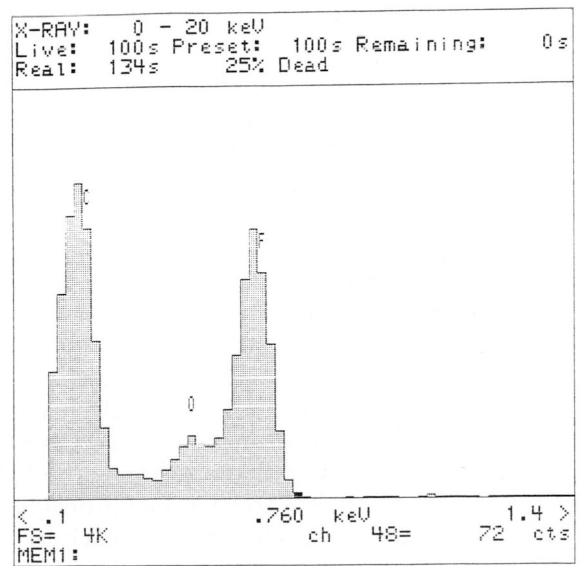

Fig. 8. The carbon and fluorine peaks are obvious in this energy-dispersive X-ray analysis of material taken from excised ureter following STING

(carbon) and 0.677 keV (fluorine). This pattern has been used in the identification of PTFE in granulomata and foreign body debris (Malizia et al. 1984; Wenig et al. 1990).

6 Discussion

As described earlier, PTFE contains the non-biodegradable C–F bond, so that it is not altered in the tissues in the same way as other foreign substances. It is therefore extremely durable. Although PTFE evokes a local macrophage response, these cells are unable to digest the PTFE and may instead carry it to distant sites. Interest has also centred on the long-term effects of injected PTFE in respect of tumour induction and diagnostic problems which may arise in the clinical situation.

6.1 Granuloma Formation

There appears to be some confusion over the meaning of the word "granuloma" in the context of PTFE injection. To the pathologist it means a collection of histiocytes some of which may be giant cells. There may or may not be necrosis depending on the underlying cause. Using this definition the reaction to PTFE is correctly described as a foreign body granuloma or foreign body reaction. This term does not infer any sinister properties.

Interestingly, Charnley (1963) in his description of the most destructive PTFE particles, extruded from prosthetic hip sockets, used the term "caseous" to describe the inflammatory mass. To the surgeon, the word "granuloma" may suggest a chronic inflammatory process, perhaps the result of an infective agent such as tuberculosis or unknown causative factors such as Crohn's disease or sarcoidosis. There is a justifiable fear of damage and destruction of tissue which, when allied to risk of progressive disease, indicates the need for specific remedial measures such as antimicrobial chemotherapy or surgical excision. The granulomata which form in response to injected PTFE particles seem to be remarkably static and not subject to extension or progression except in the mechanical and physical situation of the hip, or if some extrinsic factor such as trauma, ulceration or infection occurs in the anatomical region of the implant. It should also be understood that the clinical effect sought by the implantation is dependent on "space occupation". By the end of the first week, following resorption of glycerine, the injected mass might not be of sufficient size to maintain the clinical effect were it not for the immigration of macrophages and ultimate formation of foreign body giant cells. The inertness of the PTFE and its inability to be wetted probably accounts for the minimal fibroblastic response an excess of which would clearly be undesirable.

6.2 Migration of PTFE

WARD and WEPMAN's 1964 study was the first to address the problem of migration specifically. Using cats as the experimental animal, they compared differences in the tissue responses following retropharyngeal injection of PTFE paste and tantalum. The PTFE paste used initially was made using 6 to 12-μm particles. This was later changed to paste made using 50 to 100-μm particles. Examination of lymph nodes in the drainage area following 6 to 12-μm particle implantation revealed extensive migration with considerable numbers of particles lying in the peripheral sinuses. The change to 50 to 100-μm particles, whilst dramatically reducing the number of particles seen in nodes, did not abolish migration. In the case of vocal cord PTFE injection KIRCHNER et al. (1966) showed in dogs, the larynxes of which were serially sectioned following sacrifice, an absence of migration or extrusion. However, BOEDTS et al. (1967) drew attention to the presence of PTFE particles in a peri-arterial lymphatic vessel and a small artery. They stated that the 20–60 μm size of smallest capillaries could allow spread of 6 to 12-μm PTFE paste and the smaller particles of 50 to 100-μm PTFE paste. They did not find PTFE particles in what is described as the "various organs" examined.

On the other hand, in one of the largest series of cases presenting human histopathological data, DEDO and CARLSÖÖ (1982) noted no evidence of PTFE particles in lymphatics or blood vessels of the 12 cases described.

Concern has been expressed that the PTFE would migrate to distant sites such as the lung. This was indeed described in animals by MALIZIA et al. (1984). They noted widespread dissemination of the particles in continent female dogs and male monkeys after peri-urethral (2 ml) injection of PTFE. In all the animals PTFE particles were found as 0.1 to 1.0-cm aggregates at the injection sites irrespective of the time interval since injection. However, particles were also demonstrated in pelvic nodes and lungs, particularly in animals examined after 10 months. In the lungs the particles were free within alveoli, blood vessels or bronchi; many particles were in the interstitium and some were subpleural. At the injection site there was little reaction to the PTFE particles when studied 70 days after injection. By 10 months histiocytes had phagocytosed the outer particles and coalesced into giant cells, forming a so-called Polytef granuloma. Four animals with PTFE apparently inside histiocytes in the pulmonary interstitium had a foreign body giant cell reaction to the material. A similar foreign body reaction was found in pelvic nodes in two of the long-term animals but another five animals had a minimal reaction in their lymph node sinusoids. X-ray microanalysis was also used to demonstrate fluorine in samples from distant organs such as lung or kidney, confirming that the particles were indeed PTFE. In view of these findings, MALIZIA et al. urged caution regarding the continued use of periurethral injection in patients.

ELLIS et al. (1987), using intracordal injection of dogs in an experiment designed specifically to look for migration, consistently found PTFE particles in both the ipsilateral and the contralateral cervical lymph nodes but reported no evidence of spread to mediastinal and aortic nodes, brain, lung, liver, spleen and kidney.

There has been one report on the formation of a laryngeal polyp (Stone and Arnold 1967) and several reports on the formation of "tumour-like" nodules in the tissue external to the larynx and in proximity to the thyroid (Stone et al. 1970; Rubin 1975; Walsh and Castelli 1975; Stephens et al. 1976; Wenig et al. 1990). It is generally agreed that this represents a complication of the initial injection technique due to a combination of injection of excessive quantities of PTFE and incorrect anatomical placement of the needle at the time of injection, rather than a phenomenon of migration.

A more disturbing case report of the effect of PTFE migration to the lungs was published by Claes et al. (1989). A young woman whose urinary incontinence had been treated by peri-urethral PTFE injection on three occasions during the previous 3 years was admitted to hospital with fever of unknown origin. Despite a normal chest X-ray, bronchoscopy revealed signs of inflammation of the right upper lobe. Biopsies of this lobe contained intravascular particles of doubly refractile PTFE with characteristics identical to smeared PTFE. There was no inflammatory reaction to this material histologically but broncho-alveolar lavage fluid contained 30% lymphocytes. Her fever responded to a short course of steroids and the response persisted when this treatment was discontinued. The authors recommended that PTFE paste should be used with caution, particularly in young patients, until its long-term effects are really known.

In summary, there seems to be no doubt that migration of PTFE particles does occur. It is more likely to occur when richly vascularised regions such as the peri-urethral or retropharyngeal area are injected. In these areas the quantities of PTFE paste required to obtain the described clinical effect are also considerable and this no doubt contributes to the risk of spread. In contrast, provided that the initial injection is technically correct, the defined anatomy of the vocal cord or ureter, combined with the relatively small quantities of PTFE paste used, would suggest that the risk of migration from these sites is minimal.

6.3 Carcinogenesis

The first description of the tissue reaction to PTFE was given by Le Veen and Barberio in 1949. Noting its chemical inertness, they compared its tissue response to a number of other plastics. Attempting to make plastics as reactive as possible within tissue, they argued that they should be ground as finely as possible. They were unable to produce fine injectable suspensions of a number of the plastics, including PTFE, used in their study. In the case of PTFE they sectioned thin slices off a solid rod of polymer using a technique similar to that for cutting paraffin sections in a microtome. The slices were then placed into the peritoneal cavity of dogs. The maximum duration of the experiment was 70 days, by which time the PTFE showed the least inflammatory and fibrous tissue response of any of the plastics used. There was no evidence of neoplasia. They did advise caution in the use of the new polymer, pointing out that tumours had been induced in laboratory animals by certain plastics.

The induction of neoplasia in laboratory animals following long-term exposure to plastics was already known and had been reported in 1941 by TURNER. Experimenting with tumour induction in rats, TURNER implanted a Bakelite disc coated with carcinogenic agents and used a non-coated Bakelite disc as a control. A sarcoma was found around the uncoated disc in a control animal 23 months following implantation. Repetition of the experiment using uncoated discs in 12 rats yielded sarcomas in three of the eight animals, which survived 18 months.

Oppenheimer and colleagues, wishing to produce hypertension in rats by wrapping cellulose film (cellophane) around one kidney, incidentally observed that several rats developed sarcomas in the neighbourhood of the cellophane (OPPENHEIMER et al. 1948). Subsequent investigation by Oppenheimer's group (OPPENHEIMER et al. 1953a, b, 1955) and others confirmed that a wide range of plastics including cellophane, Dacron, Ivalon, Kel F ($CClF_3$), nylon, polyethylene, polymethyl methacrylate, polyvinyl chloride, Saran, Silastic and PTFE were capable of inducing sarcomatous tumours in small laboratory rodents (in rats more so than in mice), if they were implanted into the body in the form of thin film. The possibility that plasticisers, stabilisers, release agents and colourants could in any way be causative was ruled out by insistence on the use of products manufactured to exceedingly pure standards. Oppenheimer's group also noted that removal of the film less than 6 months after embedding resulted in no tumours being formed. Beyond 6 months, removal of the film implant still resulted in tumour formation which could be abolished only if the "capsular" tissue that surrounded the film was removed at the same time as removal of the film (OPPENHEIMER et al. 1957).

The importance of the physical form of the plastic in the initiation of tumours was also stressed. In one experiment tumours were produced in 8 of 34 rats using film, in 6 of 32 animals using perforated material but in only 1 of 387 using powdered material (OPPENHEIMER et al. 1961). RUSSEL et al. (1959) also showed that the size of film implant was important in determining the numbers of tumours which could be induced. OPPENHEIMER et al. (1955) postulated that breakdown of polymer within the body, although extremely minute in degree, might cause build-up of free radicals and thus induce tumour. ALEXANDER and HORNING (1959) pointed out, however, that no chemical reactions were possible under normal physiological conditions in which PTFE could break down, yet it was carcinogenic in thin sheet form. They considered that local anoxia was more likely to cause tumours.

At the time when PTFE paste was first introduced by ARNOLD (1962), it was known that tumour induction by PTFE was species specific, exposure time dependent and a feature of the physical form of polymer. Most subsequent investigators using PTFE paste in either experimental or clinical material have been aware of these findings and have looked specifically for evidence of neoplastic change in or near the area of injection.

There have been a number of reports of experimental injection of PTFE paste into animals including rats, cats, dogs and piglets (ARNOLD 1962; HARRIS and CARLETON 1965; KIRCHNER et al. 1966; TOOMEY and BROWN 1967; MALIZIA et al. 1984; PURI and O'DONNELL 1984; ELLIS et al. 1987). None have reported evidence of malignant transformation, although the majority of the experiments were of relatively short duration.

There are now a number of histological descriptions of injected PTFE in the human (Table 1). In none of these has there been any evidence of neoplasia. Clinical confusion of the nodules occasionally produced in the thyroid area by migration of PTFE paste with thyroid neoplasia is well recognised (WALSH et al. 1975; SANFILIPPO et al. 1980; WILSON and GARTNER 1987; WENIG et al. 1990). In urological practice there have been two cases of tumour-like swelling sufficient to cause urinary tract obstruction in one case (BOYKIN et al. 1989) and a vaginal nodule in the other (FERRO et al. 1988), but these both proved to be PTFE granulomas.

There are only three recorded examples of malignancy adjacent to a PTFE implant (DEWAN 1992). One of these was a single case of fibrosarcoma adjacent to an aortic graft implanted 10 years previously (MONTGOMERY 1982). A chondrosarcoma was reported in the vocal cord in a patient who had had a PTFE implant 6 years earlier (HAKKY et al. 1989). LEWY (1976) reported a carcinoma adjacent to a vocal cord implant in his review of 1139 cases. In none of these cases was a definite cause and effect relationship to PTFE implantation demonstrated. Apart from the cases mentioned above, neoplasia has not been described in the many clinical series, some detailing thousands of patients, reporting on the use of PTFE in otorhinolaryngological or urological treatments (DEWAN 1992). In the longest human follow-up described to date, no tumour was found 16 years after vocal cord injection (DEDO and CARLSÖÖ 1982).

The initial experiments in rodents showing a relatively high incidence of tumour induction may have caused unwarranted fears of malignancy when PTFE was subsequently used in clinical practice. There is, to date, little evidence to suggest that PTFE particles, in the size and shapes suitable for injection, are associated with malignant change. However, injection of PTFE paste into the vocal cord of an elderly patient paralysed by metastatic carcinoma, who may be expected to live a few months, is a different situation from its use in the ureter of a young child who might be expected to survive for 60–70 years following the procedure. The need for careful long-term clinico-pathological follow-up of all human cases in which PTFE has been injected and is likely to persist in situ for many years thereafter cannot be overemphasised.

6.4 Diagnostic Problems

To a practising histopathologist, the identification of a foreign body granuloma containing masses of doubly refractile crystals should not prove to be an insuperable problem. It may, however, be less easy to identify the particular crystal which is causing the reaction. Clearly there is no substitute for an accurate and complete clinical history which should clearly point to the lesion following or being associated with one of the procedures in which PTFE paste is used.

On the other hand, the clinician may be confronted by genuine problems. This can be well illustrated by referral to the case reported by WALSH and CASTELLI (1975). A 42-year-old male presented with hoarseness found to be due to left vocal cord paralysis. No causative factors could be elucidated and an elective PTFE paste injection was carried out 3 months following onset with good clinical improvement. His hoarseness returned shortly thereafter and a 3 x 2 cm hard mass was noted in the left paratracheal area. Thyroid scan revealed a cold nodule. Biopsy examination of the mass was being considered when he developed small bowel obstruction found on subsequent laparotomy to be due to adenocarcinoma of the ileum. At autopsy, following his death some 8 months later, the "thyroid nodule", for which at the time of presentation a diagnosis of thyroid cancer had been considered in the absence of known primary tumour, proved to be a PTFE granuloma caused by extension of PTFE particles through the cricothyroid membrane, presumably at the time of injection.

There have been a number of clinical presentations in which the tissue response to PTFE has been displaced from the original area of injection, raising the problem of polyps, nodules or tumours. These have been noted in the cases of vocal cord (STONE and ARNOLD 1967; STONE et al. 1970; WALSH and CASTELLI 1975; LEWEY 1976; WENIG et al. 1990), urethra (FERRO et al. 1988; BOYKIN et al. 1989), and ureter (O'HARA and HILL 1990).

Normally PTFE is radiolucent and thus not amenable to diagnosis using conventional radiological techniques. Whilst ultrasonography is of some use, PTFE can be visualised using magnetic resonance imaging technology, which may be of importance in the long-term follow-up of implants (KIRSCH et al. 1990).

7 Conclusion

There are several important considerations regarding the clinical use of injected PTFE. The local reaction is desirable if the techniques are to be successful. The granulomatous response to this biologically inert substance may occasionally expand the nodule at the injection site with the possibility of functional impairment. A second problem relates to migration to distal sites, particularly the lungs, the type of response elicited and its significance. Thirdly, in view of the known carcinogenic effects of certain physical types and forms of plastic, there is a need to assess the long-term risk of carcinogenesis following implantation of finely dispersed PTFE. Whilst its use seems established in certain situations, there is clearly a need for continuing clinicopathological surveillance of its behaviour.

References

Alexander P, Horning ES (1959) Observation on the Oppenheimer method of inducing tumours by subcutaneous implantation of plastic films. In: Wolstenholme GEW, O'Connor M (eds) Carcinogenesis mechanisms of action. CIBA Foundation Symposium. Churchill, London, pp 12–25

Altermatt HJ, Gebbers JO, Sommerhalder A, Vrticka K (1985) Histopathologische Befunde in der Rachenhinterwand acht Jahre nach Behandlung einer Voluminsuffizienz mit Tefloninjektion. Laryng Rhinol Otol 64: 582–585

Arnold GE (1955) Vocal rehabilitation of paralytic dysphonia. I. Cartilage injection into a paralyzed vocal cord. Arch Otolaryngol 62: 1–17

Arnold GE (1961) Vocal rehabilitation of paralytic dysphonia. VI. Further studies of intracordal injection materials. Arch Otolaryngol 73: 290-294

Arnold GE (1962) Vocal rehabilitation of paralytic dysphonia. Technique of intracordal injection. Arch Otolaryngol 76: 358–368

Banks RE (1988) Teflon touches gold. Chem in Britain 24: 453–454

Barry WB (1965) Experimental observations upon reconsruction of the nasal dorsum. Laryngoscope 75: 1320–1333

Billmeyer FW (1962) Textbook of polymer science, 2nd edn Wiley, New York, pp 423–424

Birmingham Reflux Study Group (1983) Prospective trial of operative versus non-operative treatment of severe vesicoureteric reflux: two years' observation in 96 children. Br Med J 287: 171–174

Blocksma R (1963) Correction of velopharyngeal insufficiency by silastic implant. Plast Reconstr Surg 31: 268–274

Boedts, D, Roels H, Kluyskens P (1967) Laryngeal responses to Teflon. Arch Otolaryngol 86: 562–567

Boykin W, Rodriguez FR, Brizzalara JP (1989) Complete urinary obstruction following urethral polytetrafluoroethylene injection for urinary incontinence. J Urol 141: 1199–1200

Brown S (1989) Open versus endoscopic surgery in the treatment of vesicoureteral reflux. J Urol 142: 499–501

Brünings W (1911) Über eine neue Behandlungsmethode der Rekurrenslähmung. Verhandl Ver Deutsch Laryng; 18: 95–151

Carlsöö B, Dedo HH, Gustafsson H (1983) Ultrastructure of Multinuclear giant cells of a human vocal cord Teflon granuloma. Arch Otorhinolaryngol 283: 205–208

Charnley J (1961) Arthroplasty of the hip. A new operation. Lancet 1: 1129–1132

Charnley J (1963) Tissue reactions to polytetrafluoroethylene. Lancet II: 1379

Charnley J (1979) Low friction arthroplasty of the hip. Theory and practice. Springer, Berlin Heidelberg New York pp 6–7

Claes H, Stroobants D, van Meerbeek J, Verbeken E, Knockaert D, Baert L (1989) Pulmonary migration following periurethral polytetrafluoroethylene injection for urinary incontinence. J Urol 142: 821–822

Daicker B, Piffaretti JM, Häfliger E, Schipper J (1985) Iatrogenes Teflongranulom des Lids. (Teflonpaste, ein untaugliches Plombenmaterial für die plastische Lidchirurgie). Klin Monatsbl Augenheilkd 186: 121–123

Dedo HH (1973) Intracordal injection of Teflon in the treatment of 135 patients with dysphonia. Ann Otol 82: 661–667

Dedo HH, Carlsöö B (1982) Histologic evaluation of Teflon granulomas of human vocal cords. A light and electron microscopic study. Acta Otolaryngol 93: 475–484

Dedo HH, Urrea RD, Lawson L (1973) Intracordal injection of Teflon in the treatment of 135 patients with dysphonia. Ann Otol Rhinol Laryngol 82: 661–667

Dewan PA (1992) Is injected polytetrafluoroethylene (Polytef) carcinogenic? Br J Urolo 69: 29–33

Dewan PA, O'Donnell B (1991) Polytef paste injection of refluxing duplex ureters. Pediatr, Urol 19: 35–38

Diamond T, Boston VE (1987a) The natural history of vesicoureteric reflux in children with neuropathic bladder and open neural tube defects. Z Kinderchir 42: 15-16

Diamond T, Boston VE (1987b) Reflux following endoscopic treatment of ureteroceles. A new approach using endoscopic subureteric Teflon injection. J Urol 60: 279–280

Du Pont (i) Chemical resistance of "Teflon" fluorocarbon resins. Information bulletin T-1024. Teflon fluorocarbon resins. Du Pont Plastics. Du Pont de Nemours International S.A., Case-Postale CH-1211 Geneva 24, Switzerland

Du Pont (ii) Knowing and recognising quality in fabricated "Teflon" fluorocarbon resins. Information bulletin T-1006. Teflon fluorocarbon resins. Du Pont Polymer Products Department Du Pont de Nemours International S.A., Polymer Products department, fluoropolymers Div, CH-1211, Geneva 24, Switzerland

Editorial (1990) Granulomatous reaction in total hip arthroplasty. Lancet 335: 203–204

Ekstein H (1922) Hartparaffinjektionen in der hintere Rachenwand bei angeborenen und erworbenen Gaumendefekten. Berlin Klin Wochenschr 1: 1185–1187

Ellis JS, McCaffrey TV, Desanto LW, Reiman HV (1987) Migration of Teflon after vocal cord injection. Otolaryngol Head Neck Surg 96: 63–66
Frey P, Whitaker RH (1992) Prevention of vesicoureteric reflux by endoscopic injection. Br J Urol 69: 1–6
Ferro MA, Smith JHF, Smith PJB (1988) Periurethral granuloma: unusual complication of Teflon periurethral injection. Urology 31: 422–423
Gangal SV (1989) Polytetrafluoethylene polymers. In: Mark HF, Bikales NM, Overberger CG and Menges G (eds) Encyclopaedia of polymer science and engineering. Wiley, New York, pp 577–600
Garrett AB (1962) The flash of genius 2. Teflon. Roy Plunkett J Chem Educ 39: 288
Gebelein CG (1982) Prosthetic and biomedical devices. In: Mark HF, Othman DF, Overberger CG, Seaborg GT (eds) Encyclopaedia of chemical technology, 3rd edn. Wiley, New York, pp 275–313
Goff WF (1960) Laryngeal adductor paralysis treated by vocal cord injection of bone paste; a preliminary investigation. Trans Pacif Coast Oto-Ophthalmol Soc 41: 77–87
Goff WF (1969) Teflon injection for vocal cord paralysis. Arch Otolaryngol 90: 98–102
Goff WF (1973) Intracordal Polytef (Teflon) injection. Histologic study of two cases. Arch Otolaryngol 97: 371–373
Hakky M, Kolbusz R, Reyes CV (1989) Chondrosarcoma of the larynx. Ear Nose Throat J 68: 60–62
Harris HE, Hawk WA (1969) Laryngeal injection of Teflon paste. Arch Otolaryngol 90: 194–197
Harris HH, Carleton JS (1966) Clinical investigation of the use of RTV silastic S-5392 for paralytic dysphonia and its histological comparison to Teflon in animals. Trans Am Acad Ophthmol Otol 70: 48–58
Homsey CA (1973) Implant stabilisation. Chemical and biochemical considerations. Orth Clin North Am 4: 295–311
Homsey CA, Anderson MS (1976) Functional stabilisation of prostheses with a porous low modulus materials system. In: Williams D (ed). Biocompatibility of implant materials. Sector, London
Horn KL, Dedo HH (1980) Surgical correction of the convex cord after Teflon injection. Laryngoscope 90: 281–286
Kirchner FR, Toledo AB, Svoboda DJ (1966) Studies of the larynx after Teflon injection. Arch Otolaryngol 83: 350–354
Kirsch MD, Donaldson JS, Kaplan WE (1990) MR appearance of subureteric injection of Teflon to correct vesicoureteral reflux. J Comput Assist Tomogr 14: 673–674
Koch WM, Hybels RL, Shapshay SM (1987) Carbon dioxide laser in removal of Polytef paste. Arch Otolaryngol Head Neck Surg 113: 661–663
Lacombe A (1990) Ureterovesical reimplantation after failure of endoscopic treatment of reflux by submucosal injection of Polytef paste. Eur Urol 17: 318–320
Le Veen HH, Barberio JR (1949) Tissue reaction to plastics used in surgery with special reference to Teflon. Ann Surg 129: 74
Lewy RB (1964) Glottic rehabilitation with Teflon injection the return of voice, cough and laughter. Acta Otolaryngolog 58: 214–220
Lewy RB (1966) Responses of laryngeal tissue to granular Teflon in situ. Arch Otolaryngol 83: 355–359
Lewy RB (1976) Experience with vocal cord injection. Ann Otol 85: 440–450
Lewy RB, Millet D (1978) Immediate local tissue reactions to Teflon vocal cord implants. Laryngoscope 88: 1339–1342
Lewy R, Cole R, Wepman J (1965) Teflon injection in the correction of velopharyngeal insufficiency. Ann Otol Rhinol Laryngol 74: 874–879
Libsersa C (1952) Trâitement chirurgical de la paralysie laryngee en abduction. J Fr Otorhinolaryngol 1: 480
Malizia AA Jr, Reiman HM, Myers RP, Sande JR, Barham SS, Benson RCJ, Dewanjee MK, Utz WJ (1984) Migration and granulomatous reaction after periurethral injection of Polytef (Teflon). JAMA 251: 3277–3281
Marcellin L, Geiss S, Laustriat S, Becmeur F, Bientz J, Sauvage P (1990) Ureteral lesions due to endoscopic treatment of vesicoureteral reflux by injection of Teflon: pathological study Eur Urol 17: 325–327
Matouschek E (1981) Die Behandlung des vesikorenalen Refluxes durch transurethrale Einspritzung von Teflonpaste. Urologe [A] 20: 263–264
Mittleman RE, Marraccini JV (1983) Pulmonary Teflon granulomas following periurethral Teflon injection for urinary incontinence. Arch Pathol Lab Med 107: 611–612
Montgomery R (1982) Polytetrafluoroethylene. In Patty's industrial hygiene and toxicology, vol 2C. Wiley, New York, pp 4308–4310

Nassar WY (1977) Polytef (Teflon) injection of the vocal cords. Experience with thirty-four cases. J Laryngol Otol 91: 341–347

O'Donnell B, Puri P (1984) Treatment of vesicoureteric reflux by endoscopic injection of Teflon. Br Med J 289: 7–9

O'Hara MD, Hill CM (1990) Teflon granulomata in vesicoureteric reflux. Paediatr Pathol 10: 655-656

O'Hara MD, Hill CM, Boston VE, Brown S (1989) A histological study of vesico-ureteric Teflon granulomata. J Pathol 157: 167A

O'Hara MD, Hill CM, Maxwell P (1991) Tissue responses in Teflon granulomata. Pathol Res Pract 187: 736

Oppenheimer BS, Oppenheimer ET, Stout AP (1948) Sarcomas induced in rats by implanting cellophane. Proc Soc Exp Biol Med 67: 33–34

Oppenheimer BS, Oppenheimer ET, Stout AP (1953a) Carcinogenic effect of imbedding various plastic films in rats and mice. Surg Forum 4: 672–676

Oppenheimer BS, Oppenheimer ET, Stout AP, Danishefsky I (1953b) Malignant tumours resulting from embedding plastics in rodents. Science 118: 305–306

Oppenheimer BS, Oppenheimer ET, Danishefsky I, Stout AP, Eirich FR (1955) Further studies of polymers as carcinogenic agents in animals. Cancer Res 15: 333–340

Oppenheimer BS, Stout AP, Oppenheimer ET, Willhite M (1957) Study of the precancerous stage of fibrosarcomas induced by plastic films. Proc Am Assoc Cancer Res 2: 237

Oppenheimer ET, Willhite M, Danishefsky I (1961) Observation on the effects of powdered polymer in the carcinogenic process. Cancer Res 1: 132–134

Plunkett RJ (1986) The history of polytetrafluorethylene discovery and development. Polym Prep Am Chem Soc Div Polym Chem 27: 485–487

Pohris E, Kleinsasser O (1987) Stenosis of the larynx following Teflon injection. Arch Otorhinolaryngol 244: 44–48

Politano VA (1982) Periurethral polytetrafluoroethylene injection for urinary incontinence. J Urol 127: 439–442

Politano VA (1992) Transurethral Polytef injection of post-prostatectomy urinary incontinence. Br J Urol 69: 26–28

Politano VA, Small MP, Harper JM, Lynne CM (1974) Periurethral Teflon injection for urinary incontinence. J Urol 111: 180–183

Puri P (1990) Endoscopic correction of primary vesicoureteric reflux by subureteric injection of polytetrafluoroethylene. Lancet 335: 1320–1322

Puri P, Guiney EJ (1986) Endoscopic correction of vesicoureteric reflux secondary to neuropathic bladder. Br J Urol 58: 504–506

Puri P, O'Donnell B (1984) Correction of experimentally produced vesicoureteric reflux in the piglet by intravesical injection of Teflon. Br Med J 289: 5–7

Report of the International Reflux Study Committee (1981) Medical versus surgical treatment of primary vesicoureteral reflux: a prospective international reflux study in children. J Urol 125: 277–283

Rethi A (1954) Stimmbandfüllung in Fällen von nichtarbenbedingten Glottisspalten. Monatsschr Ohrerh 88: 295–300

Rubin HJ (1965a) Intracordal injection of silicone in selected dysphonias. Arch Otolaryngol 81: 604–607

Rubin HJ (1965b) Pitfalls in treatment of dysphonias by intracordal injection of synthetics. Laryngoscope 75: 1381–1397

Rubin HJ (1966) Histologic high speed photographic observations on the intracordal injection of synthetics. Trans Am Acad Ophthalmol Otolaryngol 70: 909–921

Rubin HJ (1975) Misadventures with injectable Polytef (Teflon). Arch Otolaryngol 101: 114–116

Russell FE, Simmers MH, Hirst AE, Pudenz RH (1959) Tumours associated with embedded polymers. J Natl Cancer Inst 23: 305–311

Sanfilippo F, Shelburne J, Ingram P (1980) Analysis of a Polytef granuloma mimicking a cold thyroid nodule 17 months after laryngeal injection. Ultrastruct Pathol 1: 471–475

Schulman CC, Pamart D, Hall M, Janseen F, Avni FE (1990) Vesicoureteral reflux in children: endoscopic treatment. Eur Urol 17: 341–317

Siegler J (1967) Rehabilitation of voice after recurrent laryngeal nerve paralysis using Teflon suspension. J Laryngol Otol 81: 1121–1129

Stephens CB, Arnold GE, Stone JW (1976) Larynx injected with Polytef paste. Arch Otolaryngol 102: 432–435

Stone JW, Arnold GE (1967) Human larynx injected with reflon paste. Histologic study on innervation and tissue reaction. Arch Otolaryngol 86: 550–561
Stone JW, Arnold GE, Stephens CB, Jackson MS (1970) Intracordal Polytef (Teflon) injection. Histologic study of three further cases. Arch Otolaryngol 91: 568–574
Swanson SAV, Freeman MAR (1977) The scientific basis of joint replacement. Pitman Medical, London, pp 71–75
Toomey JM, Brown BS (1967) The histological response to intracordal injection of Teflon paste. Laryngoscope 77: 110–120
Turner FC (1941) Sarcomas at sites of s-c implanted Bakelite disks in rats. J Natl Cancer Inst 2: 81–83
Walsh FM, Castelli JB (1975) Polytef granuloma clinically simulating carcinoma of the thyroid. Arch Otolaryngol Head Neck Surg 101: 262–263
Ward PH (1968) Uses of injectable Teflon in otolaryngology. Arch Otolaryngol 71: 637–693
Ward PH (1985) Transcutaneous Teflon injection of the paralyzed vocal cord: A new technique. Laryngoscope 95: 644–649
Ward PH, Wepman JM (1964) Pharyngeal implants for reduction of air space in velopharyngeal insufficiency. I. An experimental study. Ann Otol Rhin Laryngol 73: 443–458
Ward PH, Goldman R, Stoudt RJ (1966) Teflon injection to improve velopharyngeal insufficiency. J Speech Hear Disord 31: 267–273
Wenig BM, Heffner DK, Johnson FB (1989) Teflonomas of the larynx and neck. Hum Pathol 21: 617–623
Williams D (1976) Stability of joint prosthesis. In: Williams D (ed) Biocompatibility of implant materials. Sector, London, pp 67–69
Wilson RA, Gartner WS (1987) Teflon granuloma mimicking a thyroid tumour. Diagn Cytopathol 3: 156–158
Wilson TG (1964) Teflon in glycerine paste in rhinology. J Laryngol 78: 953–958
Woodard JR, Rushton HG (1987) Reflux uropathy. Pediatr Clin North Am 34: 1349–1364
Wroblewski BM (1988) Wear and loosening of the socket in the Charnley low-friction arthroplasty. Orthop Clin North Am 19: 627–630
Yarington CT, Harned R (1971) Polytef (Teflon) injection for postoperative deglutition problems. Arch Otolaryngol 94: 274–275

The Pathology of Bioprosthetic Heart Valves and Allografts

H.H. SCHELD and W. KONERTZ

Current Topics in Pathology
Volume 86. Ed. C. Berry

A. Bioprostheses

1 Historical Evolution

Valve surgery continues to be a challenging aspect of current cardiac surgical practice, where each year some 30 000 patients in the United States (MILLER et al. 1987) present for what might appear to be an easy procedure: the replacement of a heart valve.

A reasonable option was initially offered by mechanical valves, but lifelong anticoagulation was a major hazard, with morbidity from anticoagulation-induced bleeding ranging from 0.5% (COHN et al. 1984) to 30% (HUME et al. 1970) per patient per year. Thus the development of biological valves followed the appearance of mechanical valves in order to minimise these problems. In July 1962 Ross carried out the first successful orthotopic allotransplantation of a fresh aortic valve, after Duran and Gunning had opened the route experimentally in the same year. In October 1962 Senning used fascia lata strips to replace the aortic valve; the risk of thromboembolism, which was at that time up to 30% with mechanical valves, became practically non-existent (SENNING et al. 1972); 5-year survival rate was 70% (ROTHLIN et al. 1977).

In 1969 Ionescu and Ross developed a supporting ring for the fascia lata strips, and from then on replacement of the mitral valve became possible. After various efforts to define the best treatment techniques for the valves to be implanted (formaldehyde vs glutaraldehyde, with or without antibiotics), it became clear that 0.625% glutaraldehyde fixation was the most appropriate (CARPENTIER et al. 1968).

In 1968 Angell also implanted glutaraldehyde-conditioned valves, but it was not until 1972 that their commercial production began. Independently and at the same time Hancock developed his own valve (COBANOGLU et al. 1987; OYER et al. 1979) and Zerbini developed another type of bioprosthetic valve, after Pigossi had used dura mater in animals in 1967. Two months later Ionescu constructed the pericardial valve, which remarkably showed the lowest thromboembolic rate at that time (0.41/100 patient-years in the aortic position, and 0.94/100 patient-years in the mitral position). Second-generation prostheses, with alterations in structural design and tissue preservation and fixation, have been introduced over the past 9 years, with anticipated improvement in long-term clinical performance (Carpentier et al. 1982, 1984; Ionescu 1986; Wright et al. 1982). They include both porcine (Carpentier-Edwards supra-annular, Hancock II, Xenomedica, Bioimplant, Biocor, Medtronic Intact) and pericardial (Carpentier-Edwards pericardial, Ionescu-Shiley low profile, and Mitroflow) valves.

1.1 Definition

A definition of bioprosthetic valves was offered by Carpentier, who defined them as "chemically conditioned xenografts, mounted on a supporting ring, whose antigenicity is reduced through the fixation. Their stability is increased by the intermolecular linking of the collagen fibers, and their durability depends on the stability of the biological material, and not on regeneration of the fibers through the recipient himself".

2 Indications for Valve Surgery

The indications for valve surgery are, among a variety of factors, relief of symptoms and/or the prevention of death or complications from the underlying disease. It is generally accepted that the long-term results are better when lesions are treated at an earlier stage.

2.1 Mitral Valve Surgery

More specifically, the indications for mitral valve surgery, due to stenosis, are NYHA class III or IV symptoms, a valve area of 1.0 cm^2 or less, and a history of systemic embolization. In mitral stenosis the left ventricle is protected by the lesion, and it is acceptable to defer surgery until the patient becomes severely symptomatic. Operative mortality ranges from 5% to 10%, depending on the condition of the patient. Before cardiac function deteriorates to NYHA class IV level, another option is offered by mitral commissurotomy with an operative mortality of 1%, when no significant mitral regurgitation and no valvular calcification are present, when the mitral subvalvular distance ratio is less than 0.12, and when young females free of hypertension (Morgan et al. 1985) are affected.

With mitral regurgitation, the indications for surgery are NYHA class III or IV symptoms and NYHA class II with (a) a left ventricular diastolic minor axis dimension of 6 cm or greater, (b) a regurgitant fraction of 40% or greater, or (c)

4 + mitral regurgitation with an ejection fraction of 60% or less, increasing ventricular volumes or regurgitant fraction, and any acute mitral regurgitation.

2.2 Aortic Valve Surgery

As far as aortic stenosis is concerned, all symptomatic patients should have an urgent operation, since a significant number of patients will have sudden death as the first clinical manifestation of their disease (FRANK et al. 1973). A peak systolic gradient of 50 mmHg or greater and a valve index of 0.5 cm^2/m^2 or less are also indications for valve replacement.

In aortic regurgitation we try to operate before left ventricular decompensation occurs. In detail we operate on patients with NYHA class III or IV symptoms, and on patients with NYHA class II symptoms and (a) a left ventricular systolic minor axis dimension of 5.5 cm or greater or (b) 3+ or 4+ regurgitation with an ejection fraction of 50% or less, increasing ventricular volumes or decreasing ejection fraction, and with any significant acute aortic regurgitation. Some authors (HURST 1982; MORGAN et al. 1985) believe that any significantly symptomatic patient should be offered an operation. Operative mortality is around 5%. The indications for surgical intervention in the paediatric age group are stenosis or insufficiency, causing right- or left-sided heart failure, and failure to thrive.

3 Haemodynamics

With a large annulus, which is usually defined as one with an aortic diameter of at least 25 mm, or a mitral diameter of at least 29 mm, haemodynamic factors are not critical, and, therefore, do not determine the selection of a type of valve prosthesis. As all valves are inherently stenotic, a smaller annulus demands superior haemodynamic performance, which makes porcine valves less attractive, the best results to date having been achieved by the St. Jude Medical (SJM) valve. The reason for this is that the right coronary leaflet contains a septal shelf of myocardium that is inflexible. As a result, the active orifice area of porcine bioprostheses is limited, and their performance is variable (WRIGHT 1979). In order to overcome unfavourable haemodynamics in the smaller sizes (19–25 mm), the right coronary cusp of the Hancock valve model 242 was replaced by a posterior cusp from another valve and a modified orifice composite valve (model 250) resulted.

CORNHILL (1977) pointed out some time ago that the many valve testing modes proposed did not accurately simulate in vivo conditions. A rather good approximation, however, was given by the so-called effective orifice areas, calculated by

Wright (1979) using the Gorlin formula (Gorlin and Gorlin 1951). So, according to the same investigator, the following order of hydrodynamic performance for the aortic position was given: first, the Hancock 250; second, Carpentier-Edwards; third, Hancock 242. Compared with mechanical valves, the Hancock 250 of equivalent size performs better than the 19-mm or 21-mm Björk-Shiley valve. Yoganathan (Woo et al. 1986) carried out similar calculations and concluded that the Carpentier-Edwards supra-annular bioprosthesis was superior to the standard model (effective orifice area 4.00 + 0.14 cm^2 vs 1.95 + 0.08 cm^2 for the 27 mm size) and to the various types of the Hancock valve.

Gabbay et al. (1984), using the pulse duplicator, showed that the Hancock and Carpentier-Edwards valves are moderately stenotic, their hydrodynamic performance being surpassed by the newer bovine pericardial valves, which are equal to the St. Jude Medical valve, the prosthesis that currently exhibits the lowest transvalvular gradients and the largest effective orifice areas (Gabbay et al. 1980). Wright (1979) noticed that, with the porcine valves, peak transvalvular gradients tend to be lower than mean gradients because of valve leaflet inertia, which may also be responsible for the fact that in vivo calculated orifice areas are always less than those approximated in vitro, and much less than the potential orifice area, calculated by planimetry, as noted by others (Craver et al. 1978; Johnson et al. 1978; Lurie et al. 1977).

In an in vivo comparison of porcine and pericardial valves in the aortic position, Cosgrove et al. (1985) concluded that the Carpentier-Edwards standard as well as the supra-annular model had inferior hydrodynamic performance to the pericardial valves. Similar results were also published for the mitral position (Becker et al. 1980; Horstkotte et al. 1983). Further, in a prospective randomised study of 100 patients, published by Khan et al. in 1990, it was demonstrated that the haemodynamics of the Hancock Modified Orifice valve, as reflected by mean gradients, valve areas, and valve resistances, was superior to the Carpentier-Edwards prosthesis in the 19–21 mm sizes. Additionally, mean gradients were also significantly lower for the Hancock 23, although differences in valve areas were not significant at the P=0.05 level. The authors were, however, cautious enough to note that further studies might be needed to assess the magnitude of the significance of these findings clinically. Overall, the bioprostheses might be said to exhibit satisfactory haemodynamics, comparable to the haemodynamics of the mechanical valves (Horstkotte et al. 1983). These are, however, flow dependent, since they fully open only at high flows.

4 Morbidity

In attempting to define guidelines for reporting morbidity after bioprosthetic valve replacement, we agree with others (Edmunds et al. 1988) and suggest the following definitions.

4.1 Structural Valve Deterioration

Primary tissue failure of bioprostheses is considered to be any change in valve function resulting from an intrinsic abnormality that causes stenosis or regurgitation, such as wear, stress fracture, calcification, leaflet tear or stent creep. It is probably their most prominent complication, and has been adequately addressed in the literature, though without much attention to practical problems (ANTUNES et al. 1984; CURCIO et al. 1981; GARDNER et al. 1982; GEHA et al. 1979; JAMIESON et al. 1989; MILLER et al. 1982; SILVER et al. 1980; THANDROYEN et al. 1980).

Primary tissue failure is generally defined as valve incompetence or stenosis, with degenerative changes, confirmed on gross and histological examination of the explanted valve, and without any clinical, bacteriological or histological evidence of infection (Fig. 1).

The prediction of Carpentier in 1976 that "at the end of 10 years the valve failure rate will be 20%" has proven accurate despite more enthusiastic attitudes. According to MAGILLIGAN (1987), the percentage of all valves free of degeneration was 97% at 5 years, 72% at 10 years and 69% at 12 years, the difference between the aortic and mitral positions not being significant ($P > 0.438$). The only risk factor for degeneration reaching statistical significance ($P < 0.001$) was age; for patients over 35 years old the freedom of degeneration was 80% at 10 years, although mitral valves tended to be at greater risk ($P > 0.089$).

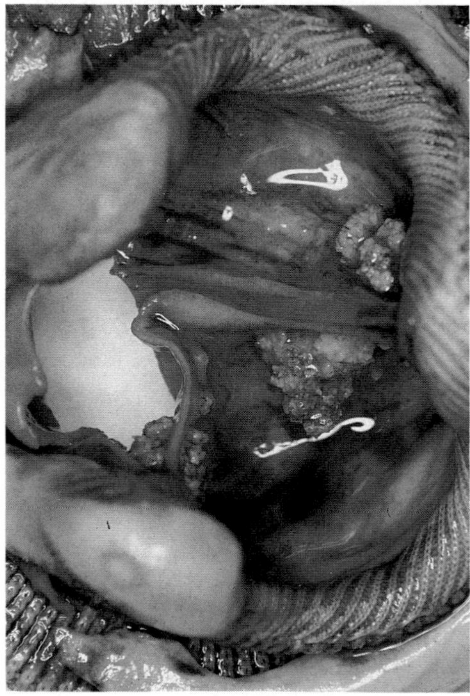

Fig. 1. Calcification with leaflet disruption in a Hancock bioprosthesis, explanted 12 years after mitral valve replacement in a 59-year-old female patient (B.R.)

Primary tissue failure is manifested as calcification and cuspal tears often due to commissural stress at the attachment to the stent; it occurs more often in the mitral position, or at both valve sites.

4.1.1 Calcification

Calcification has further been subdivided into intrinsic calcification, which involves cuspal collagen, fibroblasts, adipocytes and myocardial fibres of the right coronary cusp, and extrinsic calcification, related to surface thrombi and infective vegetations (Ferrans et al. 1980). Many investigators (Schoen et al. 1983) have appeared to consider these processes as different phenomena (Fig. 2).

Factors that promote calcification are well recognized to be youth (Fiddler et al. 1983), chronic renal disease (Hartz et al. 1986), infection (Knight et al. 1984) and mechanical stress (Stinson et al. 1977). Factors that retard calcification include prolonged storage in glutaraldehyde (Schryer et al. 1986), warfarin (Stein et al. 1985), blockage of the formation of the calcium-binding amino acid γ-carboxyglutamic acid (Menarche et al. 1986), addition of heparin–protein complex to glutaraldehyde (Rygg et al. 1986), decreasing mechanical stress by low-pressure fixation (Wright et al. 1982) and by newer stent configurations (Carpentier et al. 1982), local controlled release of diphosphonate (Levy et al. 1987), and the addition of surfactant to the fixation process (Carpentier et al. 1984; Lentz et al. 1982).

Interestingly enough, the mode of failure depends on the position of the valve. For mitral porcine bioprostheses, cusp stiffening and valve stenosis resulting from

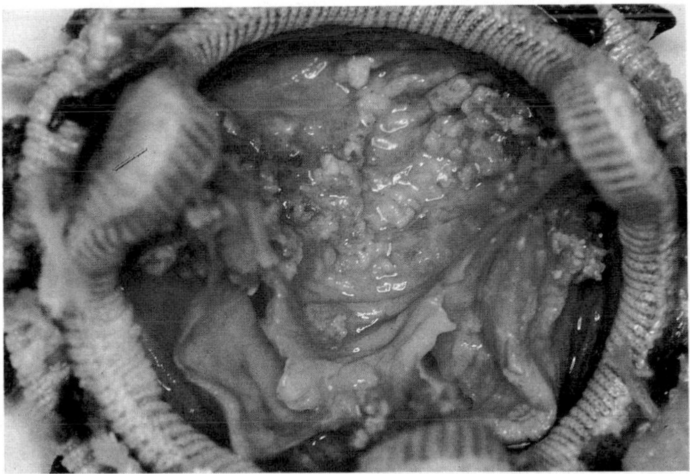

Fig. 2. Extensive calcification with moderate fibrosis and regressive changes in a Xenomedica A bioprosthesis, which was explanted 6 years after aortic valve replacement in a 43-year-old male patient (M.H.)

calcification predominate, while incompetence dominates in the aortic position (BORTOLOTTI et al. 1985). The probability of being free from primary tissue failure is similar for patients with aortic or mitral valve replacement (GALLUCCI et al. 1986). According to recent data published by MILANO et al. (1988), durability of the porcine valves is quite acceptable up to 8 years, becoming questionable beyond this time, when the actuarial curve of freedom from primary tissue failure drops progressively. Again, when evaluating durability of the bioprostheses we need to be specific (porcine vs pericardial), since in a large series of 1593 patients it was shown that in the mitral position durability of the pericardial valves was significantly less than that of their porcine counterparts (PELLETIER et al. 1989), the reoperation rates at 6 years being 68% in the former group 92% in the latter ($P < 0.001$). Thus the advantage of the larger valve areas and lower gradients of pericardial aortic valves, especially in smaller sizes, is offset by their limited durability. However, overall patient survival after up to 6 years was similar for both, which might be partly attributed to the higher early mortality in the porcine group (9%) when compared with the pericardial valve group (5.2%).

4.2 Non-structural Dysfunction

By non-structural dysfunction is meant any abnormality resulting in stenosis or regurgitation at the valve that is not intrinsic to the valve itself; examples are entrapment of pannus or suture, paravalvular leak, inappropriate sizing and clinically important haemolytic anaemia.

4.3 Thromboembolism

Thromboembolism is defined here as any valve thrombosis or embolus exclusive of infection. It includes any new, permanent or transient, focal or global neurological deficit (exclusive of haemorrhage) and any peripheral arterial emboli, unless proved to have resulted from another cause (such as atrial myxoma). Patients who do not awaken postoperatively or who awaken with a stroke or myocardial infarction are excluded (EDMUNDS et al. 1988). Any myocardial infarction that occurs after operation is arbitrarily defined as a thromboembolic event in patients with known normal coronary arteries or those who are less than 40 years of age. It is one of the most serious complications of valve replacement, since it suddenly and unexpectedly compromises an asymptomatic or clinically substantially improved patient.

Low thrombogenicity of bioprostheses is thought to be their main advantage over mechanical valves (Fig. 3). However, there are certain difficulties in interpreting the data on which this assertion is based as they are obtained from various investigators. For results to be truly comparable, they must be reported as both

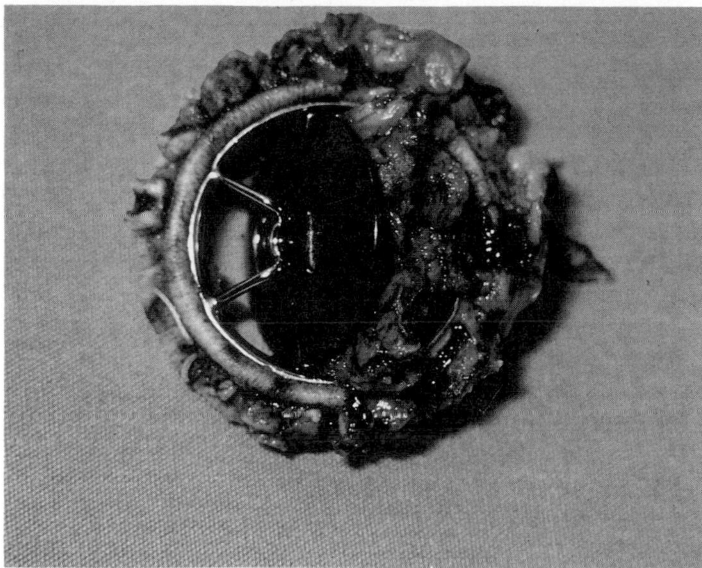

Fig. 3. Thrombosis of a Björk-Shiley valve, 5-years after valve replacement

the linearized rate and the actuarial rate (EDMUNDS 1982; McGOON et al. 1984). Some patients undergoing isolated aortic valve replacement will be in chronic atrial fibrillation, which alone is associated with a 30% incidence of thromboembolism (COHN 1979). A basic conclusion is that the incidence of thromboembolism with the porcine prosthesis in either the aortic or the mitral position without anticoagulation is the same as that with the best mechanical valves with anticoagulation (EDMUNDS 1982; MARSHALL et al. 1983). The observation of NUNEZ et al. (1982, 1984), who suggest that prophylaxis with antiplatelet agents may be as effective as warfarin in preventing thromboembolism, allows us to suspect that it might be a random event.

LYTLE et al. (1989) worked up 1689 consecutive patients who underwent isolated replacement of the aortic valve and drew some interesting conclusions. They found the hazard function for the combined rate of occurrence of myocardial infarction, stroke and peripheral thromboembolism to be constant for patients with either bioprostheses or mechanical valves throughout the follow-up period, as were the hazard functions for fatal and non-fatal bleeding complications. After careful classification of patients according to valve–anticoagulation status, using univariate testing, they were able to show that patients with bioprostheses who were not receiving warfarin had the best early and late event-free survival, while patients with bioprostheses who were receiving warfarin had equivalent survival rates to patients with mechanical valves who were also receiving oral anticoagulants. They thus agree with other investigators (BLOOMFIELD et al. 1986) in that patients with bioprosthetic valves in the aortic position should not receive warfarin beyond 6–8 postoperative weeks, unless non-valve-related indications for anticoagulation exist. The available literature is, however, confusing since the incidence of thromboembolism with aortic bioprostheses is greater in the first 3 months after operation in some series (DOUGLAS et al. 1984; GALLUCCI et al. 1982; IONESCU et al. 1982; OYER et al. 1984) but not in others (BLOCH et al. 1982; JANUSZ et al. 1982; MAGILLIGAN et al. 1985) and there are no data to indicate that oral anticoagulation during this period significantly reduces the incidence of thromboembolism (BLOOMFIELD et al. 1986; JOYCE et al. 1984; ZUSMAN et al. 1981). Likewise, there is not enough evidence to justify the long-term use of platelet inhibitory drugs in that setting, and in the absence of data to the contrary, we conclude that most patients with aortic bioprostheses are probably best managed postoperatively without either warfarin or platelet inhibitors. Furthermore, the role of these groups of drugs is unclear in the presence of risk factors such as atrial fibrillation, concomitant mitral disease, a history of embolus or a recent embolus (BLOOMFIELD et al. 1986; COHN et al. 1984; FARAH et al. 1984; MILLER et al. 1987).

The reported incidence of thromboembolism is greater in patients with bioprostheses in the mitral position [84% freedom from thromboembolism at 10 years vs 88% for the aortic position, according to TEPLY et al. (1981)]. Again, however, the efficacy of long-term use of warfarin is unclear. The risk factors named above for the aortic position are associated with increased thromboembolism in most series but not in all (BRAIS et al. 1985; GONZALEZ-LAVIN et al. 1984; VEJLSTED et al. 1984). Careful evaluation of available evidence allows us to conclude that, with the possible exception of patients with combinations of atrial fibrillation, atrial thrombus and previous embolism, long-term warfarin can no longer be recommended for patients with bioprostheses in the mitral position although immediate postoperative anticoagulation would still be needed.

To summarize, all bioprostheses are constantly thrombogenic. Aortic allografts in the aortic position are the only valvular prostheses without a tendency to thrombosis and thromboembolism (KIRKLIN AND BARRAT-BOYES 1986). The fact that most patients survive many years without a thrombotic event reflects the dynamic equilibrium between the constant thrombotic stimulus of the prosthesis and the defence mechanisms which continuously maintain the fluidity of blood.

4.4 Endocarditis

Data from ROSSITER et al. (1978), based on 1347 patients, suggested that there was no difference in the mortality rates regarding prosthetic valve endocarditis with bioprosthetic or Starr-Edwards valves. The only finding of statistical significance was a 2.5 times higher incidence of valve endocarditis in the aortic compared with the mitral position. EGLOFF et al. (1980) found the same incidence of endocarditis among recipients of mechanical and biological valves for aortic valve replacement. Later IVERT et al. (1984) recorded that, in the first 6 months after surgery, the risk of valve endocarditis was higher in patients with mechanical valves than in those with porcine valves; thereafter, both groups experienced a similar rate of infection. In the current literature the following pathogens have been identified as causative of prosthetic valve endocarditis: streptococci, *Staphylococcus aureus* and *epidermidis*, enterococci, *Enterobacter, Pseudomonas aeruginosa, E. coli, Listeria monocytogenes, Serratia marcescens, Actinobacillus actinomyces, Candida* and Phycomycetes. Atypical infections with mycobacteria pathogenic for the pig but not for man have also been described. Furthermore, Libman-Sacks endocarditis in a 19-year-old girl suffering from systemic lupus erythematosus has been reported (LEDINGHAM et al. 1988). In contrast with mechanical valves, valve endocarditis on the bioprosthesis may result in structural changes in the collagen that shorten survival of the valve (BILLINGHAM et al. 1979; FERRANS et al. 1978). Echocardiography (especially by the transoesophageal route) has proved to be a very powerful non-invasive diagnostic tool for the detection of endocarditis, where vegetations and leaks can be visualized satisfactorily (ALAM et al. 1979; REUL et al. 1985; TEOH et al. 1990).

As far as medical therapy of prosthetic valve endocarditis is concerned, MAGILLIGAN (1987) performed univariate and multivariate logistic analyses and concluded that the only predictor of failure of medical therapy was the presence of endocarditis on the aortic valve ($P < 0.035$). Freedom from endocarditis in his group was 94% (+ 1.0 SE) at 5 years and 89% (+ 1.6 SE) at 10 years. How devastating valve infection can occasionally be has been shown recently by the reported performance of heart transplantation in a patient with intractable prosthetic valve endocarditis after three previous valve replacement procedures (DISESA et al. 1990).

4.5 Haemolysis

Bioprostheses are very seldom the cause of intravascular haemolysis in contrast to mechanical valves (MYERS et al. 1978; RHODES and MCINTOSH 1977). The reasons are believed to be the central blood flow, and the slow closure of the valve. Haemolysis seems to appear only in those instances where there is a leak endocarditis or perforation of the prosthesis (Fig. 4).

4.6 Heart Rupture

A rare complication of mitral valve replacement through a bioprosthesis is rupture of the posterior wall of the left ventricle (BORTOLOTTI et al. 1980; GEROULANOS 1985; WILD et al. 1980). The reason seems to be a disproportion between the relatively high profile of the prosthesis and a too small left ventricle. Here a lower profile valve would be advantageous (LIOTTA et al. 1978).

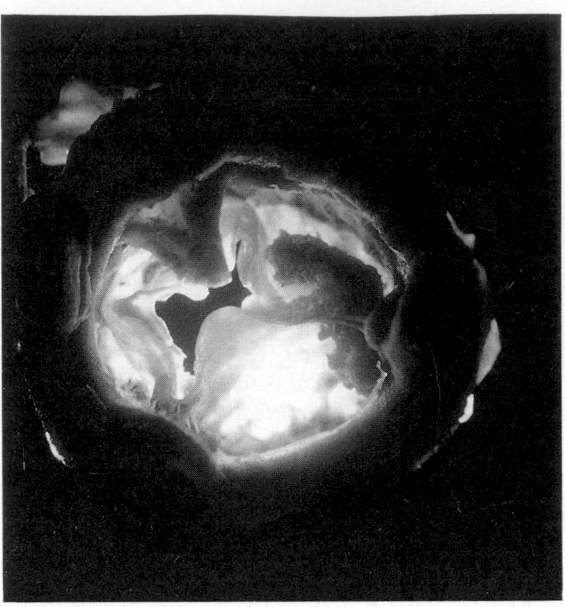

Fig. 4. Bioprosthesis with extensive chronic, lymphomononuclear inflammation, and marked degenerative changes (dystrophic calcification) extending to tissue necrosis, causing haemolysis in a 72-year-old female patient 11 years after mitral valve replacement (W.U.)

5 Pathology

5.1 Durability

Bioprostheses are generally thought to offer lower thromboembolic rates and freedom from coagulation-related abnormalities at the cost of limited durability. There is a calculated risk of reoperation and an inferior haemodynamic performance in the smaller sizes. Although they contribute to a better quality of life, initial optimism regarding their wider use has been somewhat clouded by the occasionally reported high risk of reoperation, which is due to the urgency of a second operation often performed due to sudden deterioration (timely planned reoperation has an acceptable risk). A bioprosthetic valve may start to tear slowly, but by the time the damage is recognized as a serious complication, the patient is often rushed to the hospital in profound failure and is operated upon under conditions that represent catastrophic failure (GEHA 1987). However, other groups (BORTOLOTTI et al. 1985; MILANO et al. 1989) using the Hancock valve have not found this to be true.

From longitudinal studies (HAMMOND et al. 1987) it would appear that at 10 years from operation the advantages and disadvantages of biological and mechanical valves are approximately even. Bioprostheses look better in the first 5 years, and mechanical valves in the second 5. HAMMERMEISTER et al. (1987) have also shown that 5 years following implantation, freedom from valve-related complications was significantly greater for bioprostheses in both the aortic and the mitral position and thus the use of bioprosthetic valves seems to be properly restricted to older patients with a life expectancy up to 10 years or to women of child-bearing age. Certain other groups of patients with contra-indications to anticoagulant therapy or non-compliance with it will also benefit (MAGILLIGAN et al. 1989). Some investigators have suggested that porcine bioprostheses last longer in the aortic than in the mitral position (BOLOOKI et al. 1983; COHN et al. 1984; WARNES et al. 1983), whereas others with large series of patients, which extend beyond 10 years, do not share this opinion (GALLO et al. 1986; GALLUCCI et al. 1986; HAMMOND et al. 1987; MAGILLIGAN 1987).

Recent data confirm that survival after aortic valve replacement is more patient related than prosthesis related (MILANO et al. 1989; MITCHELL et al. 1986). In their series of 506 patients who underwent replacement with Hancock standard, Björk-Shiley and Lillehei-Kaster prostheses and were followed up for 15 years, MILANO et al. found no difference in operative and late mortality rates and comparable actuarial survival rates at 15 years with the three types of prostheses. Moreover, the incidence of prosthesis-related deaths was similar, even if the cases of sudden death observed in groups with the Björk-Shiley and Lillehei-Kaster prostheses were included (MILANO et al. 1989). It would seem, then, that 35% of recipients of bioprostheses will have to undergo reoperation by 10 years (PERIER et al. 1989), an incidence frequently reported in the literature (Gallo et al. 1986; MAGILLIGAN et al. 1983, 1985; SCHOEN et al. 1983), with an operative mortality of 4% for replacement of Carpentier-Edwards or 5.5% for Hancock bioprostheses (PERIER et al. 1986, 1989 – a risk similar to that of primary operations. Additionally, no difference was observed in the rate of structural valve deterioration between the Carpentier-Edwards and Hancock prostheses (BOLOOKI et al. 1986; COBANOGLU et al. 1987; NISTAL et al. 1986; PERIER et al. 1989), with an exception offered by the work of HARTZ et al. (HAMMOND et al. 1987). This suggests that the deterioration of the Carpentier-Edwards valve was less frequent than that of the Hancock valve, but the study had a shorter follow-up.

5.2 Morphological Changes

Morphological changes occur in bioprosthetic tissues during glutaraldehyde pretreatment and other valve fabrication steps, including near-complete loss of surface endothelium (porcine valve) or mesothelium (pericardial bioprostheses), autolytic disruption of connective tissue cells, collagen bundle loosening and loss of ground substance (FERRANS et al. 1978, 1980). During glutaraldehyde-induced cross-linking, porcine aortic valves are usually preloaded by a hydrostatic back pressure (mimicking diastole), which locks the valve structure into a geometric configuration in which both corrugations and crimp are fully straightened. Thus, stresses must be absorbed by the collagen fibres themselves. Cusps may thus not open smoothly, and the series of kinks induce mechanical stresses with the resulting buckling of the fibrosa contributing to mechanical failure. Following implantation, changes are to be expected, since the cusp blood interface is not a natural biological surface (Akins et al. 1979; Alam et al. 1979). Collagen is the most important structural element (American Association of Tissue Banks 1987) and as bioprostheses have no synthetic or renewal mechanism to replace their collagen, it is gradually degraded by proteolysis or mechanical damage, and time-dependent pathological processes, including calcification are seen (Angell et al. 1976). Deposition of inflammatory cells is characteristic, together with infiltration of cellular and proteinaceous blood elements and the formation of a fibrous sheath of host origin (pannus) which grows as an extension of the tissue healing the sewing ring. Small thrombotic deposits form, there is penetration into the substance of the prosthesis by proteins and other constituents of plasma, and generalized architectural homogenization, with connective tissue disruption, mineralization and, occasionally, lipid accumulation. In pericardial valves, the above processes may be accentuated, with additional changes occurring. Since the edges of these valve cusps are cut, rather than natural edges, collagen bundles at the edges tend to splay apart during function, allowing host cells and fluid to enter the cuspal tissue with resultant cuspal stiffening and stenosis. Moreover, progressive cuspal stretching ("sagging") has been demonstrated, which leads to leaflet deformation and valvular incompetence. These changes have been observed and documented microscopically and offer the possibility of understanding and perhaps interfering with some of the events associated with valve failure. Carpentier believes that fatigue-induced lesions, which appear histologically as areas of collagen degeneration and elastic fibre fragmentation, are inevitable, due to the basic nature of the bioprosthesis (Carpentier in a discussion of Stinson et al. 1977).

An insight into the morphological substrate of primary tissue failure was given by the work of Pansini et al. (1990), who studied porcine valves extracted from the same patient from the mitral and aortic positions. After having studied 15 patients, they could not demonstrate that bioprostheses degenerate earlier and more extensively in the mitral rather than in the aortic position. Calcification was slightly heavier in the mitral position, an interesting but not statistically significant difference. The degree of creep was, however, significantly greater in the mitral position. Warnes et al. (1983) demonstrated heavier calcification on the mitral valves, where Cipriano et al. (1984) with ten cases and Bortolotti et al. (1987) with seven cases could find no difference between failing bioprostheses in the mitral and the aortic position.

5.3 Calcification

Calcification (Figs. 1, 2) is of paramount importance, since it is the most frequent cause of failure of the bioprostheses fabricated from glutaraldehyde-pretreated porcine aortic valves or from bovine pericardium (Carpentier et al. 1969; Fishbein et al. 1977; Schoen et al. 1984; Valente et al. 1985). The promising experimental work of Levy et al. (1987) reports the use of diphosphonates as an efficacious means of arresting calcification. They probably act either by binding to developing hydroxyapatite crystals and restricting further crystalline growth or by formation of polynuclear complexes with calcium. They have been used clinically in the treatment of metabolic bone diseases, and the authors suggest that optimum dosage is about 10 mg/kg per 24 h (which avoids adverse effects on epiphyseal development and overall growth) when they have to be initiated within 48 h of valve implantation.

6 Children

Children, as candidates for valve surgery, comprise a unique population, with peculiarities that need to be addressed. Cardiac valve replacement in children has now become safer, but is justified only in the presence of advanced cardiac failure or severe haemodynamic impairment. Early intervention is encouraged to prevent the development of irreversible myocardial and pulmonary vascular damage and subsequent sudden death (NUDELMAN et al. 1980; SCHACHNER et al. 1984). Furthermore, interestingly enough, children have shown a striking return to normal heart size and function following valve replacement, a change which can also occur after a second valve is inserted during their growing years (SCHACHNER et al. 1984).

Bioprostheses, however attractive an alternative they may offer, are considered by most authors as undesirable; most surgeons prefer mechanical valves. This policy is further reinforced by promising results of surgeons using St. Jude medical valves without subsequent anticoagulation and without episodes of thromboembolism (PASS et al. 1984). The requirement for excellent haemodynamic characteristics is another limiting factor in childhood.

Microscopically, extensive fragmentation of collagen with focal heavy calcification and degeneration correlate with the high incidence of relatively early failure of porcine xenograft valves in children [20% in 25 children followed for 10–54 months (GEHA et al. 1979)].

7 Pregnancy and Childbearing

The hypercoagulable state that accompanies pregnancy, warfarin embryopathy (BORTOLOTTI et al. 1982; DEVIRI et al. 1985; LANG et al. 1985; NUNEZ et al. 1983), the haemorrhagic complications of heparin and the inadequacy of antiplatelet agents in providing protection (ROTHLIN et al. 1977) make bioprostheses a particularly attractive alternative for women wishing to have children. Pregnancy has been shown to be well tolerated, the rate of spontaneous abortion [16.2% (BADDUKE et al. 1991)] falling well within the range seen in the general population (15% – 20%). Among other unknown factors, however, altered calcium metabolism and the profound effect pregnancy has on the maternal cardiovascular system may contribute to the aggressive calcification and early and accelerated rate of prosthetic valve deterioration sometimes seen in pregnancy. This requires close monitoring and planned reoperation before haemodynamic compromize appears [reoperation rate of 59% for pregnant as compared to 19% for non-pregnant women, with an overall reoperative mortality of 8.7% (BADDUEK et al. 1991)].

8 Indications for Use of Bioprosthetic Valves

Obviously, the choice of valve substitute is dependent on matching patient characteristics, taking into account life-style, to valve characteristics in order to minimise morbidity and mortality, including that due to reoperation. Valve replacement with bioprostheses continues to be indicated in:

1. The elderly [preferably in the aortic position if the annulus is 25 mm or greater, since in the mitral position there is a high incidence of atrial arrhythmias, necessitating anticoagulation, and a real possibility of perforation of the left ventricular wall by the struts of the valve (MORGAN et al. 1985)]
2. Patients with a history of cerebral, gastrointestinal or other bleeding, including epistaxis
3. Women who are pregnant or wish to have children
4. Physically active patients
5. Patients who are not expected to show complete compliance with an anticoagulation regimen.

In children bioprostheses function well and for a long period when placed in the pulmonary and tricuspid valve positions (DUNN 1981; ILBAWI et al. 1986). In other positions, for unknown reasons, bioprosthetic valves are alarmingly less durable in children than in adults; thus HUMAN et al. (1982) reported that less than 10% of valves survive beyond 5 years, while according to WILLIAMS et al. (1982) 58.5% are free of valve failure 5 years postoperatively, and according to SCHAFF et al. (1984) 41% require reoperation within 5 years.

Occasionally bioprostheses have been used as valve conduits, i.e. left atrium to left ventricle (LAKS et al. 1980; LANSING et al. 1983; WRIGHT et al. 1981). Their ability to operate silently, which makes the stigma of cardiac disease less apparent to others, is particularly appreciated by sensitive young patients. Hypertension, sickle-cell anaemia, chronic renal insufficiency and an abnormal calcium metabolism are contra-indications for the implantation of bioprosthetic valves.

Ten years without anticoagulation are not only socio-economically important; they also imply a better quality of life. In these patients, where the calculated risk of reoperation is small, a bioprosthesis might be the first choice. However, it should not be forgotten that "durable valves are limited by thromboembolism, and non-thrombogenic valves are limited by durability" (MCGOON et al. 1984).

B. Allografts

9 Historical Background

In 1952 LAM et al. first published experimental data on aortic valve allografts. It was 1956 before MURRAY reported the first clinical use of allograft aortic valves, which he had transplanted to the descending aorta in patients with aortic valve regurgitation. The first cases of orthotopic aortic valve replacement with allografts were reported by BARRAT-BOYES (1964) and ROSS (FONTAN et al. 1976). The early implantation technique, a running free-hand suturing technique with two suture lines, was published by BARRAT-BOYES (1965) and is still in use today. In these early days allograft valves were used for aortic and mitral valve disease (MURRAY 1956); however, results in the treatment of mitral valve disease were disappointing and reconstruction of the mitral valve or other replacement devices showed superior performance in the long term (FONTAN et al. 1976; ROSS et al. 1979). The use of allograft valves in correcting congenital heart disease, for replacement of the pulmonary valves or for reconstruction of the right ventricular outflow tract (KIRKLIN et al. 1987) is beyond the scope of this communication, and we concentrate here on the allograft valve as an aortic valve replacement.

Early allograft transplants were performed with freshly harvested valves. They were implantated soon after harvest, and no blood group matching or pre-implantation processing of the valve was performed. The haemodynamic performance and durability resulted in the liberal use of these valves (BARRAT-BOYES 1969). Limitation of availability, however, led to the introduction of several storage techniques with the intention of creating tissue banks. Chemical processing of the valve was performed not only to increase storage time but also to avoid donor-transmitted disease. These early storage and/or sterilisation techniques ranged from freeze drying, irradiation and glutaraldehyde pretreatment to antibiotic sterilization with prolonged storage at 4°C (BODNAR et al. 1990). Unfortunately, the clinical performance with respect to durability was negatively influenced by all of these processing maneuvers. Consequently, the early enthusiasm for allograft valves faded. Disappointing results with other valve devices, prosthetic or bioprosthetic, led to renewed interest in allograft valves which was further boosted by the excellent long-term results from O'BRIEN et al. (1987b), who reported 92% of all patients free of valve-related complications 10 years after surgery. These outstanding results were obtained with cryopreserved viable allografts.

10 Harvesting and Storage

Adequate techniques of pre-implantation processing and storage made the growth of tissue banks possible (ANGELL et al. 1976). In the initial allograft experience outlined above, only fresh aortic valves were used, causing considerable logistic and supply problems. Apart from local hospital tissue banks, in Europe an organization similar to "Eurotransplant" (which takes care of the distribution of organs for transplantation in Western Europe) – Bioimplant Services, Leiden – represents a major tissue resource.

10.1 Donor Selection

Donor criteria for Bioimplant Services (1991) are as follows:

1. Donor age: under 55 years, with no minimum age
2. Living donors: explanted hearts of heart or heart–lung transplant recipients
3. Heart-beating donors: hearts from subjects for multiorgan donation where the heart, for whatever reasons, cannot be used for transplantation
4. Post-mortem donors: subjects who have been dead not longer than 12 h

Contra-indications are as follows:

1. Valvular disease
2. Severe infections (including positive serology for HIV and HB_sAg)
3. Evidence of myocarditis or endocarditis
4. Malignancies, except for primary brain tumours
5. Collagen diseases, e.g. Marfan syndrome

Valves from heart-beating donors generally are removed in the operating theatre, which improves sterility considerably and should also, in the presence of a local tissue bank, shorten donor valve ischaemic time. Alterations of the valve caused by prolonged ischaemia are a major concern in shipping non-processed valves over long distances or taking hearts from the mortuary. From a logistic standpoint it is nearly impossible to obtain heart valves from deceased patients within the first 12 h after death, but some surgeons allow longer ischaemic times although recent research has shown a decline in fibroblast viability after 8–12 h (Louis et al. 1991). Results obtained with the use of non-viable allograft heart valves are still superior than after using other available prosthetic devices, and some centres accept cadaver valves up to 72 h post-mortem (Stelzer and Elkins 1989).

10.2 Procurement of the Valve

The heart for heart valve removal ideally should be obtained under sterile conditions in an operating room. In the mortuary as clean a technique as possible should be used. The dissection of the allograft valve from the heart in an aseptic environment, preferably under a laminar flow cabinet, has been described in detail elsewhere (KIRKLIN and BARRAT-BOYES 1986). In brief, the aorta will be dissected, keeping the valve ring and the anterior mitral leaflet intact. A few millimetres of the coronary arteries remain attached. After careful inspection of the valve to ensure its structural integrity, the valve is measured. Adequate vascular tissue is obtained for microbiological investigation, which can take up to 6 weeks. At Bioimplant Services, Leiden, cryopreservation of the valve will be performed within 24 h after dissection of the allograft valve. The allograft is frozen at a controlled rate down to –190°C and stored in the vapour phase of a liquid nitrogen container. Other protocols prescribe 24 to 72 h storage in antibiotic solution prior to freezing (KIRKLIN and BARRAT-BOYES 1986). The allograft is ready for implantation when donor blood cultures and virology are negative and tissue and medium are sterile.

10.3 Storage

Today most allograft valves are cryopreserved. After controlled freezing the valve is maintained in the gaseous phase of liquid nitrogen at a storage temperature between –150°C and –190°C depending on engineering details of the storage container (LANGE and HOPKINS 1989). This article will not deal with the complex physical – chemical interactions within the tissue which occur during freezing and thawing. However, prior to freezing so-called cryprotective agents such as dimethylsulphoxide (DMSO), glycerol or ethylene glycol are added to the tissue culture medium. [VAN DER KAMP and NAUTER (1979) found that a 10% DMSO concentration provided the highest number of viable fibroblasts.] Long-term allograft storage with maintenance of fibroblast viability requires storage of the frozen tissue below the "glass transition point" of the freezing solution, which is at about –120°C (BANK and BROCKBANK 1987). Few changes occur below this temperature – it has been estimated that mammalian embryos stored in liquid nitrogen have a shelf life of approximately 30 000 years (BANK and BROCKBANK 1987). It is clearly extremely important to maintain a proper temperature during storage and subsequent shipping of the valve.

Alternative methods of storage include maintenance of the valve in a refrigerator at 4°C in antibiotic-enriched nutrient medium (BARRAT-BOYES et al. 1965) but storage time using this method is restricted to 3 weeks. Paradoxically, the valves maintained in the refrigerator in nutrient and antibiotic solutions are often called "fresh" valves. Their viability had been shown to decline rapidly due to cytotoxic effects of the added antibiotic (YANKAH et al. 1987).

10.4 Thawing

It has been found that the optimal rate of rewarming is dependent on the freezing conditions used (BANK and BROCKBAND 1987). For heart valves, rapid rewarming has been found to be advantageous and it is recommended that the frozen allograft be placed in 37°– 42°C fluid for rapid thawing. If glycerol is the cryoprotective agent, the valve is immersed in 37°C Ringer's lactate solution until the tissue has become soft. To remove the glycerol the allograft is rinsed in three subsequent baths of 4°C Ringer's lactate solution and kept in the last bath until the moment of implantation. In the case of DMSO cryopreservation the frozen allograft is placed in normal saline solution at 42°C. After being thawed completely the allograft is unpacked and placed in tissue culture fluid containing 10% DMSO. DMSO is removed by passing the valve through three successive rinsing steps with decreasing concentrations of DMSO, and the valve can be kept in DMSO-free culture medium until implantation (Bioimplant Services 1991).

10.5 Pre-implantation Preparation

Having a valve that has been properly trimmed before storage means that little final trimming has to be done. Careful removal of excess myocardial tissue and of the anterior mitral leaflet (if it is not to be used for the operation) should be done. Shortening the aortic cuff length if only valve replacement and not aortic root replacement is to be done is the next step. At this point of the operation it should also be clear whether to implant the valve in the subcoronary position or as a cylinder implant (the so-called miniroot technique). The former choice means that at least two coronary sinuses have to be trimmed away to allow the upper suture line to run below the coronary ostia (Fig. 5); the latter requires that at this time or during the implantation of the valve two holes have to be created for the later attachment of the coronary orifices.

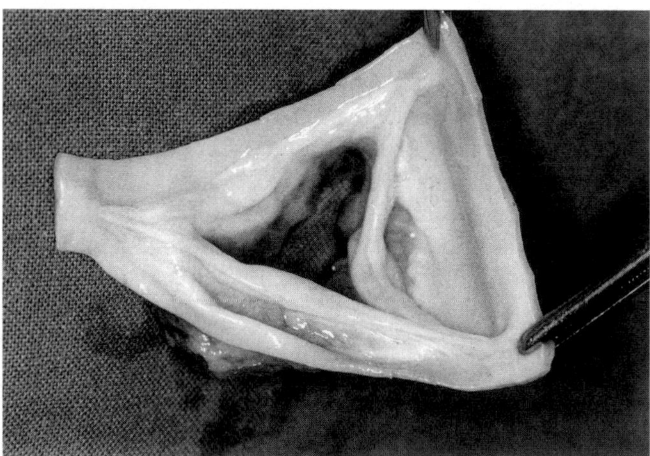

Fig. 5. Trimmed pulmonary allograft prior to implantation

11 Patient Selection and Indications for Surgery

Almost every patient requiring aortic valve replacement can benefit from an allograft valve; however, due to shortages in supply, allograft valve surgery is often restricted to younger subjects. There are also a few medical reasons why the surgeon should refrain from homograft valve implantation, e.g. connective tissue disorders, such as in patients with Marfan's syndrome. Patients with acute aortic or prosthetic valve endocarditis profit substantially from allograft valve implantation (Yankah and Hetzer 1989); see below.

Severe left ventricular dysfunction has been claimed to be a contra-indication to allograft valve replacement but it has recently been shown to be a relatively important indication, at least in very young subjects. A young patient with a failing left ventricle may profit maximally from the haemodynamic superiority of allograft valves and early survival is enhanced by the excellent hydrodynamic function of allograft valves.

At our institution exact measurement of the inner diameter of the aortic root by means of two-dimensional echocardiography precedes a planned allograft procedure. As a consequence of these measurements the valve is chosen, thawed and trimmed prior to initiation of cardiopulmonary bypass. These measures have shortened aortic cross-clamp time considerably, decreasing subsequent ischaemic damage to the myocardium.

12 Implantation

The following describes the technique currently in use at the University of Münster, Germany. In other institutions different protocols are used, for example as regards the handling of the extracorporeal circulation and myocardial protection. Implantation may also take part with different surgical techniques, and different suture material may be used. Each modification has its inherent advantages and drawbacks, so every centre should perform surgery in such a way as to obtain the most reliable results (Barrat-Boyes 1979; Konertz et al. 1991; Ross 1991). The chest is entered via a standard median sternotomy and after longitudinal opening of the pericardium the patient is placed on cardiopulmonary bypass. We routinely use normothermic cardiopulmonary bypass with high-flow (2.4–3.0 l/m^2) perfusion and membrane oxygenation. Apart from cases with severe aortic regurgitation after cross-clamping of the aorta, the heart is usually arrested by means of retrograde aortic perfusion of cold Bretschneider's HTK solution. The aorta is transected 1–2 cm above the origin of the right coronary artery. A soft-tipped thin plastic catheter is advanced into the left coronary ostium and kept in place during the whole procedure, continuously delivering cardioplegic solution. The diseased valve is excised and the aortic annulus thoroughly and carefully decalcified. The aortic annulus is measured and if the size lies within 1 or 2 mm of the chosen allograft valve, implantation can proceed; if it does not, annuloplasty has to be performed. Implantation of the valve in our institution is begun by inverting the valve into the left ventricle and fixing it; eversion of the valve is the next step. In the case of subcoronary implantation only the left and the right coronary sinus of Valsalva are excised, leaving the non-coronary sinus intact. A single commissural suspension suture at the commissure between the right and left coronary orifices is used to pull up the valve and bring it into the final position. Now a second suture is used to adapt the upper part of the valve to the native aorta just under the coronary ostia (Fig. 6). Normally the aortotomy is closed, incorporating the cranial part of the allograft in the area of the non-coronary sinus. The most important steps during the surgical procedure are proper sizing so as to avoid stretching or bulging of the valve; the former may lead to aortic regurgitation and the latter to obstruction of the left ventricular outflow tract. Orientation of the valve with regard to coronary orifices and to the sinus is especially demanding in the setting of a congenitally bicuspid aortic valve. To ensure proper cusp orientation we always perform a transverse rather than a longitudinal aortotomy, which is recommended by some surgeons (Kirklin and Barrat-Boyes 1986). The deliberate use of the so-called miniroot technique (the implant of an allograft cylinder) makes cusp orientation much easier, and for this reason it is the method of choice in our centre. After closure of the aortotomy and coming off bypass, immediate assessment of the graft function by means of two-

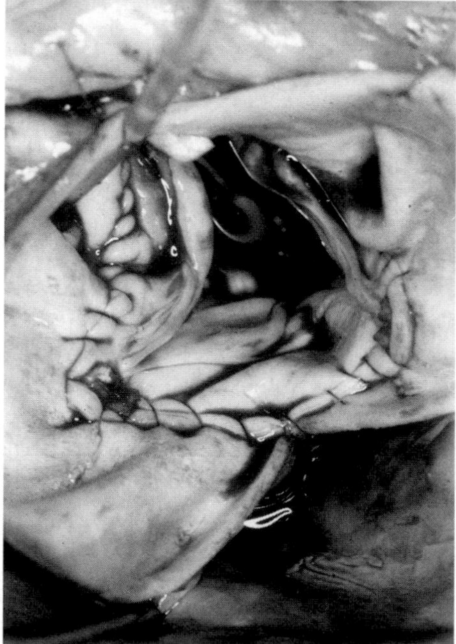

Fig. 6. Operative site after subcoronary implantation of an allograft valve prior to closure of the aortotomy

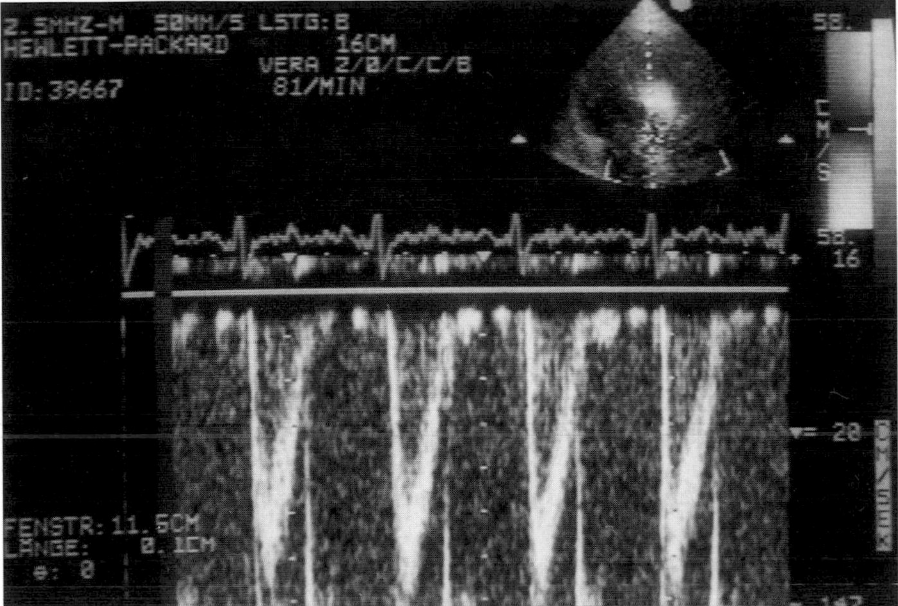

Fig. 7. Postoperative Doppler flow velocities appear normal in a patient with allograft valve replacement

dimensional echocardiography or transvalvular pressure measurements and determination of cardiac output under defined preload conditions is performed (Fig. 7).

13 Results of Surgery

13.1 Mortality

13.1.1 Early Mortality

Primary isolated aortic valve replacement has always carried a low hospital mortality. Improvements in operating techniques and a more sophisticated understanding of the conduct of cardiopulmonary bypass and myocardial protection have further lowered the operative risk. However, the trend towards operating on older and sicker patients possibly outweighs these improvements. In general, the operative risk for aortic valve replacement is at or below 2% (KIRKLIN and BARRAT-BOYES 1986). The most common mode of hospital death is postoperative acute cardiac failure, followed by haemorrhage. Elaborate analyses of incremental risk factors for hospital deaths after isolated aortic valve replacement have shown that the preoperative functional status and left ventricular function influence the operative risk (WIDEMAN et al. 1981). Greater age and pure aortic valve incompetence have also been incremental risk factors for in-hospital death after aortic valve replacement. The influence of the method of myocardial protection in obtaining good postoperative results does not need to be stressed here. Of interest is whether or not the replacement device used is a risk factor. Data from Green Lane Hospital (KIRKLIN and BARRAT-BOYES 1986) have shown that between 1976 and 1981 4.4% of the homograft recipients died early. This contrasts with an 8% –10% hospital mortality for mechanical heart valves and bioprostheses. In even larger series from 1962 to 1981 in more than 1200 patients the difference reached statistical significance ($P = 0.08$). In our own experience, even during the learning phase of allograft surgery there has been no difference between hospital mortality after allograft or bioprothestic or prosthetic aortic valve replacement (SPITAL et al. 1992). That the learning experience for the implantation technique of free-hand allograft aortic valve replacement is not necessarily associated with a higher early mortality has also been reported recently by JONES (1989). Overall early mortality in our own series with more than 70 allograft valves operated on between January 1990 and the present stands at 5.8%. In cases of elective isolated aortic valve replacement ($n = 44$) no mortality has occurred.

13.1.2 Late Mortality

According to KIRKLIN and BARRAT-BOYES (1986) the 5-year survival rate of hospital survivors of aortic valve replacement is in the range of 85%. Actuarial survival in the University of Alabama series has been 86% with the Björk-Shiley valve and 87% with porcine bioprostheses at 3–4 years (KIRKLIN and BARRAT-BOYES 1986). Modes of premature late death are related to the cardiac condition in 50% of cases. Other modes of late death are related to thromboembolism, anticoagulation-induced haemorrhage, valve thrombosis, valve failure, prosthetic valve endocarditis and paravalvular leakage. The Stanford University Medical Center series from 1964 to 1971 showed a 5-year actuarial survival of 85%, 10-year survival of 70% and 15-year survival of 55% (MILLER and SHUMWAY 1987). In these early series "fresh" aortic allografts had been used. In 1988 MCGFFIN and co-workers from Brisbane, Australia, presented outstanding long-term results with viable cryopreserved allograft aortic valves. Early mortality was 4.8%, 5-year survival was 86% and survival at 10 years was 71%. Of the late deaths after aortic valve replacement, 25% were related to the replacement device and the risk factors for premature late death were generally the same as those that influenced early mortality. In particular, preoperative left ventricular dysfunction, older age at operation, aortic regurgitation and untreated coronary artery disease are important (KIRKLIN and BARRAT-BOYES 1986).

13.2 Morbidity

In this section, the definitions of morbidity given by Edmunds and the members of the "Ad Hoc Liaison Committee for Standardizing Definitions of Prosthetic Heart Valve Morbidity" of the American Association for Thoracic Surgery and the Society of Thoracic Surgeons published in 1988 are used (EDMUNDS et al. 1988).

13.2.1 Structural Deterioration

"Any change in valve function resulting from an intrinsic abnormality causing stenosis or regurgitation is considered structural deterioration" (EDMUNDS et al. 1988). It is important to point out that an intrinsic abnormality excludes infection or valve thrombosis. A multitude of factors produce intrinsic abnormalities such as wear, stress fracture, poppet escape, calcification leaflet tear, stent creeps and disruption or stenosis of a reconstructed valve. As far as allograft aortic valves are concerned, leaflet tears or ruptures cause 8% of the total deaths late after surgery (KIRKLIN and BARRAT-BOYES 1986). These data are from earlier series, however, and there is good evidence experimentally and clinically that newer preservation techniques decrease the incidence of leaflet ruptures (JAFFE et al. 1989; O'BRIEN et al. 1987a).

13.2.2 Non-structural Dysfunction

EDMUNDS et al. (1988) define non-structural dysfunction as "any abnormality resulting in stenosis or regurgitation at the valve that is not intrinsic to the valve itself". Examples are entrapment by pannus or suture, paravalvular leak, inappropriate sizing and haemolytic anaemia. Again, thromboembolism and infection have to be excluded. According to KIRKLIN and BARRAT-BOYES (1986), paravalvular leakage was relatively common in the early allograft series but was avoided by changes in surgical technique. Inappropriate sizing may also cause non-structural dysfunction: selecting a valve too large probably causes left ventricular outflow stenosis and undersizing probably allows aortic incompetence to develop through stretching and loss of the central occlusion area. Some trivial or mild central leakage is, however, a common finding after aortic valve replacement with allograft valves. This regurgitation is not clinically detectable and is a Doppler echocardiography finding without haemodynamic or clinical relevance; it rarely progresses to clinically obvious aortic valve incompetence. Late allograft valve incompetence has been shown to be due to leaflet rupture (KIRKLIN and BARRAT-BOYES 1986).

13.2.3 Thromboembolism

Thromboembolism comprises "any valve thrombosis or embolus exclusive of infection" (EDMUNDS et al. 1988). In contrast to aortic valve replacement with bioprostheses or prosthetic valves, thromboembolic complications are a rare finding after allograft aortic valve replacement. BARRAT-BOYES (1969) has described the transient and infrequent finding of small platelet emboli in retinal vessels during the early healing phase and for this reason we anticoagulate all patients receiving allograft valves for the first 3 months after surgery. Thromboembolism has not occurred in patients with allograft valves late after surgery if the valve is free of endocarditis (KIRKLIN and BARRAT-BOYES 1986; O'BRIEN et al. 1991).

13.2.4 Anticoagulation-Related Haemorrhage

By "anticoagulation-related haemorrhage" is meant "any episode of internal or external bleeding that causes death, stroke, operation or hospitalization or requires transfusion" (EDMUNDS et al. 1988). As pointed out in the preceding section, patients are not usually on long-term anticoagulant therapy after allograft aortic valve replacement. Anticoagulation-related problems with their inherent morbidity and potential mortality are therefore unimportant in the long-term survival of allograft valve patients. An earlier series from Stanford with long-term follow-up of 1127 patients after isolated aortic valve replacement documented that 9% of late deaths were attributable to an haemorrhagic cerebrovascular accident (COPELAND et al. 1977) but all these events occurred in patients with mechanical prostheses on warfarin anticoagulation.

13.2.5 Allograft Valve Endocarditis

Replacement device endocarditis is a serious complication after aortic valve replacement (KIRKLIN et al. 1989). Risk factor analysis has shown that the use of a prosthetic heart valve and the presence of native valve endocarditis during primary surgery are the main risk factors for prosthetic valve endocarditis (IVERT et al. 1984). Allograft valves have been found to carry a low incidence of valve endocarditis and mechanical prostheses the highest. Hazard function analysis at University of Alabama (IVERT et al. 1984) showed that mechanical prostheses have a high early risk phase. The incidence of allograft valve endocarditis is constant and low over the whole time course (Fig. 8). In the presence of acute native or prosthetic valve endocarditis the allograft valve has become the valve of choice for aortic valve replacement.

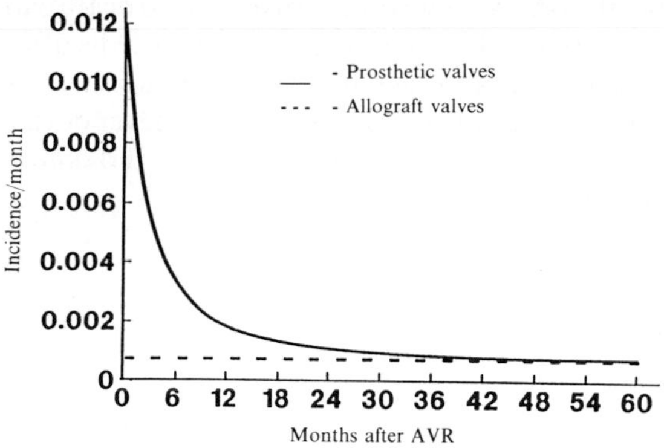

Fig. 8. Incidence of replacement device endocarditis after aortic valve replacement (AVR). (Modified from Brais MP et al. (1985)

13.3 Consequences of Morbidity

13.3.1 Reoperation

According to Edmunds et al. (1988) "Any operation that repairs, alters or replaces a previously placed prosthesis or repaired valve should be reported as reoperation". Data from O'Brien et al. (1987b) showed that 95% –97% of patients are free from reoperation 5 years after surgery. Comparison of two cohorts of patients, one with the "fresh" 4°C stored valve and the other with cryopreserved valves showed that 10 years after primary surgery 83% of the patients with "fresh" and 89% of the patients with cryopreserved allograft valves were free from reoperation. In this series the causes leading to reoperation were degeneration in 23% of the "fresh" grafts and 0.9% in the cryopreserved grafts. There was a 3% versus 2% infection incidence in the two groups and technical problems leading to reoperation occurred in 2% and 3% of the patients respectively. This shows clearly the superiority of cryopreservation methods. Similar 5-year and 10-year data have been reported by Khagani et al. (1976). In the Stanford series of Miller and Shumway (1987), 67% of patients were free from reoperation 10 years after surgery.

13.3.2 Valve-Related Mortality

Valve-related mortality is "any death caused by structural deterioration, non-structural dysfunction, thromboembolism, anticoagulant-related bleeding, prosthetic valve endocarditis or death at reoperation" (Edmunds et al. 1988). This seems to be an important issue for comparing valves of different types or in the field of allograft valve surgery when comparing different storage and valve-processing methods. Unfortunately only a few studies in the literature show the true valve-related mortality. In most studies, actuarial analysis of valve-related complications including reoperation and death is shown. However, valve-related death can probably best be evaluated by comparison of actuarial survival of patients after valve replacement with that of an age-, sex- and race-matched population. This type of analysis also makes clear that aortic valve replacement, whichever device is used, is still a palliative rather than a curative procedure (Kirklin and Barrat-Boyes 1986; O'Brien et al. 1991)

13.4 Haemodynamic Performance

The overall haemodynamic performance of the allograft aortic valve has been very satisfying. Pressure gradients across the valve are lower than with other devices. In postoperative evaluation of allograft patients aortic stenosis is uncommon. A recent Doppler echocardiographic assessment of allograft valves, however, has shown that velocities across normal functioning homograft valves are marginally higher than those in normal native aortic valves (Jaffe et al. 1989). Trivial aortic regurgitation is a relatively common finding in allograft surgery, as mentioned above. Clinically significant aortic regurgitation sometimes occurs and is due to leaflet perforation. Progression of aortic regurgitation after allograft valve replacement is infrequent and not necessarily an indication for reoperation (Jaffe et al. 1989). A recent study in which homograft valve performance was compared with performance of prosthetic heart valves in narrow aortic annuli showed the superiority of the allograft with respect to haemodynamic function (Jaffe et al. 1990).

14 Open Questions

There are many open questions regarding the universal use of allografts. The shortcut in supply could possibly be managed by increasing the donor pool from the mortuary and also by using pulmonary allografts as aortic valve substitutes (Konertz et al. 1991; Mair et al. 1993). The operation is technically more demanding than implantation of a prosthetic cardiac valve but the techniques will be learned very fast once one has started a program. The more difficult questions that still need a lot of basic research lie in the field of viability and durability.

14.1 Viability

After the pioneering work of O'Brien et al. (1987b) and their outstanding clinical series, maintenance of leaflet fibroblast viability has been postulated to be the key to the improved results. The studies of THUBRIKAR et al. (1986) have shown that the calcific deposits in aortic valves occur early in the proximity of fibroblasts. Fibroblast viability is difficult to assess and several techniques for quantification of viable cells have been proposed. Thymidine incorporation, glucose metabolism or staining techniques are among the techniques that have been used for assessment of cell viability (O'BRIEN et al. 1988; VAN DER KAMP et al. 1981). Measurements of incorporation of amino acids into valvular cells are currently the most reliable indicators of cell viability. VAN DER KAMP et al. (1981) used radiolabelled proline and methionine and clearly demonstrated that prolene is an excellent marker substance in measurement of the synthesis of matrix proteins. Cell cultures of the different components of the valve (separate culture of endothelial cells and fibroblasts) are also a very promising tool for assessment and quantitation of cell viability (O'BRIEN et al. 1988).

14.1.1 Endothelial Cells

Preservation of endothelial cell viability is very difficult and is obtained with widely varying success rates. The role of the endothelial cells in the longevity of allograft valves is not clearly understood. These cells have been claimed to be responsible for retention of proteoglycans in the matrix of valve leaflet tissue (ISHIHARA et al. 1981); the intact viable endothelial cell lining is assumed to prevent loss of collagen fibres and to protect the valvular matrix. However, viable endothelial cells express HLA antigens and thus are immunogenic (YANKAH et al. 1986).

14.1.2 Fibroblasts

O'BRIENS definition of viability (O'BRIEN et al. 1988) states "viability of valve leaflet is present when tissue culture is readily positive, biochemical assessment of glucose utilization by the whole valve exceeds 16 mg/dl/24 hrs. and when histologic examination confirms the appearance of leaving cells in the leaflet. It is the fibroblast not the endothelial cell which is assessed for viability." These connective tissue fibroblasts are responsible for the production of intercellular matrix in heart valves and their viability has been directly linked with long-term valve durability (ARMIGER et al. 1983; GAVIN et al. 1973; O'BRIEN et al. 1988; VAN DER KAMP and NAUTER 1979). Thus most viability tests are directed to establish fibroblast viability and a number of tests that have been used in the past have proved to be inadequate or semiquantative (BROCKBANK and BANK 1987). An effective way to study protein synthesis in tissues quantitatively is to use isotopic uptake coupled with autoradiography. In this way MCGREGOR et al. (1976) were able to demonstrate that the viability of heart valves stored at 4°C in antibiotic nutrient solution was severely impaired after 2 weeks. VAN DER KAMP et al. (1981), using the same technique, showed that approximately 88% of human heart valve fibroblasts were viable after slow freezing and rapid thawing.

14.1.3 Non-viable Allograft Valves

At the beginning of allograft surgery, ROSS (1962) and BARRAT-BOYES (1964) used aseptically procured valves that were implanted within 3 weeks. Our understanding of valve viability indicates that some of these valves were viable and others were not, depending on the storage time. Between 1960 and 1970 a variety of chemical methods for sterilization, including formaldehyde, ß-propiolactone, chlorhexidine, freeze drying and ethylene oxide sterilization, had been used (HOPKINS 1989a). All these valves were non-viable and had to be removed within a few years after implantation, due to leaflet calcification and rupture. However, BODNAR et al. (1990), in a recent study of 639 operative survivors after isolated aortic valve replacement, were not able to show any difference in the primary tissue failure rates between freeze-dried and irradiated or ethylene oxide-sterilised valves or any other methods of sterilization. This led them to question the whole concept of the importance of viability in allograft valves. Regardless of whether viable or non-viable valves are transplanted, allograft valve replacement of the aortic valve is still superior to any other currently available replacement device in terms of haemodynamics, valve-related complications or valve-related deaths (O'BRIEN et al. 1991).

14.2 Durability

It has been postulated that viability is the key to increased durability, a concept which has been questioned recently (BODNAR et al. 1990). Other factors responsible for valve durability may be of mechanical or immunological origin.

14.2.1 Mechanical Factors Influencing Durability

It has been suggested that valve durability after free-hand implantation of allograft valves is increased when compared with stent-mounted valves, which has recently been confirmed by ANGELL and co-workers (1990, 1991), who were able to demonstrate superior durability of the free-hand allograft valve. There is also experimental evidence that the durability of porcine valves is increased when they are kept inside the native aortic root instead of mounting the valve on a frame (DRURY et al. 1986). Another indication that mechanical factors or stress factors play an important role in preservation of valve function is the clinical finding that the allograft valve on the right ventricular outflow tract has increased longevity compared with the valve in the aortic position (ROSS1988).

The persistent distensibility (Fig. 9) of the aortic root and changes in leaflet stress related to leaflet orientation and position have both been claimed to be

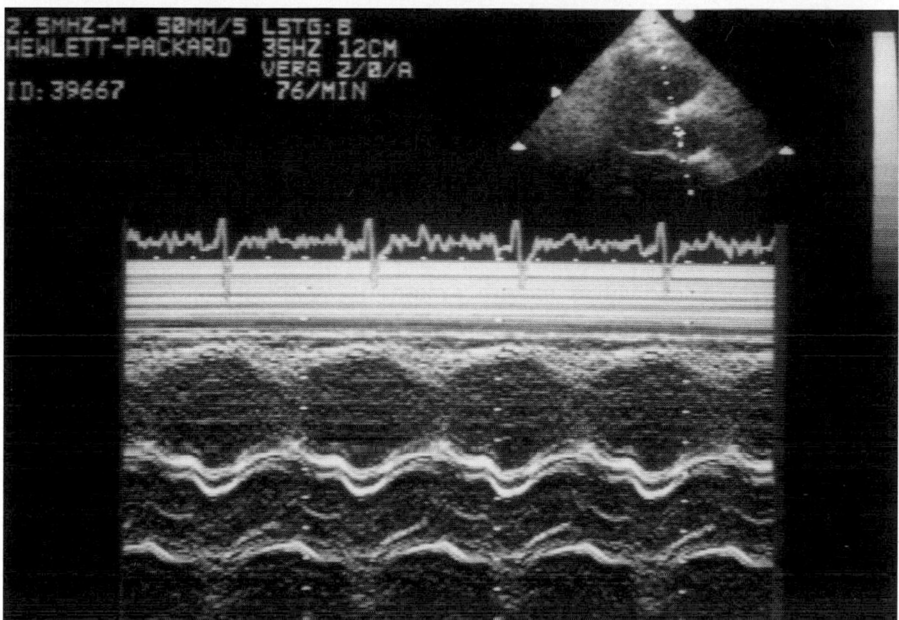

Fig. 9. Post-operative M-mode echocardiography demonstrating persistent distensibility of the aortic root

responsible for the superior performance of unstented, free-hand implanted allograft valves (ANGELL et al. 1991).

14.2.2 Immunological Factors

Work in the field of organ transplant immunology has shown that the endothelial cell is the first immunological contact of the recipient with the donor. Experimental investigations from YANKAH et al. (1987) showed that after valve leaflet transplantation in a rat model, sensitization within RT1 compatible and incompatible strain combinations takes place. The absence of endothelial cells in nonviable grafts has been shown to alter the expression of HLA antigen and to mitigate immunological attack on the valve; however, allograft tissue is foreign and there is no reason why it should be free from immunogenicity (HOPKINS 1989b). In the clinical setting this problem is difficult to investigate due to the complexity of the HLA system, but some centres have suggested immunological manipulations such as transplantation of ABO and/or HLA compatible valves or low-dose immunosuppression (KWONG et al. 1967; YANKAH et al. 1987). The long-term consequences of these interventions remain to be established. The unsolved questions of allograft immunology are among the least understood and most fascinating issues in allograft surgery.

14.3 Fresh or Cryopreserved Valves?

Today most surgeons involved in allograft surgery believe that fibroblast viability is the main factor for the improved durability of allograft valves (O'BRIEN et al. 1987a). Others have renewed their interest in the evaluation of non-viable valves, as outlined above. According to O'BRIEN et al. (1987b) one should refrain from using the term "fresh" for 4°C stored valves which may be viable within a couple of days after harvest and be dead at 5 or 6 days. Some cryopreservation methods may also produce dead valves and other methods are able to maintain fibroblast and even endothelial cell viability. It is clearly important that every valve bank establishes some form of assessment of viability of the valves (BROCKBANK and BANK 1987) and the terms "fresh" or "cryopreserved" should not be used as descriptions of viability. O'BRIEN et al. (1987b) proposed the following classification:

1. Non-viable, 4°C-stored allograft aortic valve
2. Viable, 4°C-stored aortic allograft valve (if implanted within 4 days of procurement)
3. Non-viable, cryopreserved allograft aortic valve
4. Viable, cryopreserved aortic valve

The message from this should be that any series dealing with long-term results of allograft valve replacement should indicate the status of the valve with respect to viability at implantation.

14.4 Other Options Beyond Allograft Aortic Valves

We have recently started a trial using pulmonary allografts for aortic valve replacement and found them a very reliable and, in the short term, very durable device (KONERTZ et al. 1991). Long-term evaluation of the valve continues but the wider use of pulmonary allografts should be able to increase the number of available allografts 2–2.5 times. In nearly every heart one can explant a normal pulmonary valve, while aortic valves are damaged or unacceptable in about 30%–50% of the cases (ROSS 1987).

Another interesting replacement device that is currently under investigation in a limited clinical trial is the use of stentless porcine bioprostheses. In our experience these have shown a better haemodynamic performance than the stent-mounted bioprostheses or prosthetic heart valves (KONERTZ et al. 1992). However, this study started in mid 1991 and is still ongoing. Information on the durability and the long-term performance of these valves is currently unavailable; however, there is good evidence from the allograft experience and from experimental data that stent mounting decreases the durability of bioprostheses or allografts (ANGELL et al. 1991). Improved durability above that of conventional bioprostheses is anticipated.

Acknowledgements. We gratefully acknowledge the assistance of Dr. John D. Mantas and Marlies Hagemann in the preparation of the manuscript.

References

Akins CW et al. (1979) Preoperative evaluation of subvalvular fibrosis in mitral stenosis: a predictive factor in conservative vs. replacement surgical therapy. Circulation 60 (Suppl I): I-71–I-76

Alam M et al. (1979) M-mode and two dimensional echocardiographic features of porcine valve dysfunction. Am J Cardiol 43:502–509

American Association of Tissue Banks (1987) technical manual for tissue banking. AATB, Arlington, Va.

Angell JD et al. (1976) A fresh viable human heart valve bank – sterilization, sterility testing and cryogenic preservation. Transplant Proc 8 (Suppl I): 127–141

Angell WW, Maguire PJ (1990) The effect of stent mounting on tissue valves. Circulation 82 (Suppl III): 763

Angell WW et al. (1991) Effect of stent mounting on tissue valves for aortic valve replacement. J Cardiac Surg 6 (Suppl): 595–599

Antunes MJ et al. (1984) Performance of glutaraldehyde-preserved porcine bioprosthesis as a mitral valve substitute in a young population group. Ann Thorac Surg 37: 387–392

Armiger LC et al. (1983) Histological assessment of orthotopic aortic valve leaflet allografts: its role in selecting graft pretreatment. Pathology 15: 67–73

Badduke BR et al. (1991) Pregnancy and childbearing in a population with biologic valvular prostheses. J Thorac Cardiovasc Surg 102: 179–186

Bank HL, Brockbank KGM (1987) Basic principles of cryobiology. J cardiac Surg 2 (Suppl): 137–143

Barrat-Boyes BG (1964) Homograft aortic valve replacement and aortic incompetence and stenosis. Thorax 19: 131–150

Barrat-Boyes BG (1965a) A method for preparing and inserting a homograft aortic valve. Br J Surg 52: 847–856

Barrat-Boyes BG (1969) Aortic homograft valve replacement: a longterm followup of an initial series of 101 patients. Circulation 40: 763-769

Barrat-Boyes BG (1979) Cardiothoracic surgery in the antipodes. J Thorac Cardiovasc Surg 78: 804-822

Barrat-Boyes BG et al. (1965) Homograft valve replacement for aortic valve disease. Thorax 20: 495–500

Becker RM et al. (1980) Hemodynamic performance of the Ionescu-Shiley prosthesis. J Thorac Cardiovasc Surg 80: 613–620

Billingham ME et al. (1979) Bacterial infection in implanted porcine heterografts. A histopathologic and ultrastructural study. In: Sebening F, Klövekorn WP, Meisner H, Struck E (eds) Bioprosthetic cardial valves. Eberl, Immenstadt, p 281

Bioimplant Services (1991). Heart valve transplant manual, part 2. Leiden

Bloch G, Voulse PR, Poulain II et al. (1982) Mid- and long-term evaluation of porcine bioprosthetic valves; a 6 year experience. In: Cohn LH, Gallucci V (eds) Cardiac bioprostheses, Yorke Medical Books, New York, pp 70–76

Bloomfield P et al. (1986) A prospective evaluation of the Björk-Shiley, Hancock, and Carpentier-Edwards heart valve prostheses. Circulation 73: 1213–1222

Bodnar E et al. (1990) Nonviable aortic homografts. In: Bodnar E (ed) Surgery for heart valve disease. ICR London, pp 494–500

Bolooki H et al. (1983) Failure of Hancock xenograft valve. Importance of valve position (4 to 9 year follow up). Ann Thorac Surg 36: 246–252

Bolooki H et al. (1986) Comparison of long-term results of Carpentier-Edwards and Hancock bioprosthetic valves. Ann Thorac Surg 42: 494–499

Bortolotti U et al. (1980) Left ventricular rupture following mitral valve replacement with a Hancock bioprosthesis. Chest 77: 235–237

Bortolotti U et al. (1982) Pregnancy in patients with a porcine valve bioprosthesis. Am J Cardiol 50: 1051–4

Bortolotti U et al. (1985) Results of reoperation for primary tissue failure of porcine bioprostheses J. Thorac Cardiovasc Surg 90: 564–569

Bortolotti U et al. (1987) Long-term durability of Hancock porcine bioprosthesis following combined mitral and aortic valve replacement: an 11-year experience. Ann Thorac Surg 44: 139–144

Brais MP et al. (1985) Ionescu-Shiley pericardial xenografts: follow-up of up to 6 years. Ann Thorac Surg 39: 105–111

Brockbank KGM, Bank HL (1987) Measurement of postcryopreservation viability. J Cardiac Surg 2 (Suppl): 145–151

Carpentier A et al. (1968) Mitral and tricuspid valve replacement with frame mounted aortic heterografts. J Thorac Cardiovasc Surg 56: 388–394

Carpentier A et al (1969) Biological factors affecting long-term results of valvular heterografts. J Thorac Cardiovasc Surg 58: 467–483

Carpentier A et al. (1982) Continuing improvement in valvular prostheses. J Thorac Cardiovasc Surg 83: 27–42

Carpentier A et al. (1984) Techniques for prevention of calcification of valvular bioprostheses. Circulation 70 (Part 2): I165–I168

Cipriano PR et al (1984) Calcification of aortic versus mitral porcine bioprosthetic heart valves: a radiographic study comparing the amounts of calcific deposits in valves explanted from the same patient. Am J Cardiol 54: 1030–1032

Cobanoglu A et al. (1987) A tri-institutional comparison of tissue and mechanical valves using a patient-oriented definition of "treatment failure". Ann Thorac Surg 43: 245–253

Cohn LH (1979) Bioprosthetic cardiac valves – anticoagulation or not? In: Sebening F, Klövekorn WP, Meisner H, Struck E (eds) Bioprosthetic cardiac valves. Deutsches Herzzentrum, Munich, p 107

Cohn LH et al. (1984) Early and late risk of aortic valve replacement J Thorac Cardiovasc Surg 88: 695–705

Copeland JG et al. (1977) Long-term follow-up after isolated aortic valve replacement. J Thorac Cardiovasc Surg 74: 875–889

Cornhill JF (1977) An aortic–left ventricular pulse duplicator used in testing prosthetic aortic heart valves. J Thorac Cardiovasc Surg 73: 550–562

Cosgrove DM et al. (1985) In vivo hemodynamic comparison of porcine and pericardial valves. J Thorac Cardiovasc Surg 89: 358–368

Craver JM et al. (1978) Late hemodynamic evaluation of Hancock modified orifice aortic bioprosthesis. Circulation 60 (Suppl I): 93

Curcio CA et al. (1981) Calcification of glutaraldehyde-preserved porcine xenografts in young patients. J Thorac Cardiovasc Surg 81: 621–625

Deviri E et al. (1985) Pregnancy after valve replacement with porcine xenograft prosthesis. Surg Gynecol Obstet 160: 437–443

Disesa VJ et al. (1990) Heart transplantation for intractable prosthetic valve endocarditis. J Heart Transplant 9 (2): 142

Douglas PS et al. (1984) Clinical comparison of St. Jude and porcine aortic valve prosthesis. Circulation 72 (Suppl II): 135

Drury PJ et al. (1986) Distribution of flexibility in the porcine aortic root and in cardiac support frames. In: Bodnar E, Yacoub M (eds) Biologic and bioprosthetic valves. Yorke Medical, New York, pp 580–590

Dunn JM (1981) Porcine valve durability in children. Ann Thorac Surg 32: 357–368

Edmunds LH Jr (1982) Thromboembolic complications of current cardiac valvular prostheses. Ann Thorac Surg 34: 96–106

Edmunds LH, Clark RE et al. (1988) Guidelines for reporting morbidity and mortality after cardiac valvular operation. J Thorac Cardiovasc Surg 96: 351–353

Egloff L, Rothlin H, Turina M, Senning A et al. (1980) Isolated aortic valve replacement with the Björk-Shiley tilting disc prosthesis and the porcine bioprosthesis. Eur Heart J 1 (2): 123–127

Farah E et al. (1984) Thromboembolic and hemorrhage risk in mechanical and biologic aortic prosthesis. Eur Heart J 5 (Suppl D): 43

Ferrans VJ et al. (1978) Ultrastructure of Hancock porcine valvular heterografts; pre- and post-implantation changes. Circulation 58 (Suppl I): 10

Ferrans VJ et al. (1980) Calcific deposits in porcine bioprostheses; structure and pathogenesis Am J Cardiol 46: 721–734

Fiddler GI et al. (1983) Calcification of glutaraldehyde preserved porcine and bovine xenograft valves in young children. Ann Thorac Surg 35: 257–261

Fishbein MC et al. (1977) Pathologic findings after cardiac valve replacement with glutaraldehyde-fixed porcine valves. Am J Cardiol 40: 331–337

Fontan F et al. (1976) Comparative study of the Björk-Shiley valve and aortic valve homograft in mitral valve replacement. In: Kalmanson D (ed) The mitral valve. Edward Arnold, London, pp 497–503
Frank S et al. (1973) Natural history of valvular aortic stenosis. Br Heart J 35: 41–46
Gabbay S et al. (1980) In vitro hydrodynamic comparison of St. Jude, Björk-Shiley and Hall-Kaster valves. Trans Am Soc Artif Intern Organs 26: 731
Gabbay S et al. (1984) Hemodynamics and durability of mitral bioprosthesis – an in vitro study. Eur Heart J 65: 5 (Suppl)
Gallo I et al. (1986) Six to ten year follow-up with patients with the Hancock cardiac bioprosthesis. J Thorac Cardiovasc Surg 92: 14–20
Gallucci V et al. (1982) Heart valve replacement with the Hancock bioprosthesis: a 5–11 year follow-up. In: Cohn LH, Gallucci V (eds) Cardiac bioprostheses. Yorke Medical, New York, pp 9–24
Gallucci V et al. (1986) The Hancock porcine valve 15 years later: an analysis of 575 patients. In: Bodnar E, Yacoub M (eds) Biologic and bioprosthetic valves. Yorke Medical, New York, pp 91–97
Gardner TJ et al. (1982) Valve replacement in children: a fifteen-year perspective. J Thorac Cardiovasc Surg 83: 178–185
Gavin JB et al (1973) The histopathology of "fresh" human aortic valve allografts. Thorax 28: 482–488
Geha AS (1987) Long-term outcome of cardiac valve substitutes. Ann Thorac Surg 44: 566–567
Geha AS et al (1979) Late failure of porcine valve heterografts in children. J Thorac Cardiovasc Surg 78: 351–364
Geroulanos S (1985) Bioprothesen. Hans Huber, Bern.
Gonzalez-Lavin L et al. (1984) Thromboembolism in bleeding after mitral valve replacement with porcine valves: influence of thromboembolic risk factors. J Surg Res 35: 508
Gorlin R Gorlin SG (1951) Hydraulic formula for the calculation of the area of stenotic mitral valve, other cardial valves, and central circulatory shunts. Am Heart J 41: 1
Hammermeister KE et al. (1987) Comparison of outcome after valve replacement with a bioprosthesis vs. a mechanical prosthesis: initial 5 year results of a randomized trial. J Am Coll Cardiol 10: 719–732
Hammond GL et al. (1987) Biological versus mechanical valves. J Thorac Cardiovasc Surg 93: 182–198
Hartz RS et al (1986) Eight-year experience with porcine bioprosthetic cardiac valves. J Thorac Cardiovasc Surg 91: 910–917
Hopkins RA (1989a) Historical development of the use of homograft valves. In: Hopkins RA (ed) Cardiac reconstructions with allograft valves. Springer, New York, pp 3–13
Hopkins RA (1989b) Rationale for use of cryopreserved allograft tissues for cardiac reconstructions. In: Hopkins RA (ed) Cardiac reconstructions with allograft valves. Springer, New York, pp 15-20
Horstkotte D et al. (1983) Central hemodynamics at rest and during exercise after mitral valve replacement with different prostheses. Circulation 68 (Suppl II): 161
Human DG et al. (1982) Mitral valve replacement in children. J Thorac Cardiovasc Surg 83: 873-877
Hume M et al. (1970) Venous thrombosis and pulmonary embolism. Harvard Press, Cambridge, p 455
Hurst JW (ed) (1982) The heart, artery and veins. McGraw-Hill, New York.
Ilbawi MN et al. (1986) Long-term results of porcine valve insertion for pulmonary regurgitation following repair of tetralogy of Fallot. Ann Thorac Surg 41: 478–482
Ionescu MI (1986) The pericardial xenograft valve: mode of failure and possible remedial developments. In: Bodnar E, Yacoub M (eds) Biologic and bioprosthetic valves: proceedings of the third international symposium. Yorke Medical, New York, pp 245–251
Ionescu MI, Tandon AP, Saunders NR, Chidambaram M, Smith DR (1982) Clinical durability of the pericardial xenograft valve: 11 years experience. In: Cohn LH, Gallucci V (eds) Cardiac bioprostheses. Yorke Medical, New York, pp 42–60
Ishihara T et al. (1981) Occurrence and the significance of endothelial cells in implanted porcine bioprosthetic valves. Am J Cardiol 48: 443–454
Ivert TSA et al. (1984) Prosthetic valve endocarditis. Circulation 69: 223–227
Jaffe WM et al. (1989) Doppler echocardiography in the assessment of the homograft aortic valve. Am J Cardiol 63: 1466–1470
Jaffe WM et al. (1990) Rest and exercise hemodynamics of 20 to 23 mm allograft, Medtronic intact (porcine) and St.-Jude medical valves in the aortic position. J Thorac Cardiovasc Surg 100: 167–174
Jamieson WRE et al. (1989) Cardiac valve replacement in the elderly: clinical performance of biological prostheses. Ann Thorac Surg 48: 173–185
Janusz MT et al. (1982) Experience with the Carpentier-Edwards porcine valve prosthesis in 700 patients. Ann Thorac Surg 34: 625–633

Johnson A et al. (1978) Evaluation of the in vivo function of the Hancock porcine xenograft in the aortic position. J Thorac Cardiovasc Surg 75: 600-605
Jones EL (1989) Freehand homograft aortic valve replacement – the learning curve: a technical analysis of the first 31 patients. Ann Thorac Surg 48: 26–32
Joyce LD et al. (1984) Comparison of porcine valve xenografts with mechanical prostheses. J Thorac Cardiovasc Surg 88: 102–113
Khaghani A et al. (1976) Patient status 10 years or more after aortic valve replacement using antibiotic sterilized aortic homografts. In: Bodnar E, Yacoub M (eds) Biologic and bioprosthetic valves. Yorke Medical Books, New York, pp 38–46
Khan SS et al. (1990) Differences in Hancock and Carpentier-Edwards porcine xenograft aortic valve hemodynamics. Circulation 82 (Suppl IV): 117–124
Kirklin JW, Barrat-Boyes BG (1986) Cardiac surgery. Churchill Livingstone, New York, pp 421-422
Kirklin JW et al. (1987) Intermediate term fate of cryopreserved allograft and xenograft valve conduits. Ann Thorac Surg 44: 598–606
Kirklin JW et al. (1989) Surgical treatment of prosthetic valve endocarditis with homograft aortic valve replacement. J Cardiac Surg 4: 340–347
Knight JP et al. (1984) Bacterial associated porcine heterograft heart valve calcification. Am J Cardiol 53: 370–372
Konertz W et al. (1991) Pulmonalklappen-Allograft in Aortenposition – Frühergebnisse bei 30 konsekutiven Patienten. Z Herz-Thorax-Gefäßchir 5: 68–74
Konertz W et al. (1992) Technique of aortic valve replacement with the Edwards stentless aortic bioprothesis 2500. Eur J Cardiothorac Surg 6: 274–277
Kwong K-H et al. (1967) Experimental use of immunosuppression in aortic valve homografts and heterografts. J Thorac Cardiovasc Surg 54: 199–207
Laks H et al. (1980) Left atrial-left ventricular conduit for relief of congenital mitral stenosis in infancy. J Thorac Cardiovasc Surg 80: 782–787
Lam CR et al. (1952) An experimental study of aortic valve homografts. Surg Gynecol Obstet 94: 129–135
Lang RM et al (1985) Pregnancy and heart disease. Clin Perinatol 12: 551–567
Lange PL, Hopkins RA (1989) Allograft valve banking: techniques and technology. In: Hopkins RA (ed) Cardiac reconstructions with allograft valves. Springer, New York Berlin Heidelberg, pp 37–63
Lansing AM et al (1983) Left atrial-left ventricular bypass for congenital mitral stenosis. Ann Thorac Surg 35: 667–669
Ledingham SJM et al. (1988) Bioprosthetic valve excision without replacement in the tricuspid position in a patient with Libman-Sacks endocarditis. J Cardiovasc Surg 29: 356–359
Lentz DJ et al. (1982) Inhibition of mineralization of glutaraldehyde-fixed Hancock bioprosthetic heart valves. In Cohn LH, Gallucci V (eds) Cardiac bioprostheses. Yorke Medical, New York, p 306
Levy RJ et al. (1987) Prevention of leaflet calcification of bioprosthetic heart valves with diphosphonate injection therapy. J Thorac Cardiovasc Surg 94: 551–557
Liotta D et al. (1978) Experiencia clinica conjunta con bioprotesis de bajio perfil. 6 congresso nacional de cirurgia cardiaca. Guaruja, Sao Paulo, Brazil
Louis IS et al. (1991) Effects of warm ischemia following harvesting of allograft cardiac valves. Eur J Cardiothorac Surg 5: 458–465
Lurie AJ et al. (1977) Hemodynamic assessment of the glutaraldehyde preseved porcine heterograft in the aortic and mitral positions. Circulation 56 (Suppl II) 104–110
Lytle BW et al. (1989) Primary isolated aortic valve replacement. J Thorac cardiovasc Surg 97: 675–694
Magilligan DJ (1987) Porcine bioprostheses in Cardiac surgery. In: Crawford TA (ed) current heart valve Prostheses state of the art reviews, vol 1, no 2. Hanley & Belfus, INC. Philadelphia, pp 269–284
Magilligan DJ et al. (1983) Fate of a second porcine bioprosthetic valve. J Thorac Cardiovasc Surg 85: 362–370
Magilligan DJ et al. (1985) The porcine bioprosthesis valve: twelve years later. J Thorac Cardiovasc Surg 89: 499–507
Magilligan DJ et al (1989) The porcine bioprosthetic heart valve: experience at 15 years. Ann Thorac Surg 48: 324–330
Mair R et al. (1993) Aortenklappenersatz mit kryokonservierten Pulmonalklappenallografts. Thorac Cardiovasc Surg 40 (in press)
Marshall WG et al (1983) Late results after mitral valve replacement with the Björk-Shiley and porcine prostheses. J Thorac Cardiovasc Surg 85: 902–910

McGiffin DC et al. (1988) Longterm results of the viable cryopreserved allograft aortic valve: continuing evidence for superior valve durability. J Cardiac Surg 3 (Suppl): 289–296
McGoon MD et al. (1984) Aortic and mitral valve incompetence: long-term follow-up (10 to 19 years) of patients treated with the Starr-Edwards prosthesis. J Am Coll Cardiol 3: 930
McGregor CGA et al (1976) Tissue culture, protein and collagen synthesis in antibiotic sterilized canine heart valves. Cardiovasc Res 10: 389–395
Menarche P et al. (1986) Selective blockade of collagen calcium binding sites: new process to decrease bioprosthetic valvular calcification. In: Bodnar E, Yacoub M (eds) Biologic and bioprosthetic valves. Yorke Medical, New York, p 478
Milano AD et al. (1988) Performance of the Hancock porcine bioprosthesis following aortic valve replacement: considerations based on a 15-year experience. Ann Thorac Surg 46: 216–222
Milano AD et al. (1989) Aortic valve replacement with the Hancock standard, Björh-Shiley, and Lillehei-Kaster prostheses. J Thorac Cardiovasc Surg 98: 37–47
Miller DC, Shumway NE (1987) "Fresh" aortic allografts: longterm results with freehand aortic valve replacement. J Cardiac Surg 2 (Suppl): 185–191
Miller DC et al. (1982) Durability of porcine xenograft valves and conduits in children. Circulation 66 (Suppl I): 172
Miller DC et al. (1987) Ten year clinical experience in 1681 patients with one type of tissue valve. In: Starek PJK (ed) Heart valve replacement and reconstruction. Year Book, Chicago
Mitchell RS et al. (1986) Significant patient related determinants of prosthetic valve performance. J Thorac Cardiovasc Surg 91: 807–817
Morgan RJ, Davis JT, Fraker TD et al. (1985) Current status of valve prostheses. Surg Clin North Am 65: 699–720
Murray G (1956) Homologous aortic valve segments transplants. A surgical treatment for aortic and mitral insufficiency. Angiology 7: 466–471
Myers TJ et al. (1978) Hemolytic anemia associated with heterograft replacement of the mitral valve. J Thorac Cardiovasc Surg 76: 214–215
Nistal F et al. (1986) Primary tissue valve degeneration in glutaraldehyde-preserved porcine bioprostheses: Hancock I vs. Carpentier-Edwards at 4- to 7-year follow-up. Ann Thorac Surg 42: 568–572
Nudelman I et al (1980) Repeated mitral valve replacement in the growing child with congenital mitral valve disease. J Thorac Cardiovasc Surg 79: 765-769
Nunez L et al. (1982) Aspirin or coumadin as the drug of choice for valve replacement with porcine bioprosthesis. Ann Thorac Surg 33: 354–358
Nunez L et al (1983) Pregnancy in 20 patients with bioprosthetic valve replacement. Chest 84: 26–28
Nunez L et al. (1984) Prevention of thromboembolism using aspirin after mitral valve replacement with porcine bioprosthesis. Ann Thorac Surg 37: 84–87
O'Brien MF et al (1987a) A comparison of aortic valve replacement with viable cryopreserved and fresh allograft valves, with a note on chromosomal studies. J Thorac Cardiovasc Surg 94: 812–823
O'Brien MF et al. (1987b) The viable cryopreserved allograft aortic valve. J Cardiac Surg 2 (Suppl): 153–167
O'Brien MF et al. (1988) A study of the cells in the explanted viable cryopreserved allograft valve. J Cardiac Surg 3 (Suppl): 279–287
O'Brien MF et al. (1991) Allograft aortic valve replacement: longterm comparative clinical analysis of the viable cryopreserved and antibiotic 4°C stored valves. J Cardiac Surg 6 (Suppl): 534 543
Oyer PE et al. (1979) Long-term evaluation of the porcine xenograft bioprostheses. J Thorac Cardiovasc Surg 78: 343–350
Oyer PE et al. (1984) Thromboembolic risk and durability of the Hancock bioprosthetic cardiac valve. Eur Heart J 5 (Suppl D): 81
Pansini G et al (1990) Morphological comparison of primary tissue failure in porcine mitral and aortic bioprostheses in the same patient. Eur J Cardiothorac Surg 4: 431–434
Pass HI et al (1984) Cardiac valve prostheses in children without anticoagulation. J Thorac Cardiovasc Surg 87: 832–835
Pelletier LC et al. (1989) Porcine vs. pericardial bioprostheses: a comparison of late results in 1593 patients. Ann Thorac Surg 47: 352–361
Perier P et al. (1986) Decreasing operative risk in isolated valve re-replacement. In: Bodnar E, Yacoub M (eds) Biologic and bioprosthetic valves. Yorke Medical, New York, pp 333–338
Perier P et al. (1989) A 10-year comparison of mitral valve replacement with Carpentier-Edwards and Hancock porcine bioprostheses. Ann Thorac Surg 48: 54–59

Reul GJ et al. (1985) Valve failure with the Ionescu-Shiley bovine pericardial bioprosthesis: analysis of 2680 patients. J Vasc Surg 2: 192–204

Rhodes GR, McIntosh CL (1977) Evaluation of hemolysis following replacement of atrioventricular valves with porcine xenograft (Hancock) valves. J Thorac Cardiovasc Surg 73: 312–315

Ross DN (1962) Homograft replacement of the aortic valve. Lancet II: 487

Ross D (1987) Panel discussion II. J Cardiac Surg 2 (Suppl): 222

Ross D (1988) Pulmonary valve autotransplantation (the Ross operation). J Cardiac Surg 3: 313–319

Ross D (1991) Technique of aortic valve replacement with a homograft: orthotopic replacement. Ann Thorac Surg 52: 154–156

Ross DN, Shabbo FP, Wain WH et al. (1979) Longterm results of double valve replacement with aortic homografts. In: Sebening F, Klövekorn WP, Meisner H, Struck E (eds) Bioprosthetic cardiac valves. Deutsches Herzzentrum Munich, printed by Eberl GmbtH, Immenstadt/Allgäu, pp 143–151

Rossiter SJ et al. (1978) Prosthetic valve endocarditis. Comparison of heterograft tissue valves and mechanical valves. J Thorac Cardiovasc Surg 76: 795–803

Rothlin et al. (1977) Langzeitverlauf nach Aorten- und Mitralklappenersatz. Herz 2: 268

Rygg IH, Ladefoged J, Grgensen K, Elling F et al. (1986) Prevention of protein insudation and the related exterioration of bioprosthetic materials by incorporation of heparin-protein coupler. In: Bodnar E, Yacoub M (eds) Biologic and bioprosthetic valves. Yorke Medical, New York, pp. 462–478

Sanders SP et al. (1990) Use of Hancock porcine xenografts in children and adolescents. Am J Cardiol 46: 429–438

Schachner A et al. (1984) Prosthetic valve replacement in infants and children. J Cardiovasc Surg 25: 537–544

Schaff HV et al. (1984) Late results after Starr-Edwards valve replacement in children. J Thorac Cardiovasc Surg 88: 583–589

Schoen FJ et al. (1983) Long-term failure rate and morphologic correlations in porcine bioprosthetic heart valves. Am J Cardiol 51: 957–64

Schoen FJ et al. (1984) Bioprosthetic heart valve failure: pathology and pathogenesis. Cardiol Clin 2: 717–39

Schryer PJ et al. Tomasek ER, Starr JA, Wright JTM (1986) Anticalcification effect of glutaraldehyde-preserved valve tissue stored for increasing time in glutaraldehyde. In: Bodnar E, Yacoub M (eds) Biologic and bioprosthetic valves. Yorke Medical, New York, pp 471–477

Senning A, Turina M (1972) Aortic valve replacement with free fascia lata grafts. Clinical experience and late evaluation of 141 consecutive cases. In: Ionescu MI, et al. (eds) Biological tissue in heart valve replacement. Butterworths, London

Silver MM et al. (1980) Calcification in porcine xenograft valves in Children. Am J Cardiol 45: 685

Spital G et al. (1992) Aortenklappenersatz mit Pulmonalisallograft – Perioperative Komplikationen im Vergleich mit Kunstklappen. Z Herz-Thorax-Gefäßchirurgie 6: 17–21

Stein PD et al. (1985) Effect of warfarin on calcification of spontaneously degenerated porcine bioprosthetic valves. J Thorac Cardiovasc Surg 90: 119–125

Stelzer P, Elkins C (1989) Homograft valves and conduits: applications in cardiac surgery. Curr Probl Surg 26: 381–452

Stinson EB et al. (1977) Long-term experience with porcine aortic valve xenografts. J Thorac Cardiovasc Surg 73: 54–63

Teoh KH et al. (1990) Clinical and Doppler echocardiographic evaluation of bioprosthetic valve failure after 10 years. Circulation 82 (Suppl IV): 110–116

Teply JF et al. (1981) The ultimate prognosis after valve replacement: an assessment at twenty years. Ann Thorac Surg 32: 111–119

Thandroyen FT et al. (1980) Severe calcification of glutaraldehyde-preserved porcine xenografts in children. Am J Cardiol 45: 690–696

Thubrikar MJ et al. (1986) Patterns of calcific deposits in operatively excised stenotic or purely regurgitant aortic valves and their relation to mechanical stress. Am J Cardiol 58: 304–308

Valente M et al. (1985) Ultrastructural substrates of dystrophic calcification in porcine bioprosthetic valve failure. Am J Pathol 119: 12–21

Van der Kamp AWM, Nauter J (1979) Fibroblast function and maintenance of aortic valve matrix. Cardiovasc Res 13: 167–173

Van der Kamp AWM et al. (1981) Preservation of aortic heart valves with maintenance of cell viability. J Surg Res 30: 47–56

Vejlsted H et al. (1984) Clinical experience with porcine xenografts in the mitral position. Scand J

Thorac Cardiovasc Surg 18: 33
Warnes CA et al. (1983) Comparison of late degenerative changes in porcine bioprostheses in mitral and aortic valve position in the same patient. Am J Cardiol 51: 965–968
Wideman FE et al. (1981) The hospital mortality of re-replacement of the aortic valve. Incremental risk factors. J Thorac Cardiovasc Surg 82: 692–698
Wild LM et al. (1980) Left ventricular laceration due to stented prosthesis. Chest 77: 216–217
Williams DB et al. (1982) Porcine heterograft valve replacement in children. J Thorac Cardiovasc Surg 84: 446–450
Woo YR et al. (1986) In vitro fluid dynamic characteristics of aortic bioprostheses: old versus new. Life Support Systems 4: 63
Wright JS et al. (1981) Mitral valve bypass by valved conduit. Ann thorac Surg 32: 294–296
Wright JTM (1979) Hydrodynamic evaluation of tissue heart valves. In: Ionescu MI (ed) Tissue heart valves. Butterworths, London, p 55
Wright JTM et al. (1982) Hancock II – an improved bioprosthesis. In: Cohn LH, Gallucci V (eds) Cardiac bioprostheses: proceedings of the second international symposium. Yorke Medical, New York, pp 425–444
Yankah C, Hetzer R (1989) Valve selection and choice in surgery of endocarditis. J Cardiac Surg 4: 324–330
Yankah AC et al. (1986) Identification of surface antigens of endothelial cells of fresh preserved heart allografts. Thorac Cardiovasc Surg 34 (Special Issue I): 97
Yankah AC et al. (1987) Transplantation of aortic and pulmonary allografts enhanced viability of endothelial cells by cryopreservation, importance of histocompatiblity. J Cardiac Surg 2 (Suppl): 209–220
Zusman DR et al. (1981) Hemodynamic and clinical evaluation of the Hancock modified orifice bioprosthesis. Circulation 64 (Suppl II): 189

Mechanical and Other Problems of Artificial Valves

M.M. BLACK and P.J. DRURY

1 Introduction

Artificial heart valves were first used in the late 1950s and early 1960s. Following the success of these early implants, the replacement of diseased or damaged valves with prosthetic substitutes rapidly became accepted as a routine clinical procedure. During the next 30 years, the field of heart valve replacement became one of the major growth areas in cardiac surgery, and it is estimated that over 150 000 valves are replaced in the world each year. Following an initial steady increase in the number of implants, the requirement for valve substitutes in the United States and Europe is beginning to stabilise. World demand for these devices, however, continues to expand at a rate of 10% –12% per year.

There is no perfect artificial valve. Over the years, there have been many developments in valve design and several hundred different configurations have been considered. The majority of these have been abandoned due to problems discovered during preclinical evaluation (BLACK et al. 1983a). The ideal valve should be durable and efficient in terms of minimal resistance to forward flow and minimal backflow. In addition, it should not stimulate thrombosis or cause damage to the cellular or molecular components of the blood. As no artificial valve completely satisfies these criteria, the choice of a replacement is necessarily a

Current Topics in Pathology
Volume 86. Ed. C. Berry

compromise chosen to meet the needs of an individual patient. The surgeon is faced with a difficult decision when selecting an appropriate valve and comparative information on valve performance is essential if the correct choice of prosthesis is to be made.

Human heart valves are passive devices that open and close in response to changes in pressure to maintain the unidirectional flow of blood through the heart (Fig. 1). When functioning normally, they are extremely efficient, having minimal resistance to forward flow and allowing only trivial backflow when closed. In certain situations, the efficiency of the valves may be severely compromised. Pathological changes may result in a restriction of the free opening of a valve (stenosis) or loss of competence allowing backflow through the closed valve (regurgitation). In extreme cases, a valve may be both regurgitant and stenotic. Mitral and aortic valves are most frequently affected. In all instances, the work load for the heart is increased and, depending on the severity of the lesion and the ability of the heart to adapt to the increasing work, cardiac function may be compromised. For patients with severely symptomatic valve disease, valve replacement offers an improved cardiovascular function, long-term survival and quality of life (SCHOEN 1987).

2 Development of Artificial Heart Valves

Several pathological conditions result in damage to and disease of valves in the heart. Although the aetiology of these conditions is well understood, only in the last few decades have significant improvements been made in the therapeutic procedures for such conditions.

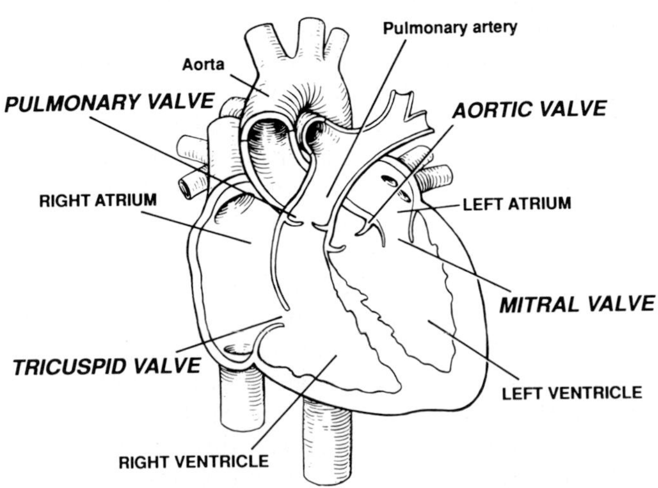

Fig. 1. The valves of the heart

In 1951, HUFNAGEL showed that synthetic materials could be tolerated in the bloodstream and that his caged-ball prosthesis, placed in the descending aorta, functioned in many patients for long periods. Three years later, Gibbon described the technique of extracorporeal circulation, which made total or partial valve replacement a viable therapeutic option (GIBBON 1954). Replacement of diseased or malfunctioning heart valves with artificial counterparts is now performed every day, and many developments have taken place in this field in the last 30 years. In the early days of valve surgery, few valve designs were available; the most common was the ball-and-cage configuration developed by the surgeon/engineer partnership of Starr and Edwards. This valve enabled many patients to enjoy a good quality of life, and although this design has been superseded by that of many newer valves, it is still in use today, more than 25 years after its introduction into clinical practice. A Starr-Edwards valve (Fig. 2) bears no resemblance to its normal biological counterpart; thus, although it was a successful replacement in many cases, it resulted in significant evidence of valve-related complications. The search for improved prostheses was therefore soon taken up by many surgical and engineering centres in the Western world.

The most obvious step was the concept of a replacement valve that more closely resembled the natural valve. Initially, the search for such a valve resulted in the use of the homograft valve, a normal human aortic valve removed at post-mortem examination and treated with appropriate antibiotics so that it could be transplanted into a suitable recipient. This technique was reported as early as 1962 (ROSS 1962). It is still used today and produces excellent long-term results. As with all organ–donor situations, the number of homografts available is severely limited, thus restricting the number of procedures that can be undertaken.

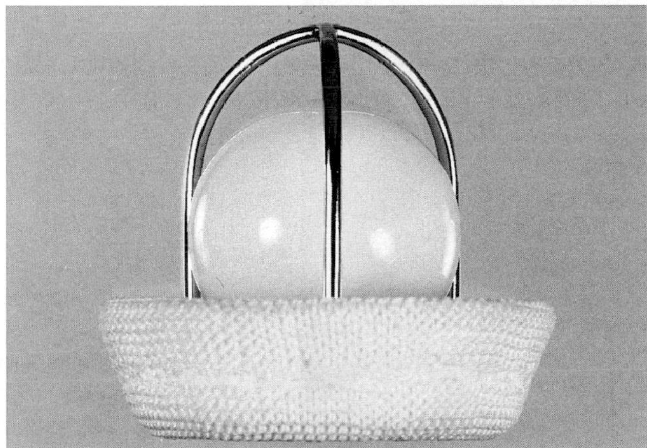

Fig. 2. Starr-Edwards aortic valve prosthesis

The largest number of valve replacements involve the use of some form of artificial valve. As already noted, there have been many developments in the design of these valves.

2.1 Mechanical Valves

Existing commercial prosthetic valves can be divided into two groups: mechanical valves, which are fabricated exclusively from materials of synthetic origin, and bioprosthetic valves, made from a combination of chemically treated animal tissue and synthetic materials. Further subdivisions may be made within these two basic categories. Mechanical valves can be of caged-ball, tilting-disc or bileaflet designs while bioprostheses can be of porcine or pericardial type (Fig. 3). Porcine

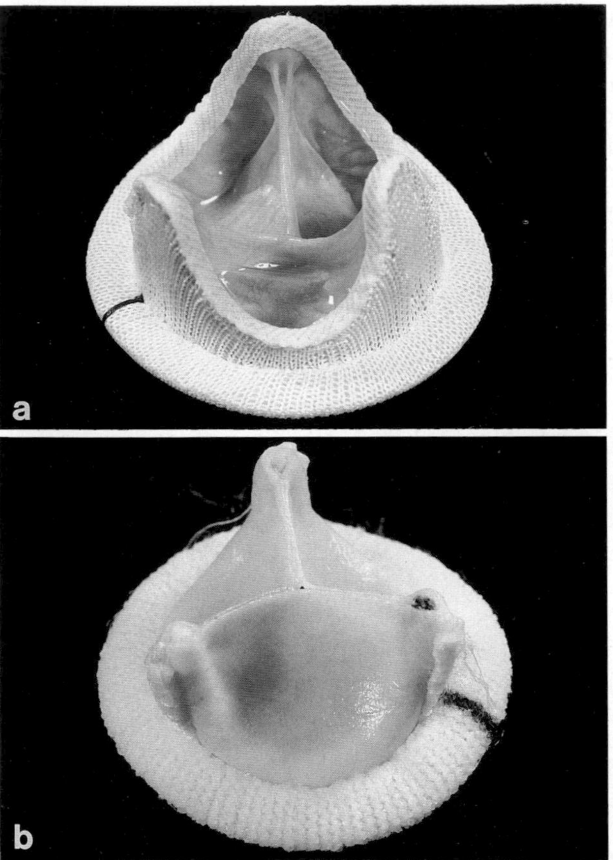

Fig. 3. a Carpentier-Edwards porcine bioprosthesis. **b** Ionescu-Shiley pericardial bioprosthesis

bioprostheses are manufactured from pig aortic valves while pericardium valves are made from bovine pericardium. In both cases, the tissue is chemically stabilised and the valve structure is supported by a frame of synthetic material.

The Starr-Edwards ball-and-cage valve (Fig. 2) was designed to solve a clinical problem in a practical way rather than to imitate the normal anatomy or the responsive function of natural valves. This form of valve replacement was first reported by STARR in 1960, and, as mentioned above, the valve is still considered a relatively safe and effective device. Since 1960 it has been modified to improve performance in terms of reduced haemolysis and thromboembolism. These changes have not affected the overall design, but have concentrated rather on the materials and techniques of its construction. Variations of the caged-ball valve have been produced, notably the Smeloff-Cutter, Magovern-Cromie and Braunwald-Cutter valves. None of these devices, nor any other designs of caged occluder valves, has displaced the Starr-Edwards valve as the preferred prosthesis in this category; even after more than 30 years of valve development, this model remains the valve of choice for many surgeons. Its durability and haemodynamic performance are well established, but the need for chronic anticoagulation therapy imposes an ever-present risk. However, it is no longer the most popular mechanical valve; its use has been superseded by use of tilting-disc or hinged leaflet valves.

The most significant development in mechanical valve design occurred in 1968 with the introduction of the Wada-Cutter tilting-disc valve (WADA et al. 1969). The design of this low-profile valve involved the concept of a freely floating disc that, in the open position, tilted to an angle depending on the design of the disc-retaining struts. The pressure drop across this valve was much lower than could be achieved with the caged-ball valve, but because of catastrophic thrombosis and wear of the Teflon disc, which produced severe valvular regurgitation or fatal disc embolisation, use of this disc was abandoned. Two new tilting-disc designs, the Björk-Shiley and

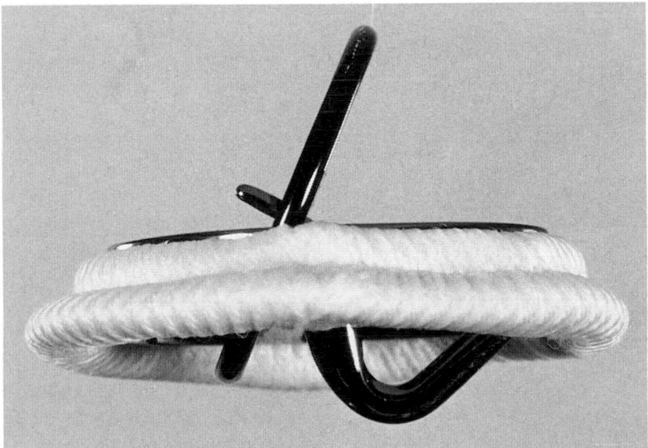

Fig. 4. Medtronic-Hall prosthesis

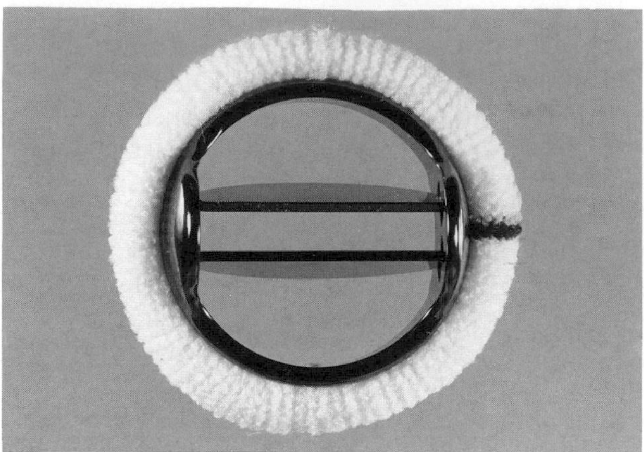

Fig. 5. St. Jude Medical bileaflet prosthesis

Lillehei-Kaster valves, which were based on the same design but incorporate a pyrolytically coated carbon disc, were introduced clinically in 1969 and 1970, respectively. In both of these valves the closed configuration allowed the occluder to fit into the circumference of the inflow ring with virtually no overlap, reducing mechanical damage to erythrocytes. Tilting-disc valves remain popular, with many various improvements having been made to the original designs. These improvements have concentrated on either alterations to the disc geometry, as in the Björk-Shiley Convexo-Concave valve, or to the disc-retaining mechanism, as with the Björk-Shiley Monostrut, the Omniscience and the Medtronic-Hall valves (Fig. 4), this last device having superseded the highly successful Lillehei-Kaster valve. An interesting development in this category of valves has been the bileaflet format, notably the St. Jude and Duromedics valves (Figs. 5, 6). These valves

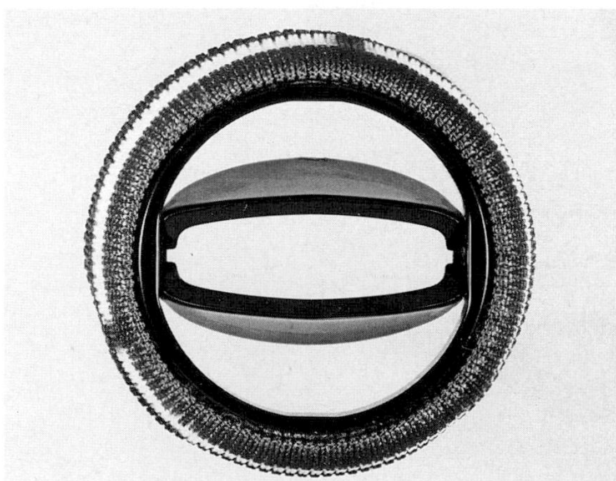

Fig. 6. Edwards Duromedics bileaflet prosthesis

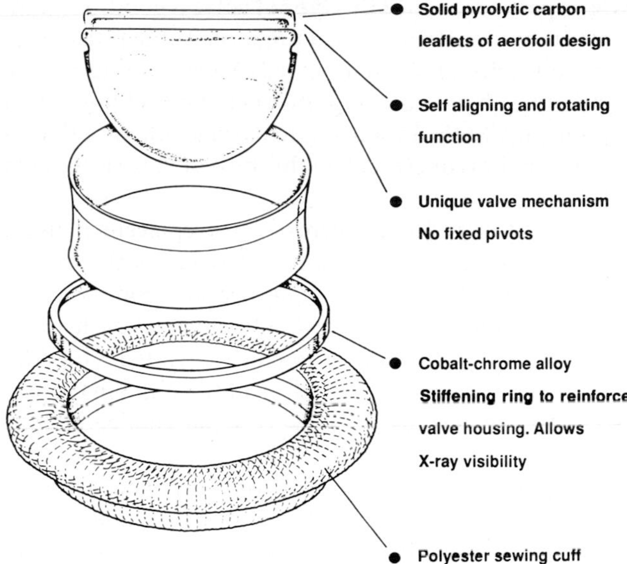

Fig. 7. Components of the Jyros bileaflet prosthesis

incorporate two semicircular, hinged, pyrolytic carbon occluders which, in the open position, provide minimal disturbance to flow.

The latest valve to join this group is the Jyros prosthesis. This valve is of bileaflet configuration and made from solid homogeneous pyrolytic carbon. The design has a number of unique features including aerodynamic geometry of leaflets and valve housing. In addition the valve mechanism does not comprise fixed pivot points but is designed such that the leaflets can rotate and have a self-aligning action which responds to blood flow. A schema of the valve components is shown as Fig. 7.

2.2 Tissue Valves

A major disadvantage associated with use of mechanical valves is the need for chronic anticoagulation therapy to prevent thrombosis and thromboembolic complications. Furthermore, the haemodynamic performance of the best mechanical valve devices differs significantly from that of normal heart valves. An alternative approach in the development of replacement heart valves was the concept of a central orifice, leaflet configuration using naturally occurring human or animal tissues.

In 1962, Ross reported the first implantation of an aortic homograft valve, that is, a human aortic valve removed from a cadaver and preserved in an antibiotic solution. The overall performance of this type of valve is good, as might be expected, because the valve is optimal from both a functional and a structural point of view. It can respond to and allow deformations in the surrounding cardiac tissue and, in the open position, enables central unobstructed blood flow. As a result, such valves are less damaging to the blood and to cardiac function than is the rigid mechanical valve. The obvious drawback to this type of valve is that the supply is limited.

In 1969, Kaiser and Hancock described a new form of valve replacement using an explanted, chemically treated, porcine aortic valve mounted on a cloth-covered metal or plastic frame (Kaiser et al. 1969). This type of valve became commercially available in 1971 as the Hancock porcine bioprosthesis. Other valves of this type have since been produced, the most popular models used in the United Kingdom being the Carpentier-Edwards and, prior to its withdrawal from the market in 1990, the Wessex Medical porcine valves (Figs. 8, 9). Less popular models include the Liotta, Xenomedica and Biocor valves.

Other biological tissues, of both human and animal origin, have been used to replace malfunctioning valves. The most noteworthy of these include human fascia lata, human pulmonary valves and bovine pericardium. The fascia lata valve was constructed at the time of operation using the patient's own living tissue. This valve was first developed by Senning in 1966, and early results were encouraging. However, by 1978 use of the valve had been discontinued for several reasons. Most important among these were the crude manufacturing technique and the observation that, in the long term, the enriched environment of total

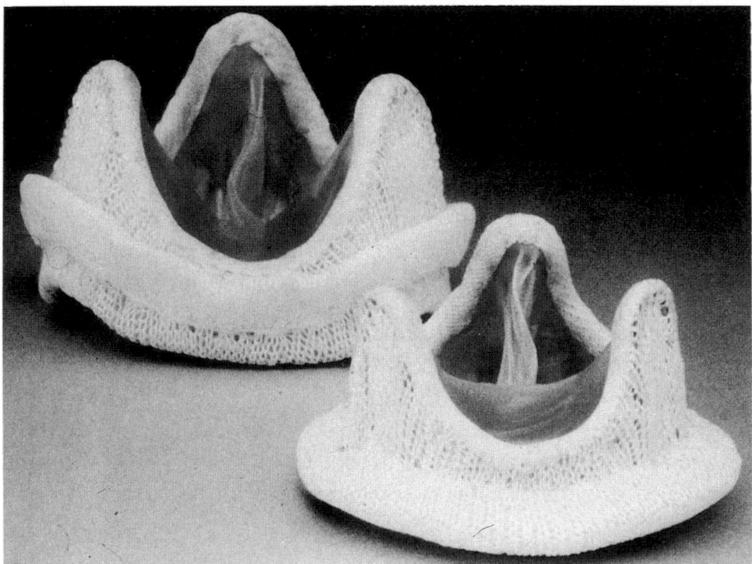

Fig. 8. Carpentier-Edwards porcine bioprosthesis showing mitral and aortic sewing cuffs

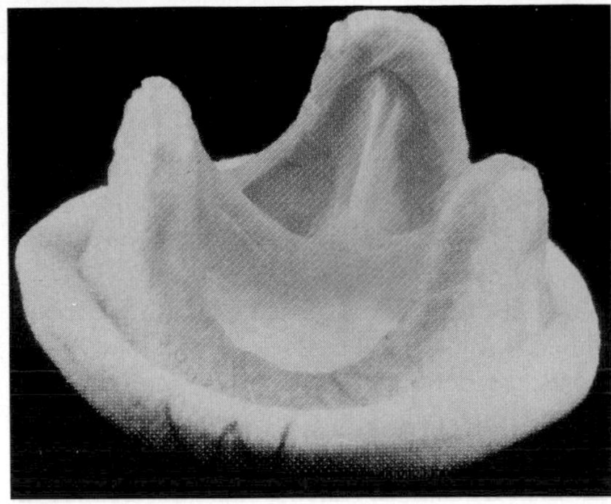

Fig. 9. Wessex Medical porcine bioprosthesis with pig pericardium trim

immersion in blood caused this living tissue to grow and distort in an attempt to conform to the stresses imposed upon it. Transplantation of a living valve from the pulmonary position to the aortic position within the same person is possible because the two valves are structurally and functionally the same. This pulmonary autograft operation was first described by Ross in 1967, and studies show that such valves remain viable and function in their new position without degenerating for as long as 13 years. The important features of this valve are that it is living, autogenous and of optimal design.

The implantation of valves constructed from bovine pericardium has been successful. Such valves are usually formed by moulding fresh tissue to a tricuspid configuration around a support frame. While firmly held in this position, the tissue is fixed with glutaraldehyde. Until its withdrawal from the market in 1987, the most popular valve of this type was the Ionescu-Shiley valve, which was introduced into clinical use in 1976.

Despite the generally satisfactory haemodynamic performance of tissue valves, recent reports on clinical experience with these valves increasingly indicate time-dependent structural changes such as calcification and leaflet wear, leading to valve failure and subsequent replacement (Lawford et al. 1987; Ferrans et al. 1978; Yoganathan 1982). The problem of valve leaflet calcification is now more prevalent in children and young adults. Therefore, tissue valves are rarely used in such patients at the present time. These problems have not been eliminated by the glutaraldehyde tanning methods so far employed, and it is not easy to see how these drawbacks are to be overcome, unless either living autologous tissue is used or the original structure of the collagen and elastin is chemically enhanced. On the latter point there is, as yet, much room for further work. For instance, the fixing of calf pericardium under tension during the moulding of the valve cusps will inevitably produce "locked-in" stresses during fixation, thus changing the mechanical properties of the tissue. A valve configuration which does not involve fixation moulding of the cusps would be advantageous.

The design of a new flexible leaflet valve, presently being developed by Black and Co-workers in Sheffield, allows the valve cusps to be formed using fully fixed, unstressed pericardium (Black et al. 1982). Furthermore, this valve is specifically designed for the mitral position and is consequently of a bicuspid form. The design also incorporates a differentially flexible frame. This allows the base ring to deform from circular in diastole to an approximate D-shape in systole, thus reproducing the physiological behaviour of the normal mitral valve annulus during the cardiac cycle.

There are also attempts to develop leaflet valves from man-made materials such as block-copolymers or modified polyurethanes (Reul 1984). The major advantages of such a valve type would be better reproducibility and cost. The currently tested valve exhibits sufficient fatigue life of more than 400 million cycles and good haemodynamics but, on the other hand, also shows severe leaflet calcification after implantation times of more than 100 days in calves. It is expected that these problems will be reduced by further modifications of the material and/or by using new materials. As with mechanical valves, much useful information can be obtained from in vitro studies such as those described in the next section. In particular, accelerated wear systems yield valuable information on the long-term durability of this type of valve relative to mechanical stressing.

3 Hydrodynamic Performance

Each type of valve demonstrates different advantages and disadvantages (Black et al. 1987a). All artificial valves present some degree of obstruction to forward flow and, hence, are less efficient than the healthy natural valve. In addition, the degree of reflux associated with certain types of prosthetic valve is often considerably greater than that of its biological counterpart. In fact, a small reverse flow is often designed into many mechanical prostheses. This enhances closure and prevents thrombus formation by providing a natural washing action.

While a true assessment of valve performance can ultimately only be obtained from the results of long-term clinical studies, the value of preclinical assessment must not be underestimated. Indeed, such tests must be regarded as an essential prerequisite to the introduction of any new valve model. One problem encountered by all valve evaluators is the difficulty of comparing data from different test centres. The major problem lies in the number of different test regimens employed; each test centre follows its own protocols. Hydrodynamic tests, including both steady and pulsatile flow studies, are useful indicators of the fluid mechanical performance of a valve. Abnormal flow dynamics may be, at least in part, responsible for a substantial number of clinical complications. However, it is important to appreciate that the interpretation of such test results must be approached with caution and their limitations recognised when extrapolating to the in vivo situation (Tindale et al. 1982).

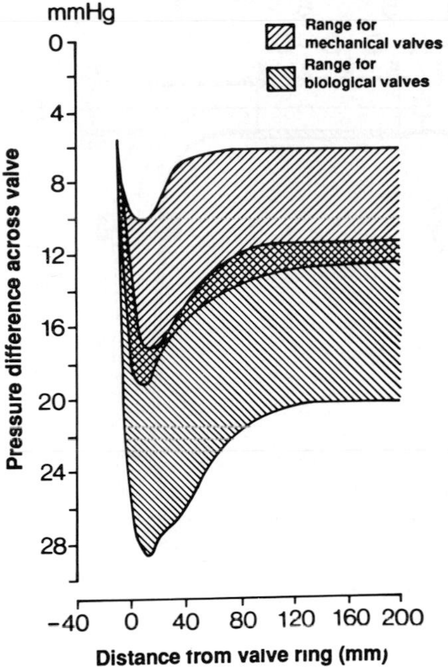

Fig. 10. Axial variation of pressure difference across mechanical and biological valvular prostheses

3.1 Steady Flow Tests

These studies, where the effects of the open valve orifice are investigated at different flow rates, are by far the simplest to perform since they do not involve the need to simulate the pulsatile nature of the cardiac cycle. The pressure difference across a valve can be measured over a range of flow rates, from which various parameters such as effective orifice area and discharge coefficient can be derived. It is essential that the sites at which pressure measurements are made both upstream and downstream of the valve are standardised (CLARK 1976). In the case of aortic valve substitutes, several downstream pressure measurements must be made at different axial locations since, due to the phenomenon of "pressure recovery", an axial variation in the measured pressure difference will occur. This phenomenon is well known in fluid mechanics from the study of flow through constricting orifices and can be explained by the interchanges between kinetic and potential energy of the fluid which occur due to the restrictive nature of the orifice. An illustration of this effect for both mechanical and bioprosthetic valves is shown in Fig. 10.

A good example of a steady flow apparatus for replacement aortic valve testing is that used in the Helmholtz Institute at Aachen (REUL and BLACK 1984) (Fig. 11). The information that can be obtained from steady flow measurements includes pressure drop across the valve (Fig. 12), effective orifice area and pressure recovery at different flow rates. Recently, several groups have introduced the use of the laser Doppler technique for the evaluation of heart valve function (BRUSS

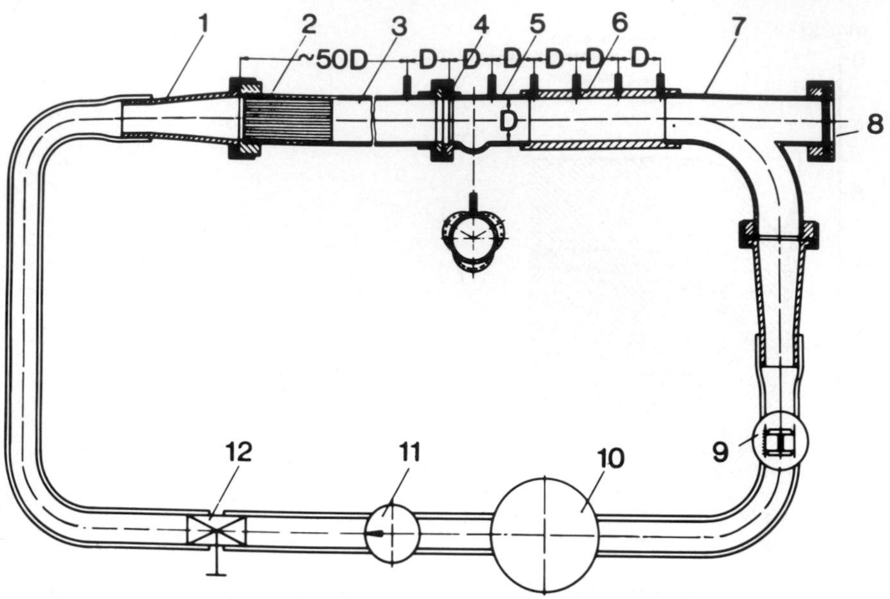

Fig. 11. Layout of a continuous steady flow valve test circuit; the test section (represented by elements *1-7)* includes flow straighteners *(2)* and simulated sinuses *(5)*; an inspection port is provided *(8)*

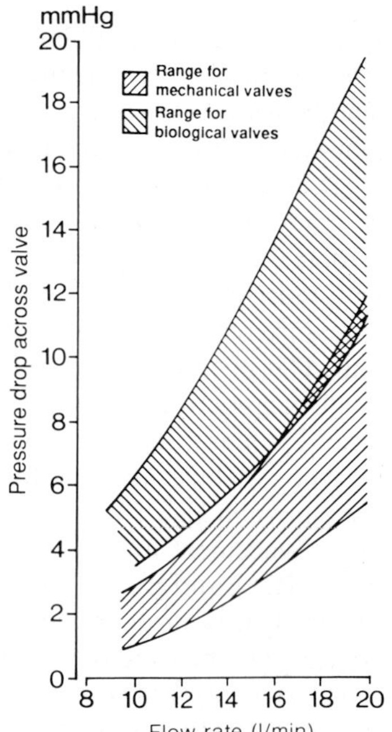

Fig. 12. Variation of pressure drop with flow rate across mechanical and biological valvular prostheses

Björk-Shiley *Monostrut*
α = 70°
Re = 6000
$\dot{V}_{PS} \widehat{=} 30$ l min
central light slit
Re = 6000
$\dot{V}_{PS} \widehat{=} 30$ l/min
shifted light slit

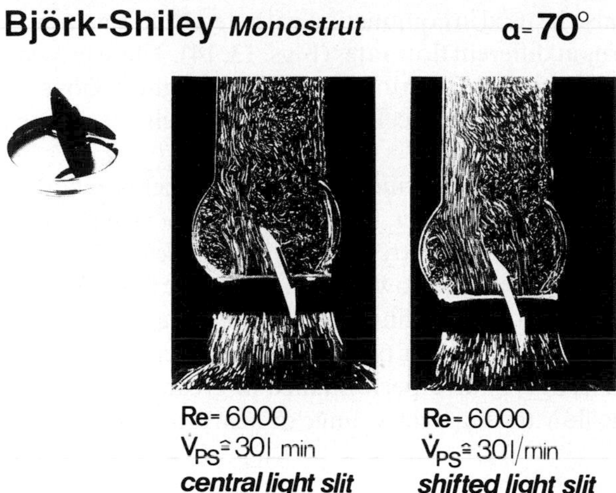

Fig. 13. Streamline visualisation during steady flow through a single leaflet disc mechanical prosthesis

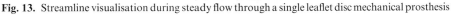

et al. 1983; YOGANATHAN et al. 1979a, b; SIMENAUER 1986). This technique yields detailed data on flow velocities and turbulence intensities. This in turn allows estimation of shear rates and turbulent stresses, which provides information on the likelihood of damage to blood cells or tissue. In general, the method is applied only to the region immediately upstream or downstream of the valve as it is not optically possible to use the laser beam within the valve itself. Furthermore, laser Doppler technology is expensive and it is tedious to chart velocity and turbulence fields point by point. Hence it is unlikely that the method will be of use for routine valve assessment. Rather, it should be available in only a few centres and should be used to answer specific design questions.

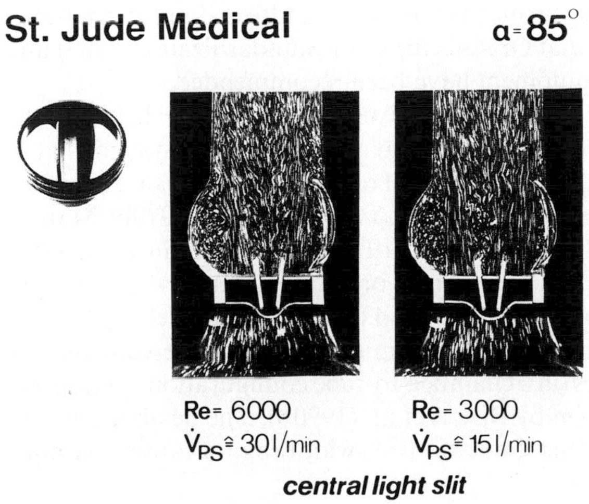

St. Jude Medical
α = 85°
Re = 6000
$\dot{V}_{PS} \widehat{=} 30$ l/min
Re = 3000
$\dot{V}_{PS} \widehat{=} 15$ l/min
central light slit

Fig. 14. Streamline visualisation during steady flow through a bileaflet mechanical prosthesis

Flow visualisation may also be used in conjunction with steady flow measurements to produce flow patterns at different flow rates (Figs. 13, 14). These provide a useful qualitative picture of the flow distribution and highlight regions of stagnation, recirculation or turbulence, where cell damage or cell–cell interactions may occur.

Pressure drop, pressure recovery and orifice area measurements relate to the obstructive properties of the valve. Laser Doppler and flow visualisation studies tell us about flow, shear and shear stress fields, which clearly have an important bearing on valve performance. However, the results of steady flow testing are not readily extrapolated to the clinical situation since they do not consider the dynamic operation of the valve or permit the assessment of valvular regurgitation. In order to investigate valve performance in greater depth, it is necessary to employ pulsatile flow testing over a range of heart rates and stroke volumes.

3.2 Pulsatile Studies

While steady flow tests provide a useful "first-line" approach, their shortcomings are obvious. Since the normal pulsatile flow of blood is not simulated, valve dynamics cannot be studied nor can the degree of regurgitation be assessed. In order to investigate performance in greater depth, a pulse duplicator, which accurately simulates the pumping action of the heart, is required.

The test conditions employed in this type of study require strict control as, once again, the results obtained may be influenced by many factors. In particular, the position of pressure measurement sites, the simulated heart rate employed, the viscosity of the test fluid and the magnitude of the simulated peripheral resistance, and hence the mean pressure in the system, all must be carefully considered. The majority of these systems operate using a test fluid of either 0.9% saline or a glycerol–water mix. All of these problems have been addressed in International Standard ISO 5840 (International Organization for Standardization 1989) and performance criteria for test equipment have been recommended.

Pulse duplicator design necessarily involves a compromise between the accurate simulation of in vivo conditions and the need for a system that is practicable for routine laboratory use. A number of different systems are available (REUL and BLACK 1984; BRUSS et al. 1983; YOGANATHAN et al. 1979b; MARTIN et al. 1978; WALKER et al. 1980; GABBAY et al. 1978; SWANSON and CLARK 1982; WIETING 1969; CHANDRAN 1985). The layout of one such system is shown in Fig. 15. The pulse duplicator is computer controlled and models the left side of the heart, enabling testing of both mitral valves (in a simple chamber-to-chamber configuration) and aortic valves (in a chamber-to-tube configuration). A detailed description of the system is given by BLACK et al. (1990b). The flexibility of this computer-driven system allows the simulation of a wide range of cardiac outputs,

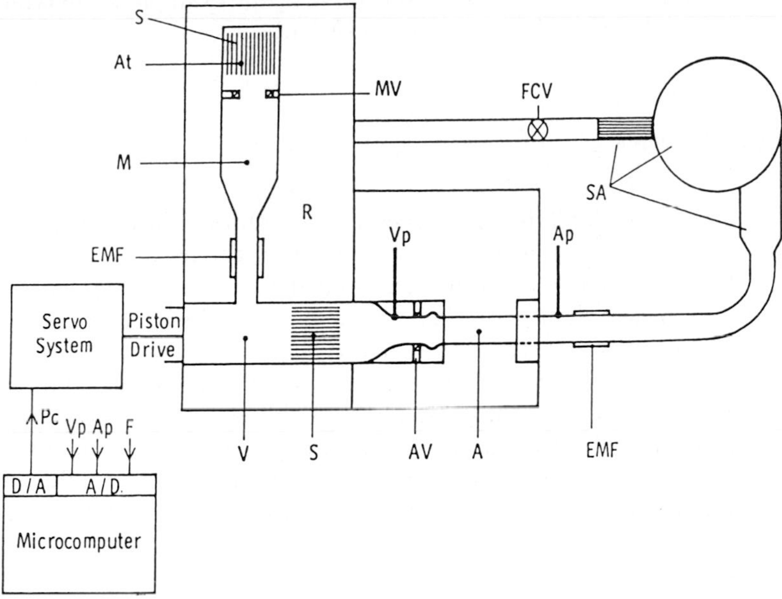

Fig. 15. Layout of the Sheffield pulse duplicator; this computer-controlled system can test both aortic *(AV)* and mitral *(MV)* valves; pressures are measured upstream *(Vp)* and downstream *(Ap)* of the valve; flows are recorded by electromagnetic flowmeters *(EMF)*; *S* = flow straighteners; *At* = atrium; *M* = mitral test section; *EMF* = electromagnetic flow meter; *Pc*-----= Signal inputs and outputs between computer and servo system; *F* = flow signal; *V* = verticular test section; *A* – aortic test section; *SA* – Systemic after load; *FCV* = flow control valve

stroke volumes and heart rates, thus enabling a valve to be evaluated over a realistic range of potential working conditions.

In the absence of a single, universally accepted index, the parameters that have been used to define valve performance are many and varied. The most commonly used are pressure difference, regurgitation and, to a lesser extent, power and energy losses through the valve (Swanson 1984; Knott et al. 1986). Functional characteristics, such as mean pressure difference during forward flow and regurgitation, give an indication of the degree of obstruction caused by the valve and the volume of reflux through the valve relative to the total forward flow. When considered together, they give an index of the total mechanical load presented to the heart by a particular valve.

Flow visualisation techniques are also applicable to pulsatile studies. Both dynamic flow patterns and the valve opening sequence may be recorded on high-speed video for subsequent freeze-frame analysis. Laser Doppler anemometry and hot-film anemometry have also been used to obtain a measure of the blood-damaging characteristics of the valve.

All of the techniques mentioned previously involve only the use of laboratory test systems. Acute animal experiments have also been performed in order to obtain "living" indicators of the behaviour of valves. A good example of this is the excellent work carried out by Hasenkam et al. (1988a,b).

3.3 In Vitro Test Results

No in-depth comparison of all the valve types across a range of heart rates and stroke volumes and across the range of valve sizes has been carried out. However, several limited studies have been performed, and these enable some general conclusions to be drawn about valve behaviour in vitro (Knott et al. 1986; Dellsperger et al. 1983; Black et al. 1990a). The types and sizes of valves tested, and combinations of cardiac output, heart rate and stroke volume used in three such studies, are given as Table 1. The range of results obtained from these studies in terms of mean pressure difference, regurgitation and energy losses are summarised as Table 2. Direct comparisons made between results obtained by different research groups must be made with caution as differences in test equipment and methodology influence the absolute values of any measurements made.

The two most common parameters used in defining the performance of a valve are pressure drop and regurgitation since these relate most directly to the behaviour of a diseased valve whether it is stenotic or incompetent. More recently, studies by Walker, Knott and Swanson have introduced the concepts of energy loss and performance indices in an attempt to obtain a single parameter to aid comparison among the various prosthetic valves (Walker et al. 1980; Knott et al. 1986). At this stage it is not clear how these factors relate to overall heart valve performance, particularly when biological phenomena such as haemolysis and thromboembolism are considered. However, they do give a measure of the work required from the heart if any particular valve is implanted and in this sense help in the interpretation of pulse duplicator results as extrapolated to the in vivo

Table 1. Details of in vitro studies on various valve types

Reference	Valve type studied	Valve size and position	Cardiac output (l/min)	Heart rate (bpm)	Stroke volume (ml)
Knott et al. (1986)	BC, TD, BL	27 (A)	3.0, 4.5, 6.5, 8.0	70	43, 64, 93, 114
Scotten et al. (personal communication)	Po, Pe	19 (A)	1.8, 3.6, 7.3, 4.3	60, 80, 120, 200	35, 55, 70, 30
Black et al. (1992)	BC, TD, BL, Pe	17, 19, 21, 23, 25, 27, 29, 31, 33 (M) (A)	2.0, 4.0, 6.0, 8.0	40, 70, 100, 120	50, 100, 28.6, 57.1, 85.7, 114.3, 20, 40, 60, 80, 42.9, 57.1

BC, ball and cage; TD, tilting disc; BL, bileaflet; Po, porcine; Pe, pericardial; M, mitral; A, aortic; N/A data not available.

Table 2. Results of the in vitro studies detailed in Table 1

Reference	Valve type	Mean pressure difference (mmHg)	Regurgitation (ml/beat)		Energy loss[b]		
			Closing	Leakage	E_C	E_L	E_S
Knott et al. (1986)	BC	8.5–32	4–1.5[a]	0–0.3[a]	1–0.3	0	10–22.5
	TD	2.0–6.5	7–2.5[a]	3–0.6[a]	1–0.6	2–0.5	2.5–5.5
	BL	1.5–5.5	6.5–2.5[a]	8.5–1.5[a]	1.5–0.7	4.5–0.7	2.5–5.5
Scotten et al. (1988)	Po	5–24	0.6–0.15	0.4–0.8	1.5–0	0.7–1.5	5–21
	Pe	2–12	1.2–0.4	0.8–1.2	2.5–1	0.6–1.5	3.5–13
Black et al. (1990a)	BC	1.0–53	2.5–0.2	6.0–0	N/A	N/A	N/A
	TD	1.0–42	7.5–0.5	10.0–0.2	N/A	N/A	N/A
	BL	1.0–42	7.5–0.5	7.5–0.8	N/A	N/A	N/A
	Pe	1.0–28	1.5–0.1	5.0–0.2	N/A	N/A	N/A

BC, ball and cage; TD, tilting disc; BL, bileaflet; Po, porcine; Pe, pericardial; M, mitral; A, aortic; N/A, data not available

[a] Results for regurgitation presented in this group are given as percentage of the stroke volume

[b] Energy losses are expressed as percentages of the mean aortic flow energy per beat. E_C, energy loss due to valve closure; E_L, energy loss due to valve leakage; E_S, energy loss due to pressure drop across valve during systole

situation. As the in vivo performance of a valve is ultimately dependent on both physical and biological factors, it is unlikely that a single parameter that can adequately predict long-term in vivo performance will be found.

At present, pulse duplicators provide the only means of initial assessment of the likely in vivo haemodynamic performance of a prosthetic valve. Laboratory testing using non-compliant, rigid-walled test chambers is bound to limit the validity of in vitro models, particularly in relation to pulsatile flow conditions.

In addition, reference has been made to the phenomenon of pressure recovery and the concomitant exchanges between kinetic and potential energies. These haemodynamic aspects appear to be significant in laboratory testing but may not be of equal importance in vivo. Flow conditions induced by the shape of the open configuration of the occluder may be more significant in terms of energy losses due to disturbed flow.

The problems produced by the use of inflexible valve frames, particularly in the plane of the orifice, have already been referred to. The significance of this phenomenon has never been assessed in vitro. This is because no pulse duplicator has adequately catered for the precise anatomical juxtaposition of the aortic and mitral valves, nor do pulse duplicators simulate the precise myocardial and major vessel compliances obtaining in the cardiovascular system.

Many of the above analyses can be enhanced by the use of computerised studies of both the haemodynamics and the mechanical behaviour of the myocardium and major blood vessels and provide interesting examples of computerised haemodynamic analysis. Such studies tend to be limited by being in only two dimensions and also by ignoring the deformability of the myocardium. On the other hand, a number of researchers have investigated the stress analysis of the myocardium in general and valve leaflets in particular. Little has been done by way of combining these two aspects as an aid to valve design. Such studies indicate the value of computer simulations of the haemodynamics associated with heart valve design. However, once again it is not clear at this stage how significant such analyses are in relation to the clinical performance of the valves.

4 Wear Testing

Inadequate long-term durability continues to be a major drawback of tissue valves, and the only universally accepted method of evaluating long-term wear is extensive routine clinical use. This has the inherent disadvantage that the durability of any particular valve, or modified design, is not known for several years. Although both mechanical and biological factors can influence valve failure, their individual effects often cannot be separated in the clinical implantation situation.

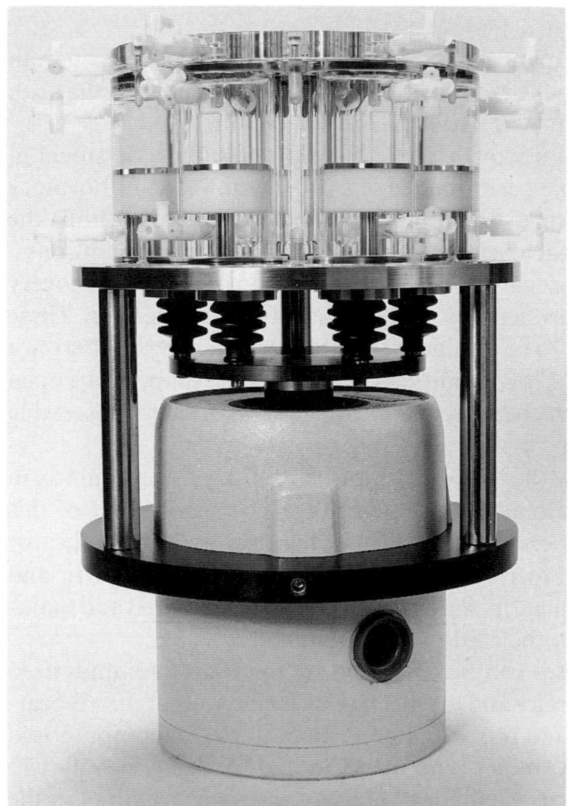

Fig. 16. The Sheffield six-chamber accelerated valve wear test system

These problems can be partially overcome by accelerated wear testing of valves in the laboratory. This technique can usually isolate the mechanical factors that may reduce the long-term durability of any prosthesis. Such test systems are designed to open and close the valve at a rate that is much greater than the average physiological value of around 70 beats/min, and with some equipment can be as high as 1600 cycles/min. In this way, 8 months of continuous running in the laboratory is "mechanically equivalent to 10 years of in vivo operation. Varying degrees of success with this approach to valve wear testing have been achieved, as assessed by comparison with results of long-term clinical findings.

The principle of operation of the Sheffield test system (Fig. 16) involves small-amplitude axial oscillations of the test valve at high frequency in a fluid medium. The inertial forces that are produced not only open and close the valve but, when correctly adjusted, can create a "physiological" closing pressure difference across the valve. This technique was first developed by Black (1973) and later modified by Martin et al. (1980). As with hydrodynamic testing, the value of accelerated wear testing depends not only on the design of the test equipment and experimental procedures, but also on careful interpretation of the results.

Although in vitro accelerated wear testing can separate some of the influences of mechanical and biological factors on valve durability, it cannot distinguish easily among the effects of tissue selection and treatment, leaflet geometry, frame design and techniques of construction. Some of these latter effects can be isolated only by extensive laboratory evaluation of the materials used in a valve's construction.

5 Theoretical Analysis

Dubini et al. (1991) and Fumero and Pietrabissa (1986) have applied computerised fluid dynamic (CFD) simulation of several different mechanical heart valve prostheses. In spite of several simplifications (the most important being the two-dimensional approach and the assumption of steady flow), the results were qualitatively in good agreement with those of in vitro studies, without requiring sophisticated testing procedures and complex devices. These workers reported that it was very important to bear in mind that the simulations, both in vitro and with the methods shown, are only aimed at permitting comparisons of different valve types of different operating conditions.

The plots generated by the simulations clearly indicate the importance of a correct fluid dynamic design of artificial heart valve prostheses in order to avoid or limit phenomena such as vortices, stagnation, recirculation and high-velocity gradients which may lead to thrombus formation and haemolysis. The results underline the major role played by local fluid dynamics and provide useful information about the most critical zones in the flow channel. It is clear that CFD analysis is a useful tool for understanding fluid dynamic phenomena and improving the fluid dynamic design of artificial heart valve prostheses.

Recent research on this topic in Sheffield has provided data on pressure drop, turbulence and velocity profiles from the CFD analysis of the Navier-Stokes equations of flow. Typical examples of these analyses are shown in Fig. 17.

A comprehensive analysis of the stress state in structural components is also an important part of the design process. In the case of bioprosthetic heart valves, this is often not completed due to the difficulty in analysing the valve leaflets. Although the widespread use of these valves has been restricted by tearing of the tissue leaflets after relatively short periods of function, they have many advantages over mechanical valves, mainly in terms of biocompatibility. The tearing is almost certainly a consequence of high stress levels. Although the exact mechanism is not fully understood, it may be a result of material fatigue and/or the formation of focal calcium. It is clear, however, that a design which gives a reduction in the stress state is likely to give an improved performance.

The stress/strain response of bioprosthetic heart valve tissue involves highly non-linear behaviour with large deformations at normal working stresses. A number of models for representing such non-linear behaviour of various biological materials have been proposed by various investigators (Tong and Fung 1976; Synder 1972; Demiray 1972). A substantial review of these analyses has been presented by Sahay (1984).

The appropriate interpretation of the stress–strain behaviour of valve leaflet material is essential if the stresses in the complete valve under load are to be calculated. The work of Trowbridge and Crofts (1987) on the mechanical behaviour of both fresh and treated bovine pericardium has contributed significantly to the development of full valve stress analysis. Various techniques involving both two- and three-dimensional methodologies have been used in the analysis of stress and deformation of leaflet valves. In the case of the two-dimensional approach, Thubrikar et al. (1980) have calculated stresses in the leaflet based on a simple cylindrical model. Alternatively, Trowbridge and Crofts (1987) have based their evaluation of leaflet stresses on the application of flat plate theory.

The assumptions made in all these analyses significantly restrict the validity of the final calculated stresses. However, Huang et al. (1990) have shown the value of a two-dimensional approach in relation to calculating the stresses at the line of attachment of the leaflet to the frame. Their solution was based on a finite element analysis. A more appropriate model of valve geometry is that of a shell structure. The simplest approach using this model is the assumption that the leaflets are subjected only to membrane stresses. In this case the assumed shell conforms with the shape of the mid-section of the valve leaflet, and it is assumed that no material stresses obtain perpendicular to the membrane surface. Several previous workers in this area, including Christie and Medland (1982), Hamid et al. (1985) and Rousseau et al. (1988) have tackled the problem using membrane elements which, essentially, model membrane stresses only.

However, in the two-dimensional analysis already referred to, bending stresses in the leaflet were found to be significant, particularly in regions of leaflet attachment to the frame (Huang et al. 1990). Such stresses give rise to both tension

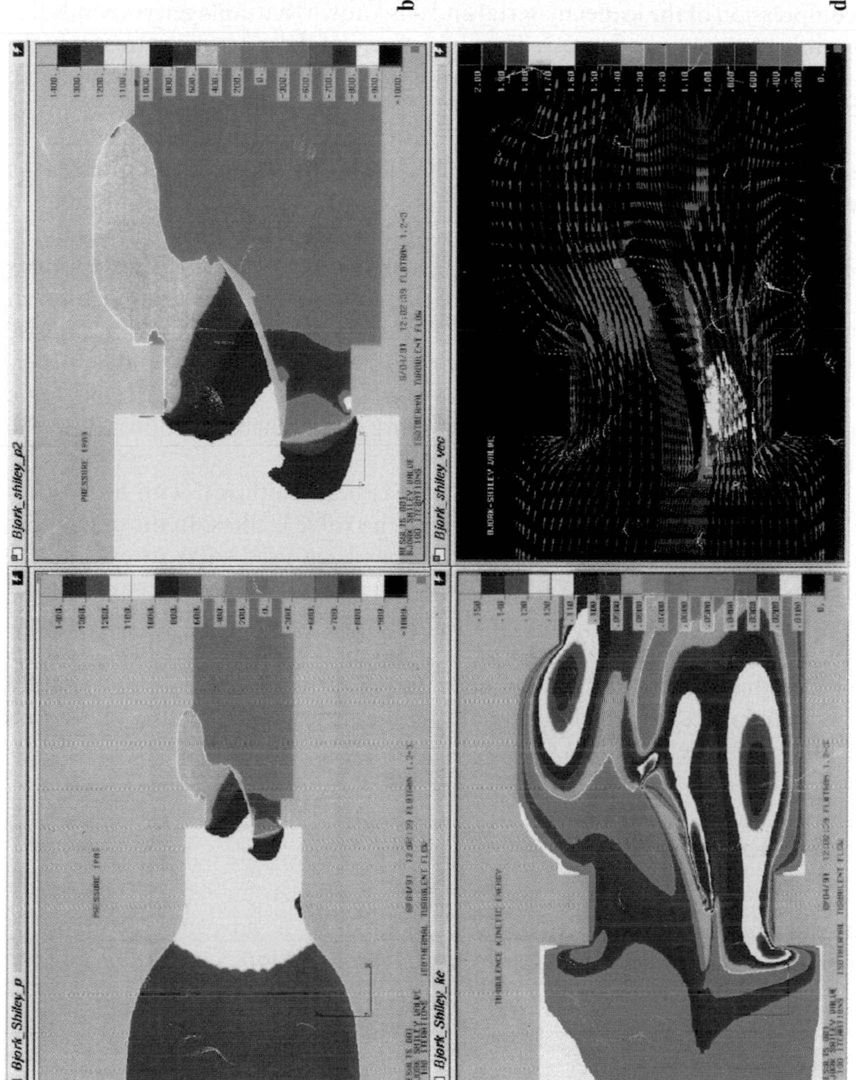

Fig. 17a–d. Computational fluid dynamic analysis of flow through a single leaflet disc valve; the figures illustrate pressure **(a,b)**, turbulence **(c)** and velocity streamlines **(d)** around the valve

and compression of the leaflet material and it is known that collagen responds less favourably to compressive stress. The importance of these bending stresses highlights the need for three-dimensional analysis of valve leaflets which allow for the variation of stress and displacement through the thickness of the leaflet.

The authors have been responsible for the development of a new design of bioprosthetic bicuspid valve for the mitral position (BLACK et al. 1986). As noted above, a two-dimensional finite element analysis of this design has been completed (HUANG et al. 1990). However, one of the authors has also been involved in the development of a three-dimensional analysis of this valve which also incorporates realistic modelling of the stress–strain behaviour of the pericardium used in constructing the valve (BLACK et al. 1986). The results of this analysis emphasise the need to include bending stresses when considering the strength and deformation of bioprosthetic valve leaflets. The development of sophisticated finite element software packages facilitates this more comprehensive approach to the determination of the stresses in valve leaflets.

In the past, bioprosthetic valve design has been empirical with little or no account being taken of the actual stresses on the valve leaflets. In the case of the Sheffield bicuspid valve, full stress analysis has been used so as to obviate the possible tearing failure of the leaflets which has occurred in other pericardial valves. As a result, in both in vitro and in vivo tests of the valve there has been no evidence of any gross material failure. The same method of stress analysis has shown that the location of high regions of stress correlate well with the position of tears found in explanted commercially available pericardial valves (LAWFORD et al. 1986; FISHER et al. 1986).

6 Clinical Experience

As already noted, the most valuable assessment of a valve's performance is obtained from the results of long-term clinical implantation. Such results must be

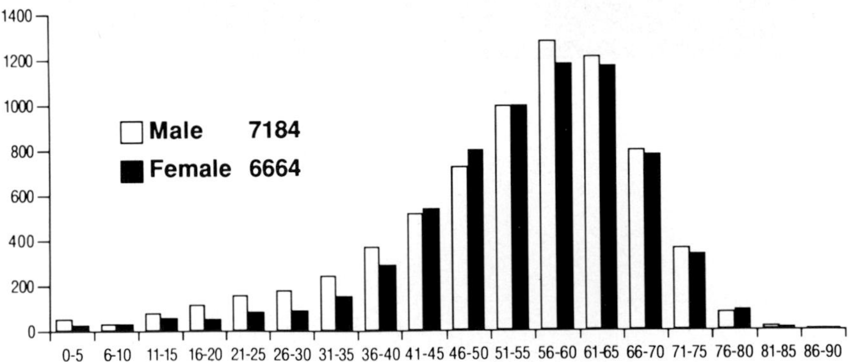

Fig. 18. Patient distribution by age and sex

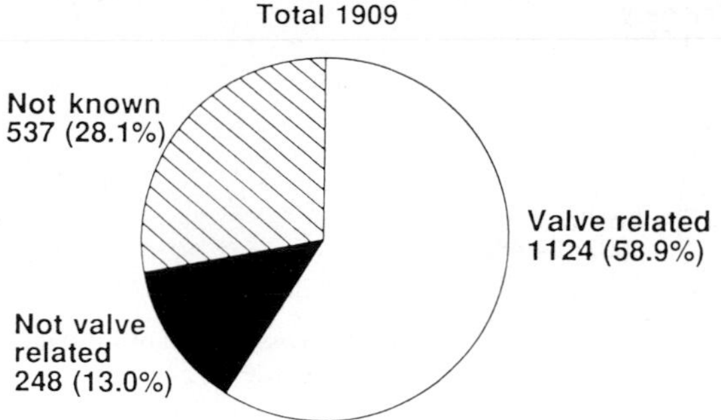

Fig. 19. Causes of patient mortality

based on data from a large number of cases. A sufficient spread of data covering all the various types of valves is unlikely to be available from any single surgical centre. In this section, details are given of the results of long-term follow-up studies on valve patients obtained from a multicentre approach.

The Multicentre Valve Study, now in its 18th year, is processing data on 16 359 valve implants in 13 852 patients. These data have been received from 22 centres involving a total of 57 surgeons. Follow-up details are available on 12 644 valves. This figure represents 77.3% of the total valve numbers. There is a maximum follow-up of 23.8 years with a mean of 4.2 years for individual valves and a mean of 4.3 years for individual patients (responders only).

The patient population is almost evenly distributed between the sexes, with 6664 females (48.1%) and 7184 males (51.9%). The age distribution of these patients, both in total and by sex, is given in Fig. 18. From this histogram it can be seen that there is no significant difference in age distribution between the sexes, and the incidence of valve replacement is a maximum for both sexes in the age group 56–60. Of the 13 852 patients in the study, 7826 (56.5%) have had a previous history of cardiac illness, of whom 3064 (39.2%) have had previous cardiac surgery. At the time of operation, 4191 (30.26%) of the patients underwent additional concomitant surgery. The majority of patients, 9607 (69.4%) were given a New York Heart Classification of either 2 or 3 prior to their first surgery in the study, while 1565 (11.3%) were graded 4 and 909 (6.6%) graded 1. The total number of deaths so far recorded is 1909; 1124 (58.9%) were valve related, 248

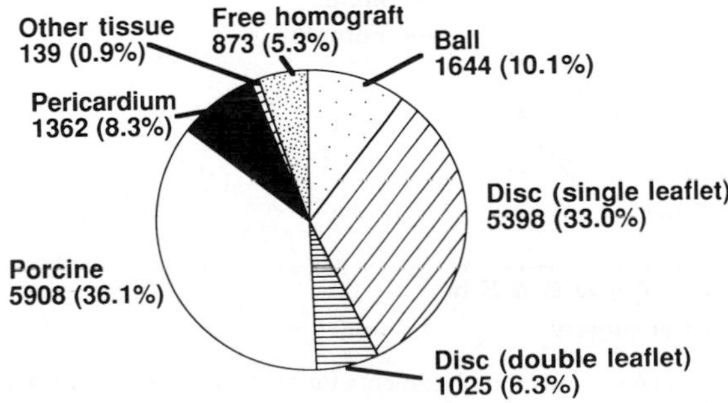

Fig. 20. Distribution of major valve types

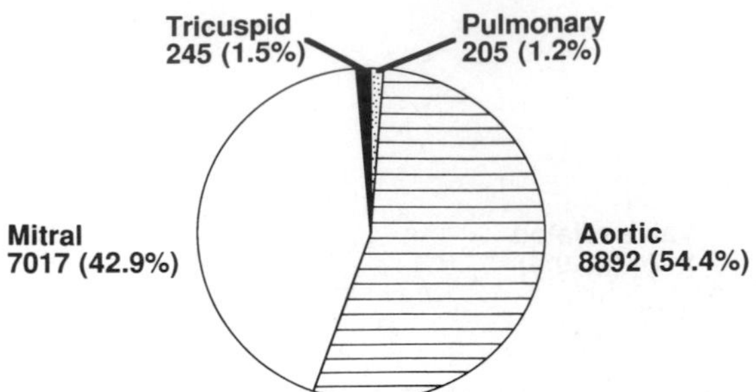

Fig. 21. Distribution of valve implantation site

(13.0%) were not and the reason for 537 (28.1%) was recorded as being unknown. These data are presented in Fig. 19.

Figure 20 shows the number of the various heart valves used according to their classification into the major groups. The majority of the valves have been either porcine (36.1%) or single leaflet disc valves (33.0%), with pericardial (8.3%) and ball valves (10.1%), and double leaflet disc valves (6.3%) and free homografts (5.3%) being used in comparable proportions. Of the 16 359 implants, 8892 (54.4%) have been in the aortic position, 7017 (42.9%) in the mitral, 245 (1.5%) in the tricuspid and 205 (1.2%) in the pulmonary (Fig. 21). There have been 13 852 patients who have had either single, double or triple valve replacement procedures. Of these, 12 113 (87.4%) have had single valve replacements, 1677 (12.1%) double and 62 (0.5%) triple valve replacements.

Figure 22 indicates the variation with age of the ratio of aortic mitral replacements for male and female patients. It can be seen that for male patients there is the expected higher ratio of aortic valve replacement. The pattern is less clear for female patients; those aged either less than 30 or greater than 65 have a higher incidence of aortic valve replacement while those aged 30–65 have a higher incidence of mitral valve replacement. The trend in valve usage is independent of follow-up period. The distribution of the major valve types by year of implant is shown in Fig. 23 and clearly illustrates the rise in proportion of bioprosthetic valve implants from 1974 to 1981. In 1981, bioprosthetic valves accounted for 65% of

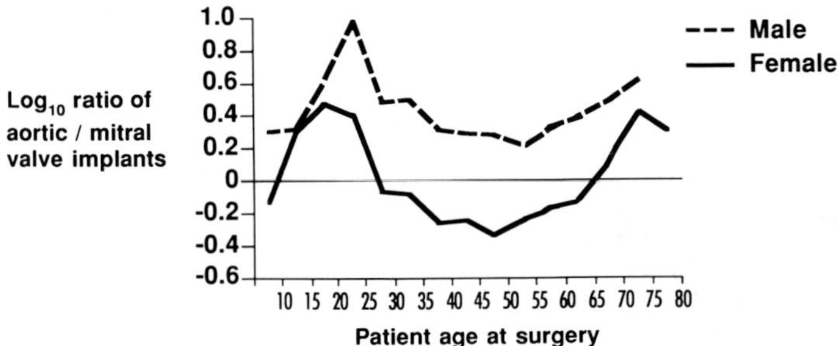

Fig. 22. Variation with age of the ratio of aortic to mitral replacements for male and female patients

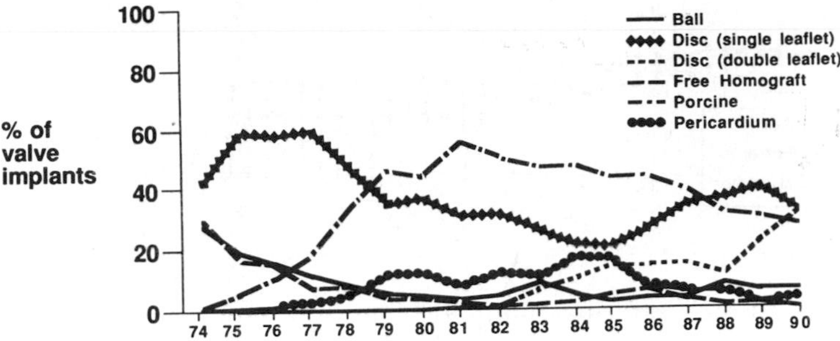

Fig. 23. Distribution of major valve types by year of implantation

all implants being recorded by the study. Since that time there has been a gradual decrease in the proportion of bioprostheses implanted with a concomitant increase in mechanical valves. However, it was not until 1987 that bioprosthetic valves became less popular than mechanical valves, that is less than 50% usage. At the present time, only 31% of the implants being recorded by the study are bioprosthetic.

6.1 Actuarial Analysis

Many different aspects of valve substitute implantation have been quantitatively assessed from the data recorded by the Multicentre Valve Study (Black et al. 1983 a, b, 1985, 1987a, b, 1990 c; Drury et al. 1986, 1987; Fessatidis et al. 1989;

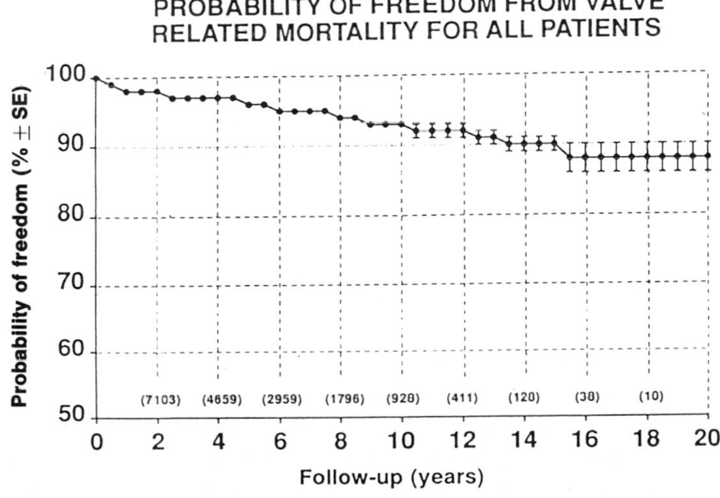

Fig. 24. Probability of freedom from valve-related mortality for all patients

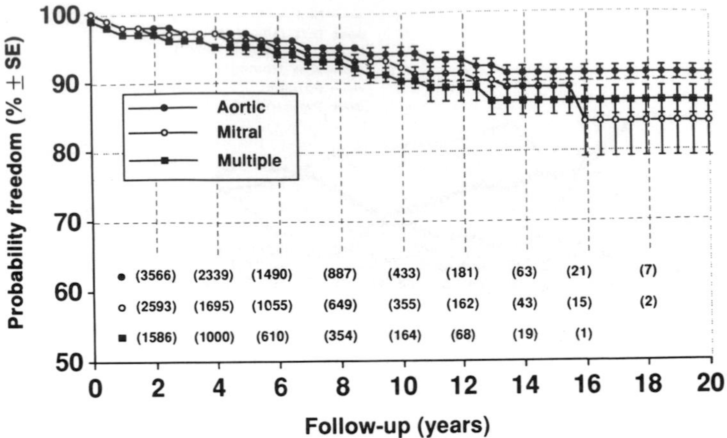

Fig. 25. Proabability of freedom from valve-related mortality after aortic, mitral and multiple valve replacement

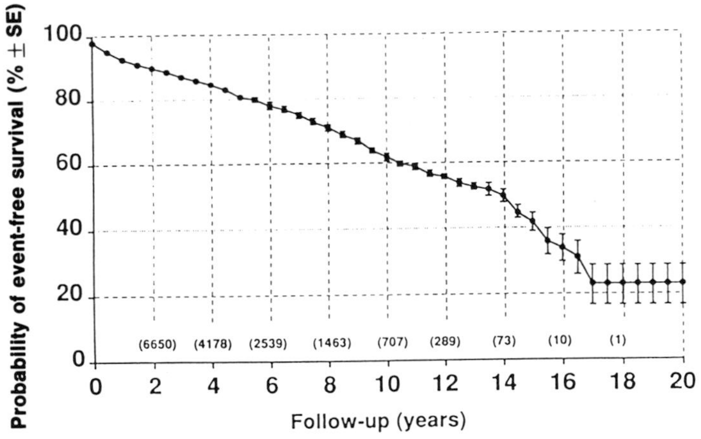

Fig. 26. Probability of event-free survival after valve replacement for all patients

Walesby 1983) and one of the major objectives of the project is the provision of comparative performance data on the various valves which predominate in routine clinical use. One of the ways in which such information may be obtained is by the use of the statistical method of actuarial analysis.

Actuarial curves of probability of freedom from valve- related mortality are shown in Figs. 24 and 25. Figure 24 gives the overall freedom from valve- related mortality following valve replacement procedures, whilst in Fig. 25 the results are divided according to single aortic, single mitral and multiple procedures. It can be

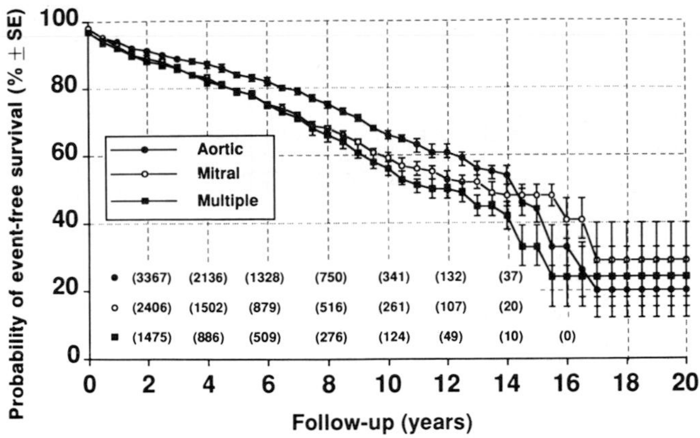

Fig. 27. Probability of event-free survival after aortic, mitral and multiple valve replacement

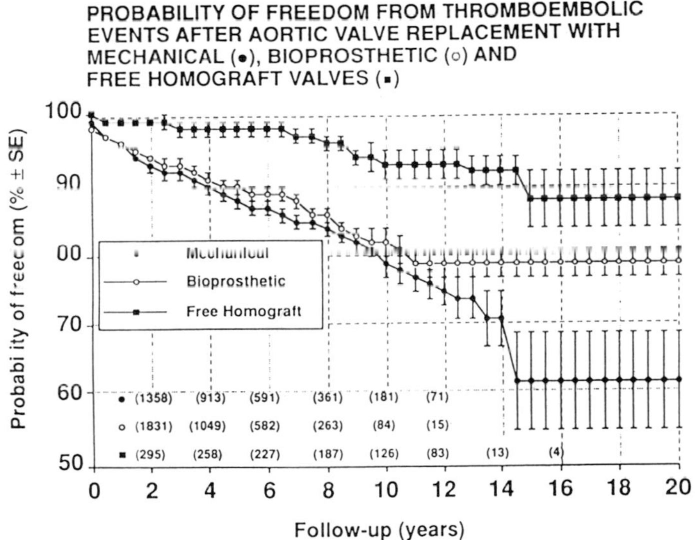

Fig. 28. Probability of freedom from thromboembolic events after aortic valve replacement with mechanical, bioprosthetic and free homograft valves

seen that at 12 years the probability of freedom from valve related mortality following these procedures is around 92% (AVR), 90% (MVR) and 89% (mVR) with an overall survival of 91%.

Actuarial curves of probability of event-free survival are shown as Figs. 26 and 27. The overall event-free survival following valve replacement procedures is given as Fig. 26, whilst in Fig. 27 the results are divided into single aortic, single mitral and multiple procedures. At 12 years, the probability of event-free survival

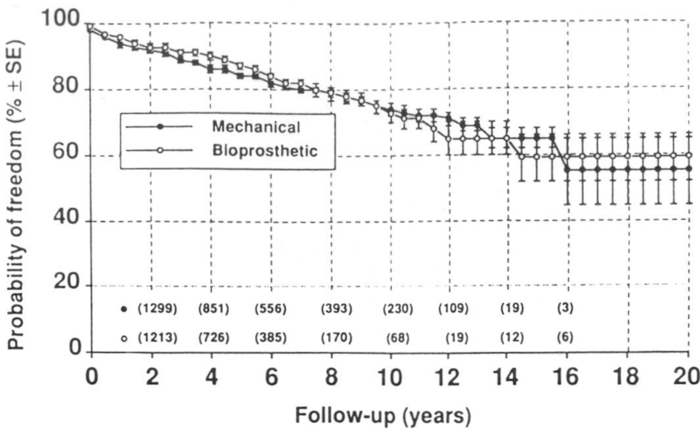

Fig. 29. Probability of freedom from thromboembolic events after mitral valve replacement with mechanical and bioprosthetic valves

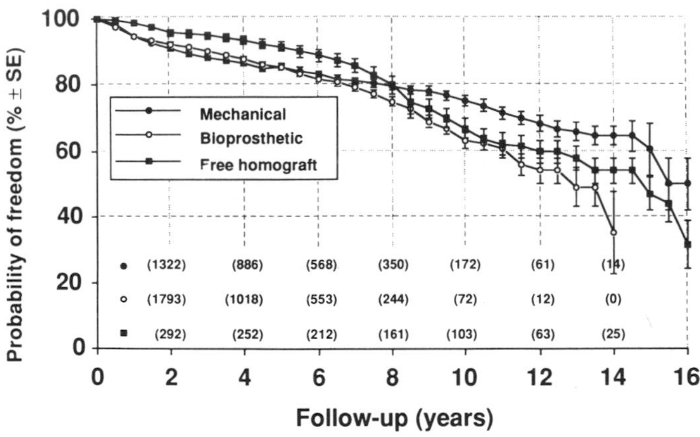

Fig. 30. Probability of freedom from valve dysfunction after aortic valve replacement with mechanical, bioprosthetic and free homograft valves

is around 59% (AVR), 52% (MVR) and 49% (mVR) with an overall event-free survival of 53%.

Actuarial curves of probability of freedom from thromboembolic events are given as Figs. 28 and 29. During 10 year's, follow-up there is no difference between mechanical and bioprosthestic valves implanted in either the aortic or the mitral position. However, in the aortic position the free homograft valve performs significantly better than the other valves over the whole of this time period.

Actuarial curves of probability of freedom from valve dysfunction are given as Figs. 30 and 31. During the first 7 years following aortic valve implantation there is little to choose between mechanical and bioprosthetic valves. Thereafter,

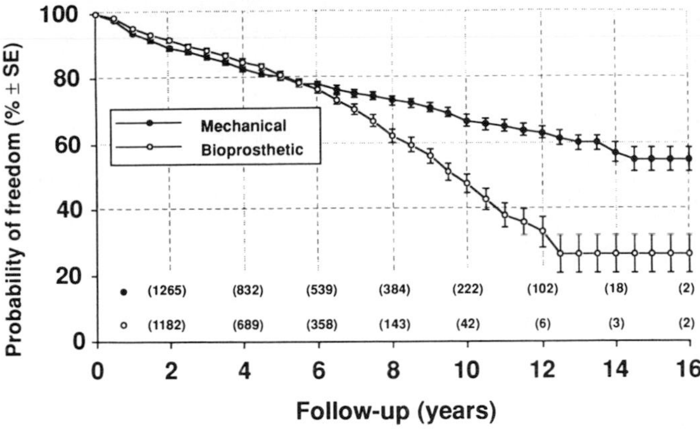

Fig. 31. Probability of freedom from valve dysfunction after mitral valve replacement with mechanical and bioprosthetic valves

there is a significant increase in the probability of valve dysfunction in the bioprosthetic valve group, so at 12 years the probability of freedom from valve dysfunction is around 54% as compared with around 66% for the mechanical group of valves. For the first 7 years the free homograft valve performs significantly better than either mechanical or bioprosthetic valves, but after 8 years it appears to perform slightly better than the bioprosthetic valve but slightly worse than the mechanical valve.

In the mitral position, once more there is no significant difference between mechanical and bioprosthetic valves for the first 7 years, but thereafter there is, again, a significant increase in the probability of dysfunction in the bioprosthetic valve group, so that at 10 years the probability of freedom from these complications is around 43% as compared with around 66% for the mechanical group of valves.

6.2 Proportional Hazards Analysis

There are a number of limitations associated with the use of actuarial analysis, two being of particular importance. First, the comparison of valve performance is made quantitatively, since it is not possible to make valid statements about the statistical significance of their difference. Second, no account can be taken of the underlying patient prognosis.

Actuarial methods estimate the survival time $S(t)$, that is, the proportion surviving beyond time t. A more informative approach is to use models of survival time which are expressed in terms of the hazard rate $l(t)$ which is directly related to $S(t)$. Figure 32 shows the estimated survival times for one set of prognostic

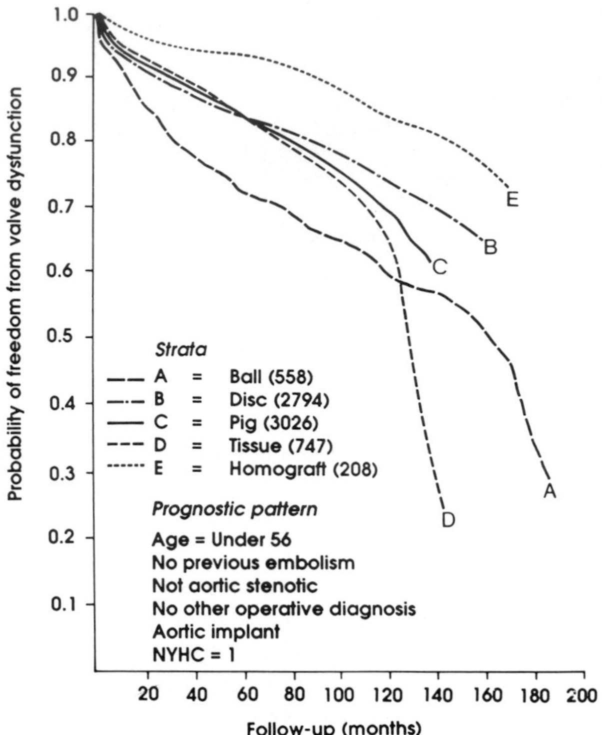

Fig. 32. Proportional hazards analysis – probability of freedom from valve dysfunction after valve replacement with the major valve types

factors. Each of these prognostic factors has a specific and significant effect on time to valve dysfunction. Many other plots like this can be produced by varying the pattern of these prognostic factors. For example, it may be more desirable to determine estimated survival times for patients with the same prognostic pattern as in Fig. 32 except that they are aged over 56, not under 56.

Figure 32 does in fact represent a slightly complicated model because rather than one survival function for a given set of prognostic factors there are five. The reason for this "stratified" model is because the prognostic factor "valve type" violated the assumption of proportionality. Proportionality means that any differences between the individual levels within a prognostic factor remain constant over time; clearly this is not the case here (the survival functions of disc, pig and tissue valves cross between 60 and 80 months).

There are many possible subsets of the data which could be analysed using the proportional hazards model. Due to the size of this study such analyses should be possible without much loss in power of the statistical tests employed.

The results of any such study using non-random data should always be treated tentatively. As with all statistical analysis based on the use of non-random data, care must always be taken in any interpretation involving behavioural prediction.

Table 3. Advantages and disadvantages of different valve types

Valve type	Advantages	Disadvantages
Mechanical	1. Long-term durability 2. Consistency of manufacture	1. Unnatural form 2. Patient usually requires long-term anticoagulant therapy
Tissue	1. More natural form and function 2. Less need for anticoagulant therapy	1. Unproven long-term durability 2. Less consistency of manufacture 3. In vivo calcification

7 Summary

This chapter has discussed the design, development, laboratory testing and clinical performance of artificial heart valve replacements. The published material on this subject is extensive and clearly this present chapter represents only a limited selection of the many topics and researchers associated with the production of clinically implantable valves. Any omissions should not be regarded as a criticism, but simply the result of economy of space.

The field is still developing and the situation regarding the advantages and disadvantages of the various types of valves as illustrated in Table 3 still obtains notwithstanding the many improvements which have been made with current designs. Valve development is, and will continue to be, closely allied to advances in our understanding of the behaviour of the materials of construction.

Ultimately, improved haemodynamic performances of the various valve configurations will result from designs based on data from computerised fluid dynamic analysis combined with finite element stress analysis according to recognised engineering design principles.

References

Black MM (1973) Development and testing of prosthetic heart valves: cardiovascular simulation and life support systems. In: Kenedi RM (ed) Perspectives in biomedical engineering. Macmillan, London, pp 21–28

Black MM, Drury PJ, Tindale WB (1982) A bicuspid bioprosthetic mitral valve. Proc Eur Soc Artif Organs 9:116–119

Black MM, Drury PJ, Tindale WB (1983a) Twenty-five years of heart valve substitutes: a review. J R Soc Med 76:667–680

Black MM, Drury PJ, Smith GH (1983b) Long-term assessment of heart valve substitutes. Life Support Systems 1:301–304

Black MM, Drury PJ, Tindale WB (1985) The clinical performance of bioprosthetic heart valves. In: Williams D (ed) Biocompatibility of tissue analogs, vol 2. CRC, Boca Raton, FL., pp 173–186

Black MM, Drury PJ, Tindale WB, Lawford PV (1986) The Sheffield bicuspid valve; concept, design and in vitro and, in-vivo assessment. In: Bodnar E, Yacoub M (eds) Biologic bioprosthetic valves. Proc 3rd Int Symp. Yorke Medical, New York, pp 709–717

Black MM, Cochrane T, Drury PJ, Lawford PV (1987a) Artificial heart valves past performance and future prospects. Cardiovasc Rev Rep 8:40–45

Black MM, Cochrane T, Drury PJ, Lawford PV (1987b) Assessing the performance and safety of artificial heart valves. Proc 9th EMBS Conference 3:1183–1184

Black MM, Cochrane T, Drury PJ, Lawford PV (1990a) A hydrodynamic model for the left side action of the human heart. Proc 12th Annual Int Conf of the IEEE, IEEE,USA, pp 535–536

Black MM, Cochrane T, Drury PJ, Lawford PV (1990c) In vitro and in vivo performance of artificial heart valves. Proc Conf on Medical and Biological Implant Technology, London. UK Liaison Committee for Services Allied to Medicine and Biology

Black MM, Howard IC, Huang X, Patterson EA (1991) A three-dimensional analysis of a bioprosthetic heart valve. J Biomech 24:793–801

Black MM, Lawford PV, Cochrane T (1992) Health equipment information bulletin. Evaluation of mechanical valve prostheses, Report no MDD/92/46 Department of Health, London

Bruss K-H, Reul H, Van Gilse J, Knott E (1983) Pressure drop and velocity fields at four mechanical heart valve prosthesis: Björk-Shiley Concave-Convex, Hall Kaster and St Jude Medical. Life Supp Syst 1:3–22

Chandran KB (1985) Pulsatile flow past St. Jude medical bi-leaflet valve: an in vitro study. J Thorac Cardiovasc Surg 89:743–749

Christie GW, Medland IC (1982) A non-linear finite element stress analysis of bioprosthetic heart valves. In: Gallagher RH, Simon BR, Johnson PC, Gross JF (eds) Finite elements in biomechanics. Wiley, New York, pp 153–179

Clark C (1976) The fluid mechanics of aortic stenosis. I: Theory and steady flow experiments. J Biomech 9:521–528

Dellsperger KC, Wieting DW, Baehr DA, Band RJ, Brugger J-P, Harrison EC (1983) Regurgitation of prosthetic heart valves; dependence on heart rate and cardiac output. Am J Cardiol 51:321–328

Demiray H (1972) A note on the elasticity of soft biological tissues. J Biomech 5:309–311

Drury PJ, Kay R, Lawford PV, Black MM (1986) Statistical reappraisal of the analysis of heart valve patient follow-up data – the estimation of valve failure rates. Life Supp Syst 4:121–123

Drury PJ, Black MM, Lawford PV, Kay R (1987) The long-term clinical assessment of heart valve substitutes. Eng Med 16:87–94

Dubini G, Pietrabissa R, Fumero R (1991) Computational fluid dynamics of artificial heart valves. Int J Artif Organs 14: 169–174

Ferrans VJ, Spray TL, Billingham ME, Roberts WC (1978) Structural changes in glutaraldehyde-treated porcine heterografts used as substitute cardiac valves. Transmission and scanning electron microscopic observations in 12 patients. Am J Cardiol 41:1159–1184

Fessatidis IT, Vassiliadis KE, Monro JL, Ross JK, Shore DF, Drury PJ (1989) Thirteen years' evaluation of the Björk-Shiley isolated mitral valve prosthesis. The Wessex experience. J Cardiovasc Surg 30:957–965

Fisher J, Reece IJ, Jack GR, Cathcart L, Wheatley DJ (1986) Laboratory assessment of the design, function and durability of pericardial bioprostheses. In: Unsworth D, Black MM, Drury PJ, Taylor K (eds) Heart valve engineering. Institution of Mechanical Engineers (IMechE), London, pp 57–64

Fumero R, Pietrabissa R (1986) Fluid dynamic models as a guide to determine prosthetic heart valve diameter. J Biomech 19:71–77

Gabbay S, McQueen DH, Yellin EL, Frater RWM (1978) In vitro hydrodynamic comparison of mitral valve prosthesis at high flow rates. J Thorac Cardiovasc Surg 76:771–787

Gibbon JH (1954) Application of a mechanical heart and lung apparatus to cardiac surgery. Minn Med 37:171–185

Hamid SM, Sabbah HN, Stein PD (1985) Finite element evaluation of stresses on closed leaflets of bioprosthetic heart valves with flexible stents. Finite Elements Anal Design 1:213–225

Hasenkam JM, Ostergaard JK, Pedersen EM, Ruben PK, Nygaard H, Schurizek BA (1988a) A model for acute haemodynamic studies in ascending aorta in pigs. Cardiovasc Res 22:464–471

Hasenkam JM, Pedersen EM, Ostergaard JH, Nygaard H, Pauben PK, Johannsen G, Schurizek BA (1988b) Velocity fields and turbulent stresses downstream of biological and mechanical aortic valve prosthesis implanted in pigs. Cardiovasc Res 22:472–483

Huang X, Black MM, Howard IC, Patterson EA (1990) A two-dimensional finite element analysis of a bioprosthetic heart valve. J Biomech 23:753–762

Hufnagel CA (1951) Aortic plastic valvular prostheses. Bull Georgetown U Med Cent 4:128–130
Kaiser GA, Hancock WD, Lukban SB, et al. (1969) Clinical use of a new design stented xenograft heart valve prosthesis. Surg Forum 20:137–138
Knott E, Reul H, Steinseifer U (1986) Pressure drop, energy loss and closure volume of prosthetic heart valves in aortic and mitral position under pulsatile flow conditions. Life Supp Syst 4(S2): 139–141
Lawford PV, Roberts K, Black MM, Drury PJ, Bilton G (1986) The in vivo durability of bioprosthetic heart valves – modes of failure observed in explanted valves. In: Heart valve engineering. IMechE, London, pp 65–74
Lawford PV, Roberts K, Black MM, Drury PJ, Bilton G (1987) The in vivo durability of bioprosthetic heart valves – modes of failure observed in explanted valves. Eng Med 16: 95–103
Martin TRP, Palmer JA, Black MM (1978) A new apparatus for the in vitro study of aortic valve mechanics. Eng Med 7:229–230
Martin TRP, Van Noort R, Black MM, Morgon J (1980) Accelerated fatigue testing of biological tissue heart valves. Proc ESAO 7:315–319
Reul H (1984) In: Planck H et al. (eds) Polyurethanes in biomedical engineering. Elsevier Science, Amsterdam, pp 257–277
Reul H, Black MM (1984) The design development and assessment of heart valve substitutes. In Bajzer, Baxa P, Franconi C (eds) Proceedings of the 2nd International Conference on Application of Physics to Medicine and Biology. Singapore, World Scientific Publishing, 99
Ross DN (1962) Homograft replacement of the aortic valve. Lancet II:487
Ross DN (1967) Replacement of the aortic and mitral valve with a pulmonary autograft. Lancet II:956
Rousseau EPM, Steenhoven AA, von Hansen JD, Huysmans HA (1988) A mechanical analysis of the closed Hancock heart valve prosthesis. J Biomech 21:543–562
Sahay KB (1984) On the choice of strain energy function for mechanical characterisation of soft biological tissues. Eng Med 13:11–14
Schoen FJ (1987) Cardiac valve prostheses: review of clinical status and contemporary biomaterials issues. J Biomed Mater Res 21:91–117
Senning A (1966) Aortic valve replacement with fascia lata. Acta Chir Scand 365B (Suppl): 17–20
Simenauer PA (1986) Test protocol: Interlaboratory comparison of prosthetic heart valve performance testing. US Food and Drug Administration, Rockville, Md.
Starr A (1960) Total mitral valve replacement: fixation and thrombosis. Surg Forum-258–260
Swanson WM (1984) Relative performance of prosthetic heart valves based on power measurements. Med Instrum 18:318–325
Swanson WM, Clark RE (1982) A simple cardiovascular system simulator: design and performance. J Bioeng 1: 135–145
Synder RW (1972) Large deformation of isotropic biological tissue. J Biomech 5:601–606
Thubrikar M, Piepgrass WC, Deck JD, Nolan SP (1980) Stresses of natural versus prosthetic heart valve leaflets in vivo. Ann Thorac Surg 30:230–239
Tindale WB, Black MM, Martin TRP (1982) In vitro evaluation of prosthetic heart valves: Anomalies and limitations. Clin Phys Physiol Meas 3:115–130
Tong P, Fung YC (1976) The stress-strain relationship for the skin. J Biomech 9:649–657
Trowbridge EA, Crofts CE (1987) Pericardial heterograft valves: an assessment of leaflet stresses and their implications for heart valve design. J Biomed Eng 9:345–356
Wada J, Komatsu S, Ikeda K et al. (1969) A new hingeless valve. In: Brewer KA (ed): Prosthetic heart valves. Charles C. Thomas, Springfield, Ill, pp 304–314
Walesby R (1983) A surgical assessment of the Starr-Edwards mitral prosthesis. Curr Med Lit 2:65–67
Walker DK, Scotten LN, Modi VJ, Brownlee RT (1980) In vitro assessment of mitral valve prosthesis. J Thorac Cardiovasc Surg 79:680–688
Wieting DW (1969) Dynamic flow characteristics of heart valves. Doctoral Dissertation, University of Texas, Austin
Yoganathan AP (1982) Prosthetic heart valves: a study of in vitro performance. Phase I final report. FDA contract no, 223-81-5000 (NTI S no. PB 83-134478)
Yoganathan AP, Corcoran WH, Harrison EC (1979a) In vitro velocity measurements in the vicinity of aortic prostheses. J Biomech 12:135–152
Yoganathan AP, Corcoran WH, Harrison EC (1979b) Pressure drops across prosthetic heart valves under steady and pulsatile flow – in vitro measurements. J Biomech 12:153–164

The Pathology of Artificial Hearts and Ventricular Assist Devices

A. Coumbe and T.R. Graham

Current Topics in Pathology
Volume 86. Ed. C. Berry

1 Introduction

Recent years have seen a huge increase in the number and scope of therapeutic procedures involving mechanical devices and the heart. Diseases of the heart which can now be treated using devices fall into four categories: valvular disease, abnormalities of cardiac innervation, congenital malformations and myocardial disease.

A large number of mechanical and biological valves are now available and valve replacement is routinely undertaken. Pacemakers of remarkable sophistication are also widely used in the treatment of conduction defects. Artificial and biosynthetic conduits and baffles are used in the correction of congenital defects and some of these topics are dealt with elsewhere in this volume. In this chapter we are concerned with the use of devices in the treatment of diseases of the myocardium.

Coronary artery bypass grafting and balloon angioplasty have made a great impact in the management of ischaemic heart disease, but both techniques are dependent on the capacity of the myocardium to recover when coronary perfusion is improved. In patients with end-stage ischaemic heart disease or cardiomyopathy, medical management can only be palliative. In such cases the options are to replace the failing heart with either an allograft or a mechanical device.

1.1 Historical Perspective

The idea of using mechanical devices to augment or substitute extrinsic mechanical energy for intrinsic ventricular energy is not a new one. Investigators at the turn of the century were designing devices for the perfusion of isolated organs. Their pumps provided a pulsatile flow similar to that of the native heart by means of various systems involving the cyclical compression of a pumping chamber. The displaced blood was then replaced by the refilling of the chambers by gravity or suction (Brodie 1903; Embly and Martin 1905; Richards and Drinker 1915).

Roller pumps that utilised metal rollers to massage rubber tubing and so propel blood in a non-pulsatile manner were described by Van Allen (1932) and DeBakey (1934) and it is true to say that the importance of pulsatile versus non-pulsatile flow in assisted circulation remains controversial. In 1933 Barcroft developed and electrically driven rotary pump and the same year Gibbs (1933) devised an artificial heart for use in dogs during pharmacological investigations.

The National Institutes of Health in the United States has been supporting the development of partial and total artificial hearts since 1963. The first successful temporary use of a pulsatile left ventricular assist device in a clinical setting was by DeBakey in 1966 (DeBakey 1971). DeVries performed the first elective clinical transplantation of a total artificial heart in 1982 (DeVries et al. 1984).

1.2 Clinical Need and Potential Applications

The advances in cardiac surgery have only been possible through the technique of cardiopulmonary bypass which allows "open heart surgery" to be undertaken. This is a technique not without risk, despite methods to enhance myocardial preservation, such as topical and systemic hypothermia and induced hyperkalaemic cardioplegia.

1.2.1 Post-cardiotomy Shock

Following otherwise uncomplicated procedures, approximately 10% of patients require reinstitution of cardiopulmonary bypass for brief periods. This is in order to overcome acute biventricular decompensation and to allow the ventricles to resume proper function to support the pulmonary and systemic circulations. Approximately 2% of patients who undergo open heart surgery develop post-cardiotomy cardiogenic shock and cannot be weaned from cardiopulmonary bypass (Pennock et al. 1983; Pae et al. 1985; Pennington et al. 1985). Conventional inotropic drug therapy and intra-aortic balloon pump counterpulsation provide adequate circulatory support in half of these patients (McEnany et al. 1978, Sanfelippo et al. 1986). The remaining 1% of patients with persisting ventricular inadequacy require more aggressive temporary ventricular support to reduce myocardial work and oxygen consumption, so allowing time for metabolic recovery of the "stunned" myocardium (Dennis et al. 1962; Pennock et al. 1979; Braunwald and Kloner 1982; Schoen et al. 1985a).

The limitations of prolonged cardiopulmonary bypass are haemolysis, protein denaturation, thrombocytopenia, the appearance of haemorrhagic diatheses and consumptive coagulopathy. In clinical terms cardiopulmonary bypass may be regarded as a controlled form of shock and as such only applicable for short periods of time. The aims of ventricular assist devices are to allow the support of patients with post-cardiotomy shock for longer periods with fewer complications.

1.2.2 Post-infarction Cardiogenic Shock

Patients who develop cardiogenic shock following myocardial infarction have a high mortality. Conventional medical treatment, inotropic agents and balloon counterpulsation are available as initial management options, but in those patients unresponsive to this, ventricular assistance may have a role. At present this role is undefined, but the extension of present criteria to include these patients appears to be reasonable and future clinical trials are warranted (Pae and Pierce 1980, 1981; Noda et al. 1989; Loisance et al. 1990; Lewis et al. 1990).

1.2.3 Acute Myocarditis

Myocarditis, be it viral, acute rheumatic or of unknown aetiology, can cause rapidly progressive heart failure. The inflammatory process is essentially reversible and often occurs in young, otherwise fit and healthy subjects. Furthermore a recent National Institutes of Health report has indicated a relatively high mortality following transplantation for acute myocarditis (O'Connell et al. 1989). Activation of the immune system associated with myocarditis is thought to promote severe graft rejection and may contra-indicate transplantation in the acute phase. For these reasons young patients with myocarditis are potentially excellent candidates for temporary mechanical circulatory assistance (Rockman et al. 1991).

1.2.4 Bridge to Transplantation

Heart transplantation is no longer "a fantastic speculation for the future" (Marcus et al. 1951) and, since the introduction of cyclosporin A immunosuppression, is widely accepted as an effective therapeutic option. However, the widespread application of transplantation is limited by several factors, the most important of which is the scarcity of donor organs. While awaiting a suitable donor heart, patients may die or suffer complications which render them ineligible for transplantation. Potential transplant recipients with severe heart failure have an average life expectancy of approximately 30-60 days (Baumgartner et al. 1979). Of those patients accepted into various transplant programmes, over 20% die per year before an organ becomes available (Copeland et al. 1985). Such patients are candidates for temporary circulatory assistance by a ventricular assist device providing a "bridge to transplantation" (Joyce et al. 1986; Pifarre et al. 1990). There are, however, difficult ethical issues involved in using scarce donor organs to transplant such patients.

1.2.5 Acute Failure Following Cardiac Transplantation

Patients may require support following transplantation for acute failure of the donor heart due to ischaemia (prolonged donor ischaemia time), reperfusion injury or hyperacute rejection (Emery et al. 1991). On occasions, patients have been bridged to retransplantation with ventricular assist devices (Loisance et al. 1987).

1.2.6 Permanent Implantation in End-Stage Failure

The potential demand for donor organs unfortunately far exceeds the availability. In the United States there are approximately 15000 potential recipients per year but only 2000 potential donors (EVANS et al. 1986). Furthermore, there are many patients with end-stage failure who are not currently candidates for transplantation. There currently exists the need for the development of mechanical circulatory assist devices for permanent implantation in the treatment of refractory heart failure. The National Heart, Lung and Blood Institute has estimated that 17000–35000 patients each year in the United States may be candidates for long-term mechanical circulatory support (Working Group on Mechanical Circulatory Support 1985).

1.3 Device Design and Configuration

The native heart beats 40 million times per year and pumps 9818 litres of blood each day. Mechanical devices must be capable of replacing this or augmenting

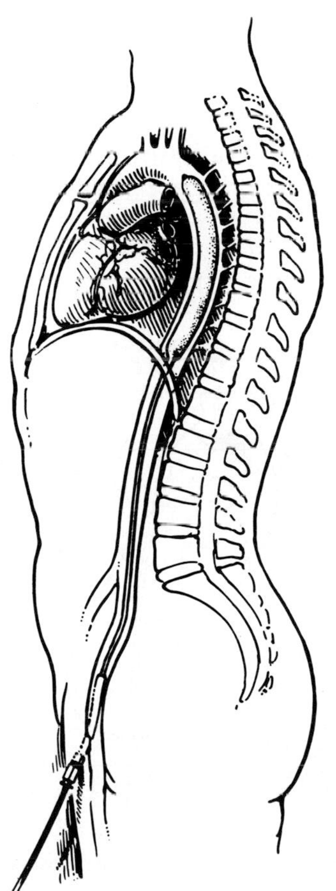

Fig. 1. Intra-aortic balloon pump showing mode of insertion via the femoral artery and siting of inflated balloon within the thoracic aorta

cardiac output to this level. The ideal properties of a mechanical assist device for the heart are that it should be a reliable pump and not require servicing. It must have a reliable and portable power source and be capable of responding to physiological demands. Most importantly, it should show complete biocompatibility both to surrounding soft tissues and to blood circulating through it. In theory an ultra-smooth biomaterial lining should be inert to the coagulation system. In practice this is not the case and an alternative strategy has been adopted which is discussed later (see Sect. 6.1).

Mechanically assisted circulation can be considered in three categories:

1. Series mechanical assistance, e.g. intra-aortic balloon pump (IABP) counterpulsation, in which all of the cardiac output passes through the native heart.
2. Parallel ventricular assistance, in which a variable proportion of the cardiac output bypasses the native heart. This may be achieved using a ventricular assist device (VAD) and either the right (RVAD) or left (LVAD) ventricle may be bypassed.
3. Mechanical replacement of the heart with a total artificial heart (TAH).

1.3.1 Intra-aortic Balloon Pump Counterpulsation

Clinically the IABP is the most commonly used mechanical assist device for patients in acute left ventricular failure. It will improve the cardiac output by up

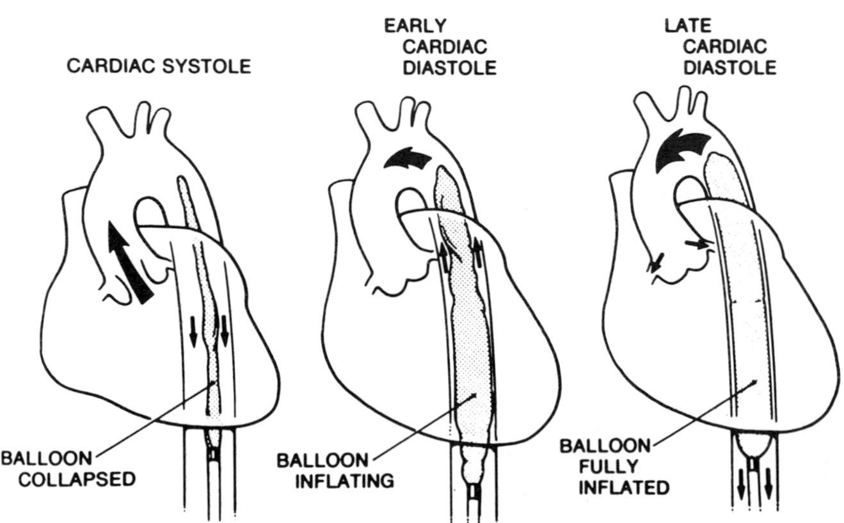

Fig. 2. The timing of balloon inflation with the cardiac cycle. Full inflation during late diastole promotes carotid and coronary perfusion as well as forward flow in the aorta

to 25%, reduce afterload, augment diastolic pressure, increase myocardial perfusion and decrease myocardial oxygen consumption. Furthermore, the use of a percutaneous route of insertion allows rapid institution of therapy and easy removal (Figs. 1, 2).

1.3.2 Centrifugal and Impeller Pumps

The blood pumps which can be used for ventricular assistance fall into two groups: the non-pulsatile impeller and centrifugal pumps and pulsatile devices with artificial chambers which are driven pneumatically or electrically. Centrifugal pumps provide non-pulsatile blood flow by utilising rotating cones to generate energy which is recovered in the form of pressure/flow work. This action is transmitted by a magnetic coupling to a drive magnet. While operating at a given constant speed, the pumps generate nearly constant pressure over a wide range of flow rates. Impeller pumps generate unidirectional flow by the action of an axial vaned impeller. These pumps cause less trauma to blood elements than conventional roller pumps (Fig. 3) and may be used for longer periods. Nevertheless, haemolysis and the need for anticoagulation are the main limitations to prolonged use.

1.3.3 Pulsatile Ventricular Assist Device

The basic elements of a pulsatile VAD are a blood sac, inlet and outlet conduits containing valves and a drive mechanism. Typically the blood sac has a volume of 50–70 ml. The valves used to maintain unidirectional flow range from standard

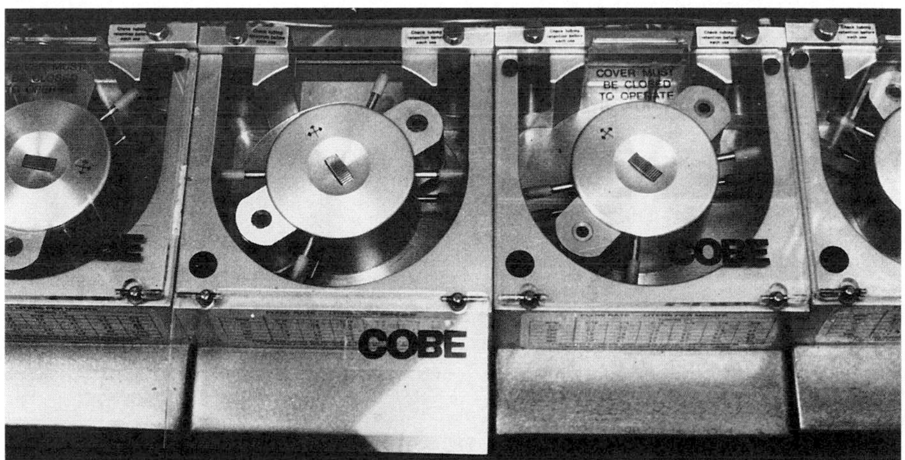

Fig. 3. Cobe roller pump

mechanical valves of the tilting-disc variety (e.g. Björk-Shiley) to pericardial, porcine and dural types. VADs work in parallel with the native ventricle, with input either from the atrium or ventricle and output returned to the great vessels (aorta or pulmonary artery). Ventricular assist pumping can support either or both systemic and pulmonary circulations (Figs. 4, 5). Simultaneously these devices unload the failing ventricle and decrease myocardial oxygen demand. Haemodynamic criteria (cardiac output; right and left atrial, pulmonary arterial and systolic aortic pressures) are used to determine which anatomical form of assistance is appropriate. Right ventricular failure may occur in isolation but more commonly is a consequence of left ventricular failure and the associated increase in pulmonary vascular resistance. Inadequacy of right ventricular function may only be revealed after institution of left ventricular mechanical support. Clinical experience to date indicates that in post-cardiotomy shock the majority of patients

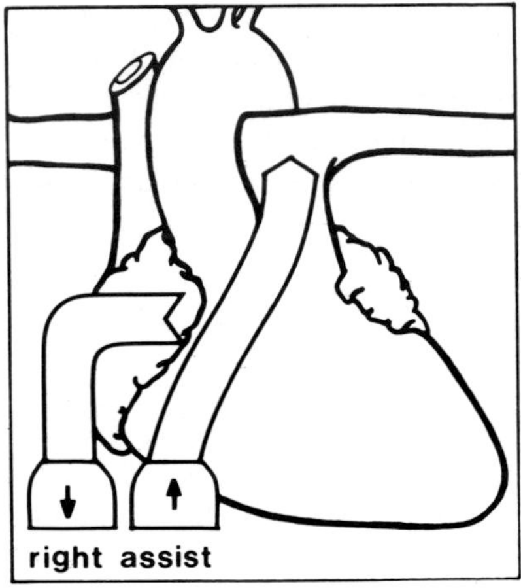

Fig. 4. RVAD insertion with inlet cannula in right atrium and outlet in pulmonary artery

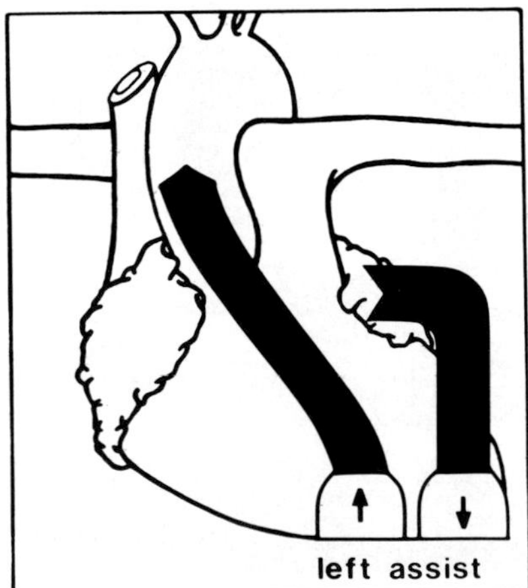

Fig. 5. LVAD insertion with inlet cannula in left atrium and outlet in ascending aorta

(80%) respond to a left VAD alone and an additional right VAD is necessary in only 20% of cases (Fig. 6) (PENNINGTON et al. 1986). Unlike IABP counterpulsation, LVADs can support the circulation fully even through episodes of supraventricular and ventricular arrhythmias, including fibrillation and asystole. The other advantage of VADs is that the native heart remains in situ with the potential for recovery. The disadvantages are the need for transcutaneous passage of cannulae or drive lines (Figs. 7, 8), anticoagulant therapy and the potential hazards of inactivation or failure of the pump.

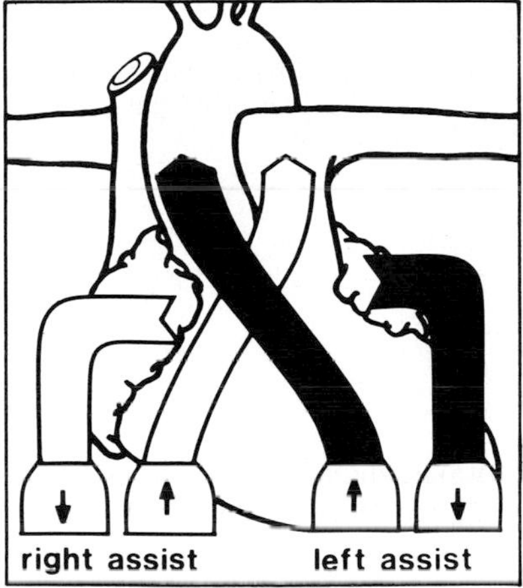

Fig. 6. Biventricular assist device insertion

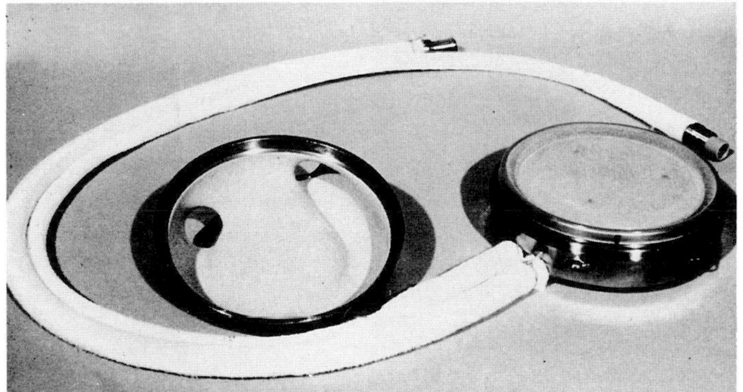

Fig. 7. ThermoCardioSystems pneumatic textured surface LVAD opened to reveal the blood-containing chamber. Attached transcutaneous monitoring and drive lines are also shown

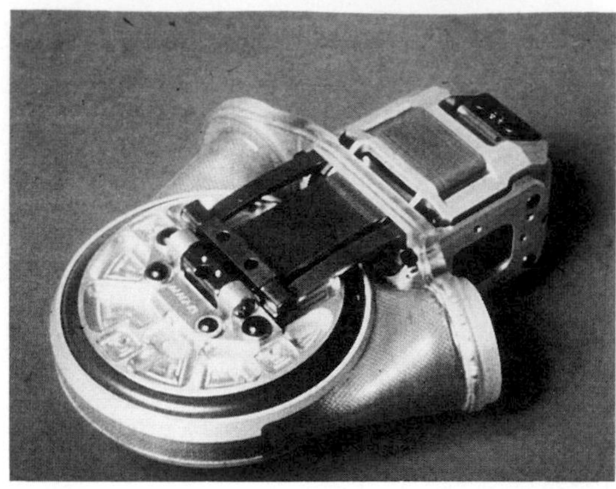

Fig. 8. Novacor Heartmate LVAD, an electrically driven blood pump. Drive lines not shown

1.3.4 Total Artificial Heart

The disadvantages of VADs also apply to the total artificial heart (TAH). Early attempts at permanent implantation of TAHs in the 1980s were plagued with complications of haemorrhage, thromboembolism, sepsis and cerebrovascular accident. No permanent implantation of TAH has been performed world-wide since April 1985 but TAHs have been widely used in clinical practice as mechanical bridges to transplantation (Fig. 9).

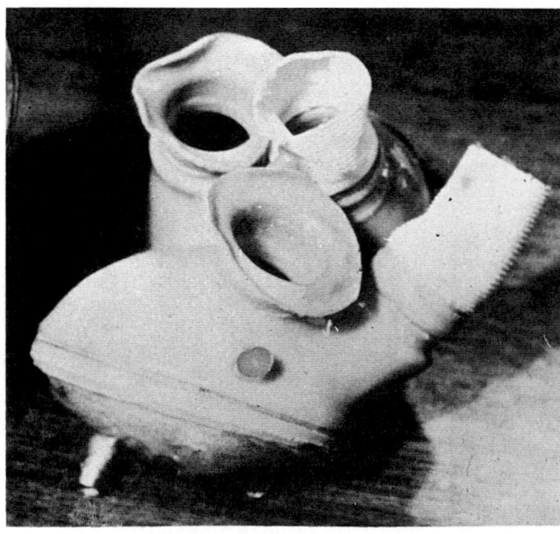

Fig. 9. Utah TAH

1.4 Biomaterials and Device Linings

In order for permanent mechanical circulatory support to become a reality, a satisfactory blood-contacting biomaterial has to be developed. These materials need to be durable and flexible surfaces as they need to move through 40 million cycles per year. They should obviously be non-toxic, non-thromboembolic and maintain haematological homeostasis.

The current choices of blood-contacting, flexible biomaterials for these devices are broadly either smooth or textured polyurethanes (PORTNER et al. 1983). The major limiting factor for long-term use remains the formation of a thin, stable biological lining within the pump (BERNHARD et al. 1978). Complications related to the use of anticoagulants have been a common finding in experimental studies using smooth surface devices (MOCHIZUKI et al. 1981; VASKU et al. 1981; HASTINGS et al. 1981; HARTMANNOVA et al. 1984). Clinical trials have also been troubled by either bleeding or thromboembolic complications, which have accounted for some early deaths (SCHOEN et al. 1982, 1985b; LEVINSON et al. 1986). Particular sites of predilection for thrombus formation have been identified, especially areas of stagnant flow within the device and around valves, but design modifications have had only limited success in reducing these (OLSEN et al. 1975; KESSLER et al. 1978; LEVINSON et al. 1986).

2 Underlying Myocardial Pathology

During insertion of an LVAD a small core of apical left ventricle may be removed to allow cannulation. This may, and indeed should, be submitted for histological examination. Such evaluation may allow some prediction to be made of the likelihood of recovery in doubtful cases. Furthermore it may uncover an unexpected diagnosis such as cardiac amyloid.

The pattern or degree of pathological changes in the myocardium may be subsequently altered by the institution of mechanical assistance.

2.1 Reversible Ischaemia and Reperfusion Injury

Studies have shown that within 60 s of onset of severe ischaemia, cardiac myocytes lose contractility and demonstrate biochemical abnormalities indicating profound derangement. Despite this rapid onset of change, cell death is not immediate but occurs only after a period of 20–30 min. Dysfunctional and severely ischaemic myocardium may thus be reversibly injured and hence viable (REIMER et al. 1983). If reperfusion occurs within the period of reversible injury, necrosis does not result and functional recovery generally occurs (KLONER et al. 1983). The return to normal may be delayed for as long as several days: prolonged post-ischaemic ventricular dysfunction or "stunned" myocardium (Braunwald and Kloner 1982, 1985). Reperfusion causes accelerated destruction of cells that are irreversibly injured, leading to a morphological pattern often called "contraction band" necrosis (Braunwald and Kloner 1985). It also changes the morphological appearance of the area of infarction. Haemorrhage is more marked and neutrophil infiltration considerably reduced (Reichenbach and Cowan 1991; Waller 1988). There is also a striking increase in interstitial and intracellular (intramitochondrial) oedema (Jennings and Reimer 1983). Experimentally a limitation of infarct size can be seen in those cases supported by LVAD compared with controls (Nishi et al. 1989; Chiang et al. 1990).

2.2 Post-cardiotomy Shock

Patients who die following cardiopulmonary bypass or during temporary cardiac assistance frequently have myocardial necrosis with or without haemorrhage and oedema (Schoen et al. 1986).

Ventricular assistance reduces the myocardial workload and oxygen consumption, so leading to a demonstrable improvement in myocardial function after 48–96 h of VAD support (Ghosh 1989). The delay in return of normal myocardial function may be due to gradual resolution of the oedema which develops as a result of myocardial salvage by reperfusion (Schaper et al. 1982). An empty, nonfunctioning ventricle recovers more slowly than a decompressed ventricle in sinus or regular ventricular rhythm with wall tension and diastolic volume reduced to normal (Lefemine et al. 1986). So although VADs are capable of completely taking over from the native ventricle, it is theoretically preferable to maintain the degree of bypass between 30% and 70%.

2.3 Myocarditis and Cellular Rejection

Both myocarditis and cellular rejection are potentially reversible processes in which there is lymphocyte infiltration, interstitial oedema and myocyte necrosis. This causes a loss of compliance and deterioration of myocardial function.

The role of immunosuppressant therapy in reversing this process is well established in rejection, but remains controversial in myocarditis. In the latter it is thought that immunosuppression causes enhanced myocardial necrosis and may retard viral clearance, so resulting in more marked pathological damage (Tomioka et al. 1986).

During recovery the improvement in systolic function is paralleled by clearing of the inflammatory infiltrate (Fenoglio et al. 1983).

3 Animal Models for Device Implantation

The very early research with artificial hearts was conducted during the 1960s on dogs. Later, adult sheep were used but were found to be an unsatisfactory model. In retrospect the failures in these early studies cannot be attributed wholly to the use of sheep and recently investigators have been re-evaluating this model (RAMASAMY et al. 1988, 1989).

The most widely used animal model for artificial heart research has been the calf. Implantation is undertaken at 3 months of age when the calf weighs 70–90 kg. The physiological demands of the calf under exercise are comparable to those of man, and haemodynamically the calf is a good corollary to man. Calves are docile, easily managed in a laboratory setting and remarkably resilient to major surgery. The cost of calves is relatively low and availability is assured. There is a large body of information and data on normal calf physiology, and responses to bypass and ventricular assistance. The use of one animal in assisted circulation research permits the easy and ready exchange of data and information between various international groups (OLSEN and MURRAY 1984). Unfortunately, long-term experiments have demonstrated several specific limitations that are unique to the calf model:

1. *Haematological differences.* The interspecies differences between human and bovine coagulation systems are sufficiently great as to make comparisons between them difficult. Fibrinogen activation and platelet stimulation is much slower in the calf than in man. Conversely, the fibrinolytic system in calves is very poorly developed.
2. *Age.* The calf is a paediatric model and so presents the problem of a growing recipient with a blood pump which cannot grow. At the time of implantation a healthy calf will gain weight at a rate of 0.6 kg per day.
3. *Calcification.* The deposition of calcium phosphate crystals on pump components has been a common problem and may be a reflection of bovine calcium homeostasis.
4. *Pannus formation.* A proliferative fibroblastic growth (pannus) forms around valves, junctions and seams in the devices. This can seriously limit the filling of the pump and so cause failure (WEIDERMANN et al. 1990).
5. *Infection.* The rumen in calves is effectively a large microbiological fermentation tank which causes transient bacteraemias.

4 Experimental Implantation at the Royal London Hospital

To evaluate some of these areas of interest, a multidisciplinary research project has been undertaken at the Royal London Hospital to evaluate an implantable, textured surface LVAD. This has involved an in vivo assessment of safety, reliability and durability, together with haematological, haemodynamic and

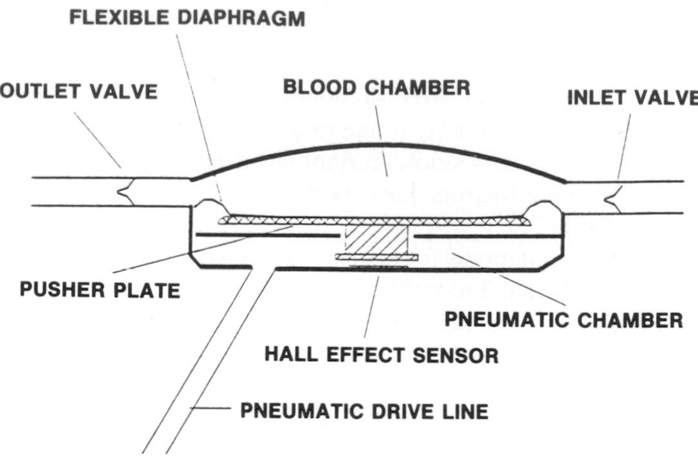

Fig. 10. Pneumatic ThermoCardioSystems LVAD shown diagrammatically in cross-section to illustrate chambers, diaphragm and conduits

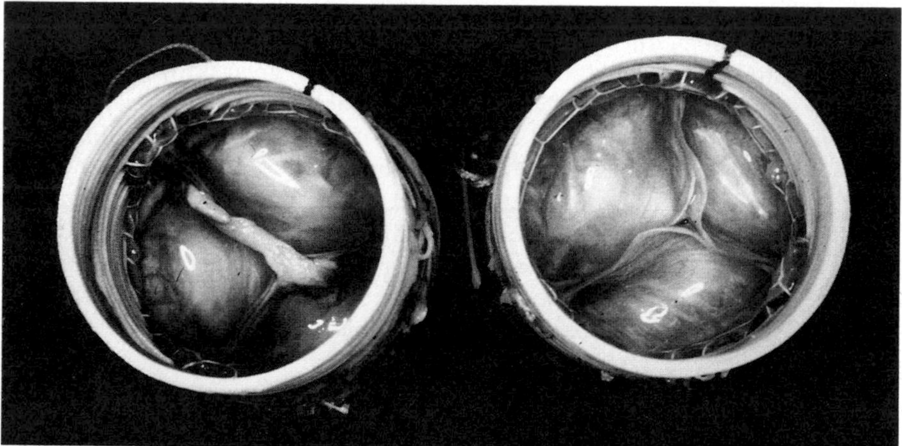

Fig. 11. Medtronic Hancock valves mounted in Dacron conduits

echocardiographic studies. The biologically induced lining and its interaction with circulating blood has also been examined.

A "pusher plate" device: the ThermoCardioSystems Model 14 LVAD (ThermoCardioSystems Inc., Boston, Mass.) was implanted in 21 calves. This is powered either pneumatically or electromechanically; in the pneumatic model, a flexible diaphragm overlying a rigid pusher plate separates the blood-containing chamber from a pneumatic chamber. A pulse of pressurised air enters the latter, moving the diaphragm across towards the static housing. The blood-containing chamber empties during this phase and valves within the inlet and outlet conduits

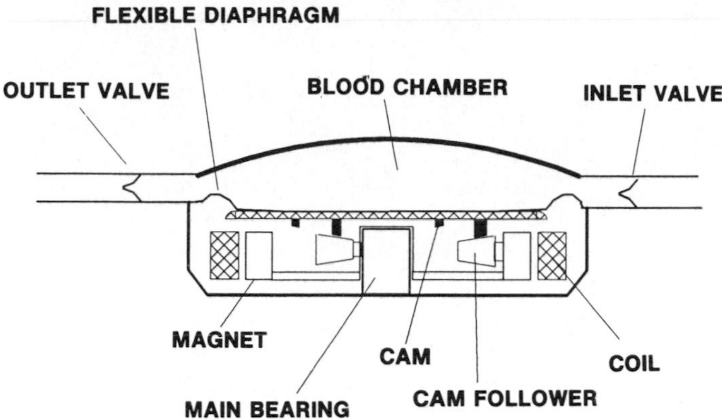

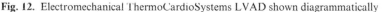

Fig. 12. Electromechanical ThermoCardioSystems LVAD shown diagrammatically

maintain unidirectional flow. During the filling phase, which is a passive process, air is vented to the exterior (Fig. 10). The conduits are Dacron (Dupont, Wilmington, Del.) tubes containing glutaraldehyde-fixed, porcine, Medtronic Hancock valves (Fig. 11; Medtronic Inc., Minneapolis, Minn.). In the electromechanical version, the pneumatic chamber is replaced by an electric motor and rotating cam (Fig. 12).

Seventeen pneumatic models and four electromechanical LVADs have been implanted in calves. This LVAD features textured blood-contacting surfaces. Sintered titanium microspheres line the static housing and an integrally textured polyurethane (Biomer, Ethicon, Somerville, NJ.) flexible diaphragm attached to the pusher plate (Fig. 13). These are designed to attract an adherent, organising coagulum which will lead to neointima formation.

The device was inserted extraperitoneally below the left hemidiaphragm. The inlet conduit was inserted through the apex of the left ventricle into the cavity of the left ventricle. It crossed the central tendon of the diaphragm to reach the device. The outlet conduit passed across the lateral diaphragm and was anastomosed to the descending thoracic aorta. The pneumatic drive line passed across the skin to the external console.

The pathological component of this study involved a full autopsy performed on each animal soon after death or the termination of the experiment. Organs, explanted device and conduits were examined macroscopically and histologically.

Devices were electively explanted at varying time periods (1–127 days, mean 48 days). Survival times are indicated by the height of the bars in Fig. 14. Ten of the devices were seeded with bovine fetal fibroblasts prior to implantation. A summary of the main macroscopic and microscopic changes is given in Table 1.

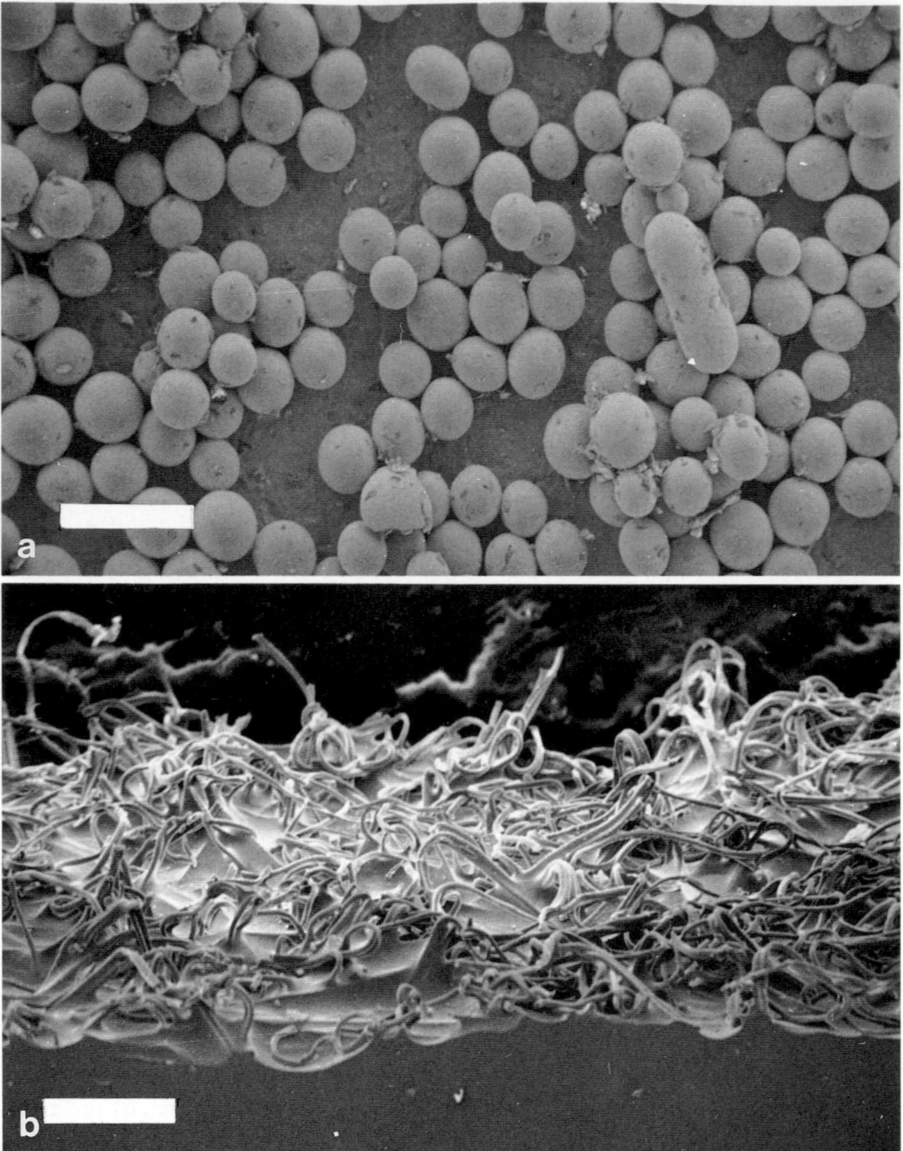

Fig. 13 a,b. Scanning electron micrographs of the textured linings in the ThermoCardioSystems LVAD. **a** Sintered titanium microspheres and **b** integrally textured polyurethane fibrils. Original magnification **(a, b)** × 100 (*Scale bar* = 200 μm)

Table 1. Main microscopic and macroscopic changes observed in calves (n=21) in which the ThermoCardioSystems Model 14 LVAD was implanted

Organ	Pathology	No.
Heart	Subendocardial haemorrhage	9
	Subepicardial haemorrhage	5
	Myocytolysis	3
	Mitral valve: recent haemorrhage	3
	Mitral valve: nodular fibrosis and haemosiderin	1
Prosthetic Valves	Endocarditis	6
	Fibrocalcification	6
	Thrombosis	1
Lungs	Septal/intra-alveolar haemorrhage	13
	Intra-alveolar haemorrhage	11
	Vascular congestion	8
	Peripheral thromboembolism	6
	Bronchopneumonia	3
	Bronchiolitis	2
	Aspirated vegetable matter	2
	Pleural effusion	1
	Haemothorax	1
	Empyema	1
	Pneumomediastinum	1
	Birefringent foreign body emboli	1
	Lung worm	1
Spleen	Longstanding infarction	3
	Recent emboli: septic	1
	Recent emboli: calcific	2
Liver	Portal tract mononuclear cell infiltrate	6
	Fatty change	4
	Acute vascular congestion	7
	Infarcts (subcapsular)	1
CNS	Infarction	1
	Septic emboli	1
	Haemorrhage into white matter	1
	Hypoxic changes in hippocampus	1
Kidney	Interstitial/periglomerular fibrosis	10
	Dystrophic calcification	10
	Hypertensive vessel changes	11
	Vascular congestion	4
	Subcapsular infarction	5
	Recent emboli: calcific	5
	Recent emboli: septic	4
	Recent emboli: birefringent	1
	Calcific concretions in renal pelvis	1

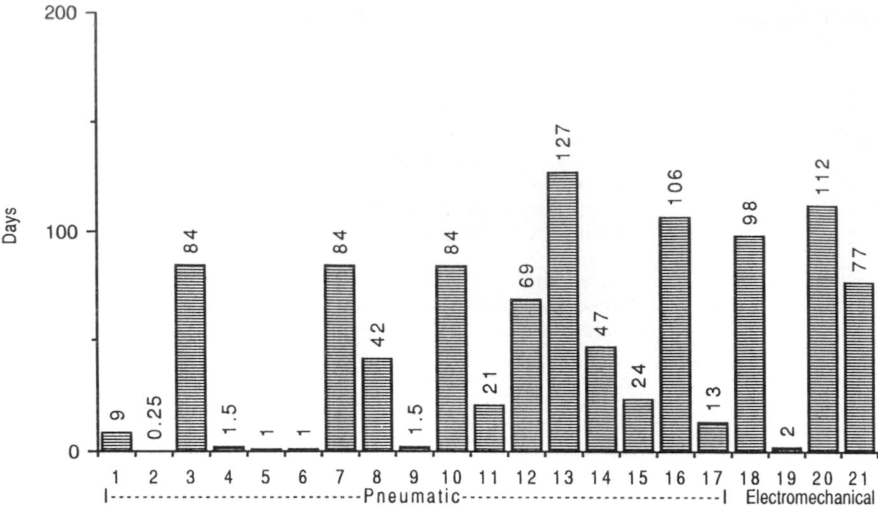

Fig. 14. Duration of LVAD implantation of calves in the Royal London Hospital study

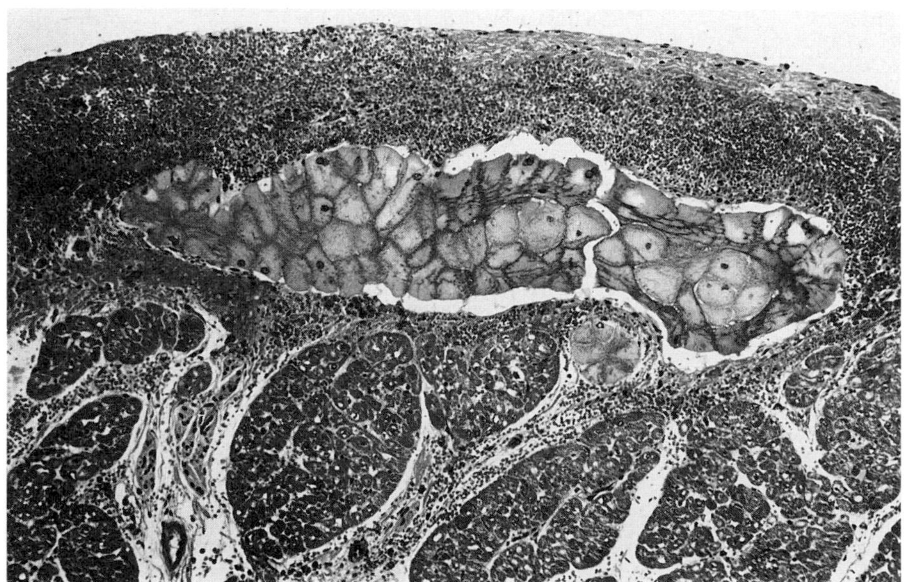

Fig. 15. Subendocardial haemorrhage surrounding large pale conducting fibres *(top)* with normal myocardium beneath. H&E, × 100

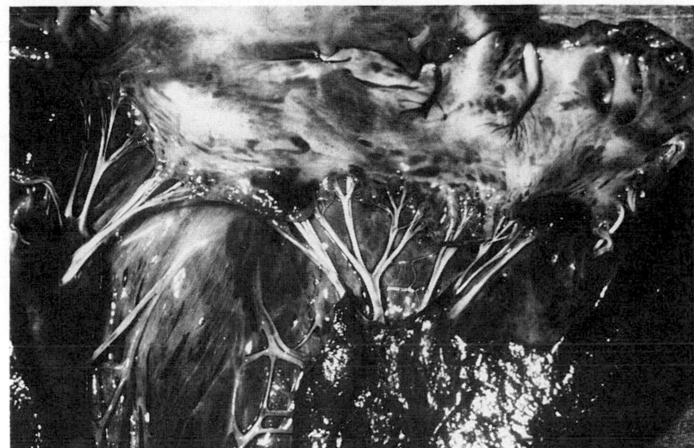

Fig. 16. Traumatic haemorrhage in mitral valve leaflets

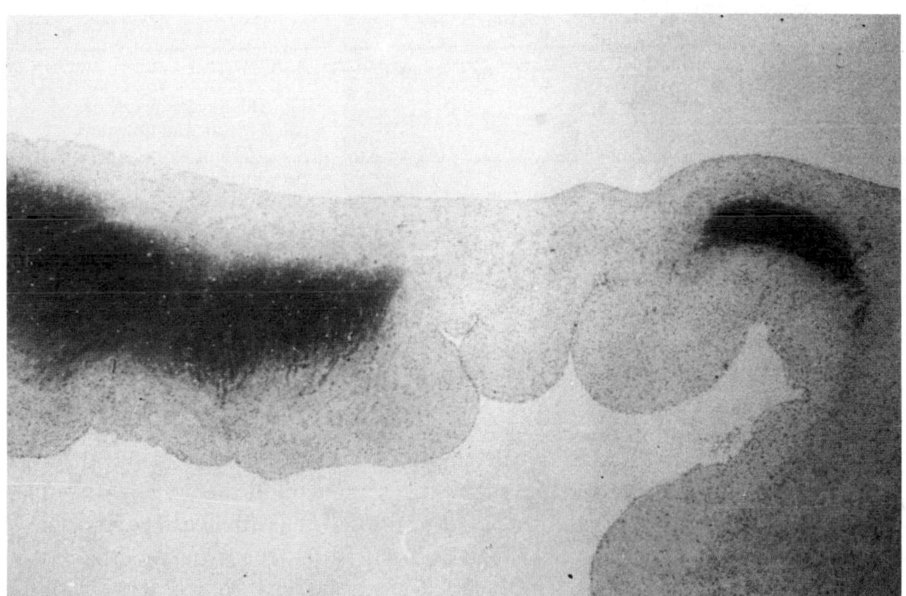

Fig. 17. Haemorrhagic mitral valve seen microscopically shows recent haemorrhage within the valve spongiosa. H&E, $\times 40$

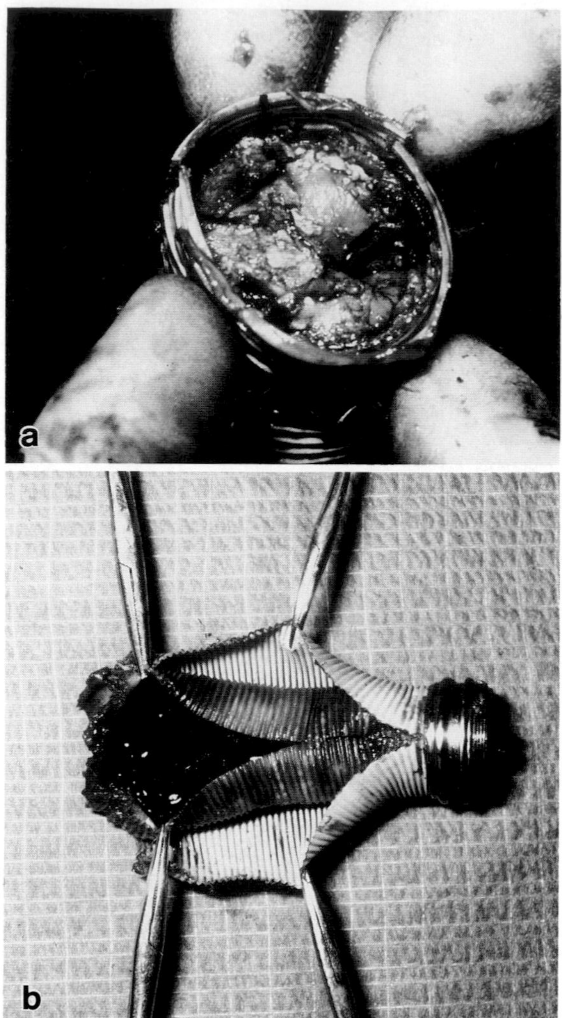

Fig. 18. Severe degree of calcification and fibrotic distortion in bioprosthetic valve **(a)** which resulted in impaired device function and ultimately occlusive thrombosis **(b)**

4.1 Cardiovascular Complications

Subendocardial haemorrhage was a common finding (n = 9). It occurred not only around the insertion of the apical cannula but extended for some distance proximally. Histologically haemorrhage was seen around the conspicuous pale conducting bundles beneath the endocardium (Fig. 15). Evidence of haemorrhage into mitral valve cusps was also seen (n = 4). Both recent haemorrhage and changes indicating previous haemorrhage were seen (Figs. 16, 17). In none of the cases did we find thrombus within the heart, haemorrhage from apical or aortic anastomoses or atrophy of the myocardium.

Varying degrees of calcification and fibrous distortion were noted to the prosthetic valves of several ($n=6$) of the longer term implants. In one case the degree of obstruction was sufficient to cause impaired device filling followed by the formation of occlusive thrombosis (Fig. 18). Superadded endocarditis intervened in some whilst in others it arose de novo ($n=6$). Peripheral emboli from these sources were seen in spleen, kidney, pancreas and brain.

Peripheral birefringent emboli were seen in only one case, a long-term unseeded implant, indicating that the device biomaterial lining had embolised. Embolised calcific debris was seen in spleen ($n=2$) and kidney ($n=5$). This could have arisen from calcified prosthetic valves or fragmented calcified neointima lining the device (Fig. 19).

The finding of haemorrhage into the mitral valves concurs with haemodynamic studies which revealed that the device can exert a negative or subatmospheric pressure within the left ventricle during the filling phase (Withington et al. 1991) Echocardiographic studies also showed that there is a reduction in volume of the left ventricle when the device is functioning (Carey et al. 1991). It would appear that this combination of factors causes the mitral valve cusps to be traumatised by the apical titanium cannula. Repeated trauma of this sort could result in fibrosis and distortion of valve leaflets causing mitral stenosis and so impair the function of long-term implants. Indeed, early fibrosis associated with haemosiderin deposition was seen in one case. Such damaged valves would also be at risk of infective endocarditits.

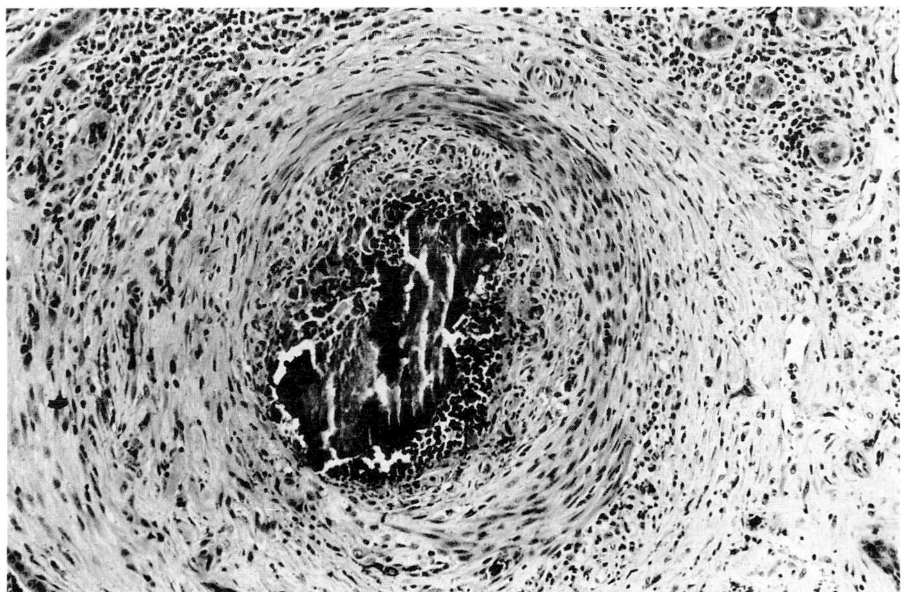

Fig. 19. Calcified debris embolus in kidney. H&E, × 100

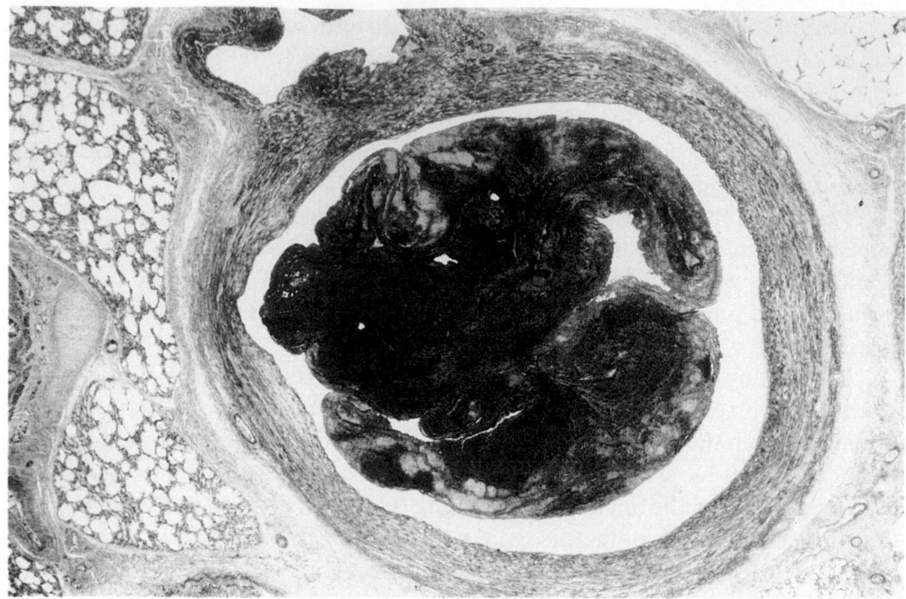

Fig. 20. Peripheral thromboembolus in branch of pulmonary artery. H&E, × 40

4.2 Pulmonary Changes

Oedema, congestion and intra-alveolar haemorrhage were common findings and are inevitable consequences of surgical handling of the paediatric lung. Bronchiolitis ($n = 2$), bronchopneumonia ($n = 3$) and aspiration of vegetable matter were also predictable postoperative complications.

In one case larval forms of bovine lung worm, *Dictyocaulus viviparus,* were seen within alveoli and distal air passages.

Small peripheral thromboemboli (Fig. 20) were seen ($n = 6$), but no large proximal fatal pulmonary emboli were observed. Pulmonary hypertensive changes were not noted in any case.

4.3 Cerebral Pathology

Pathological changes in the calf brains were relatively infrequent, comprising infarction ($n = 1$), septic embolus ($n = 1$), haemorrhage into white matter ($n = 1$) and hypoxic changes in hippocampus ($n = 1$). The low incidence of cerebral changes in part may be due to anatomical differences between the calf and man. Blood flow to the brain of the calf passes through a structure, the rete mirabile, which may serve to filter out emboli before they reach the brain.

4.4 Renal Pathological Changes

Kidneys from many ($n = 11$) of the animals with longer term implant showed a pale and thinned cortex with patchy, dark discoloration of the subcapsular cortical surface. In these cases changes were noted in interlobular arteries and arterioles: medial hypertrophy, intimal hyperplasia and significant reduction in vessel lumen diameter (Figs. 21, 22). Secondary diffuse ischaemic changes were apparent in the kidneys of these animals: interstitial and periglomerular fibrosis with dystrophic calcification and chronic inflammatory infiltrates in the interstitium (Fig. 23). Glomerular tuft collapse and ischaemia were apparent and hyalinisation of afferent arterioles was also seen. Features of accelerated or malignant hypertension, particularly fibrinoid necrosis, were not seen in any of these cases.

Subcapsular infarcts were seen in association with prosthetic valve endocarditis. These infarcts showed rather marked marginal haemorrhage, probably because the calves were anticoagulated.

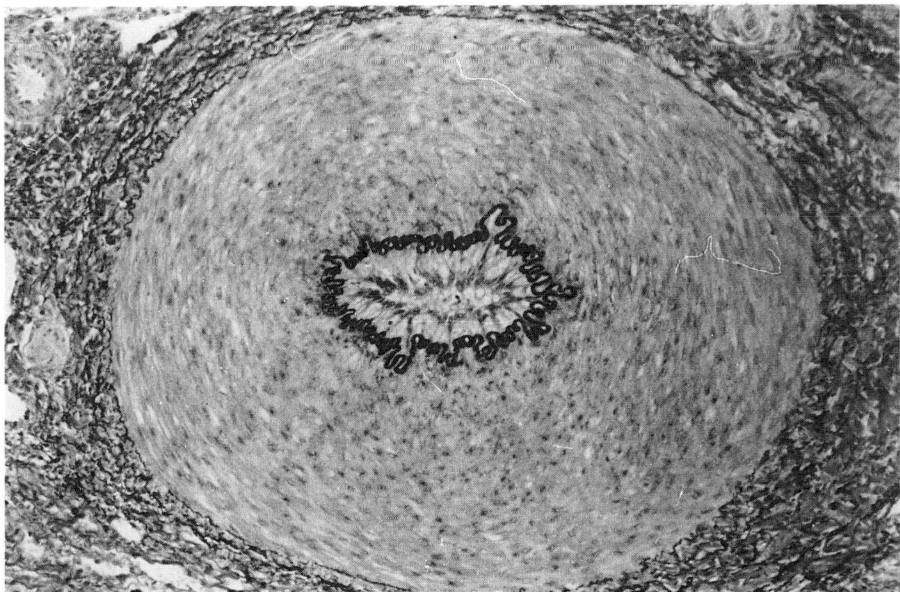

Fig. 21. Interlobular artery showing marked medial hypertrophy, intimal hyperplasia and reduction in luminal cross-sectional area. Elastin–van Gieson, × 140

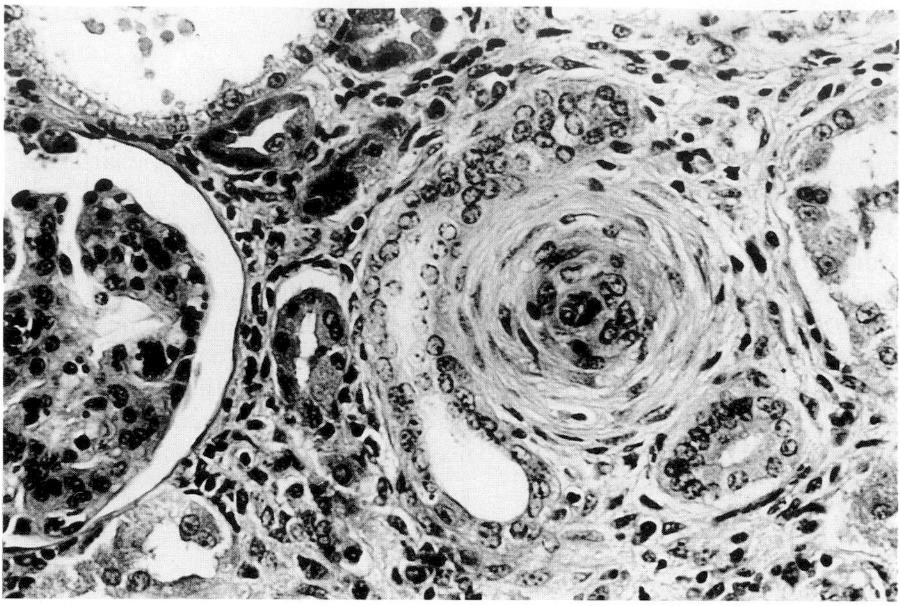

Fig. 22. Glomerulus and afferent arteriole with pronounced medial changes in the latter. H&E, × 140

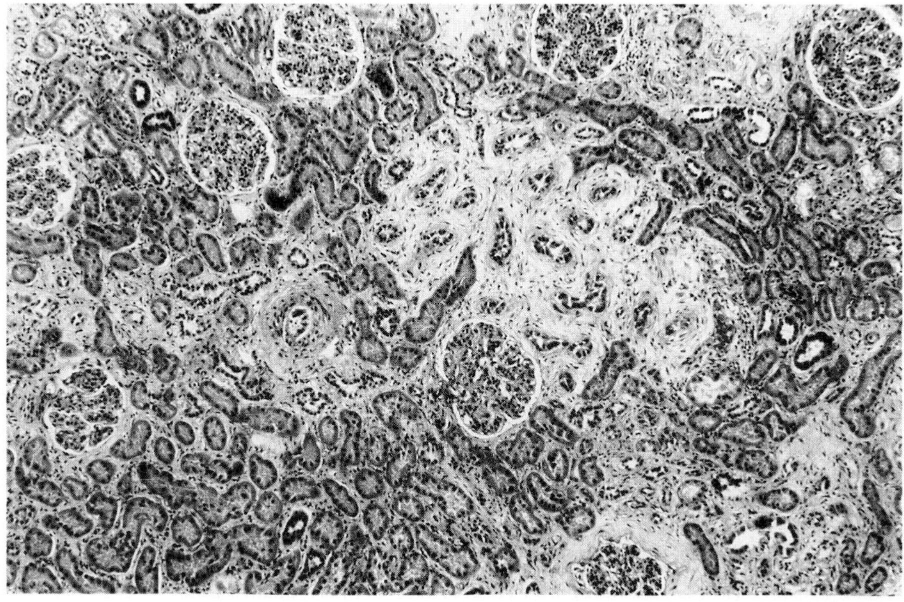

Fig. 23. Patchy interstitial fibrosis in renal parenchyma secondary to vascular changes. H&E, × 40

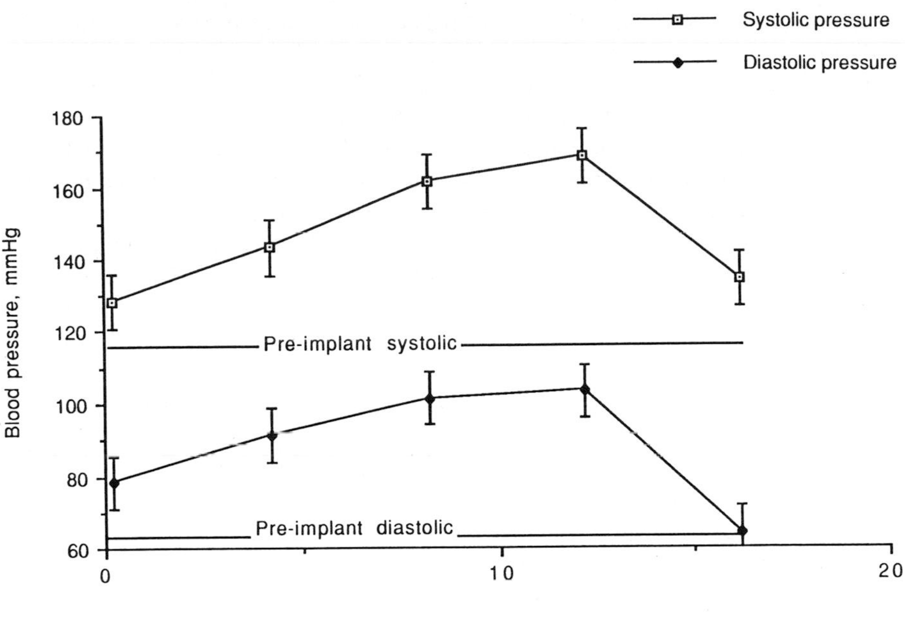

Fig. 24. Summary of long-term implant haemodynamic data

4.5 Hypertension

The haemodynamic data from the longest surviving implants are summarised in Fig. 24. There is little change in the systolic and diastolic blood pressures in the early postoperative period from the preoperatively. However, significant and sustained elevations in both systolic and diastolic blood pressures were noted in calves surviving up to and beyond 50 days (WITHINGTON et al. 1991).

Renovascular pathological changes associated with this hypertension have been a consistent complication in long-term implants. The mean duration of implantation for cases showing renovascular changes was 79 days, and for those without changes, 13.5 days. The degree of calcification observed in the kidneys is probably a reflection of a bovine paediatric model. Chronic pyelonephritis may also cause fibrosis and renal scarring but persistent urinary infections were not documented and scarring of the renal pelvis was not seen. Renal calculi were only seen in one case. Multiple peripheral thromboemboli to the renal vasculature may also cause a "flea-bitten" appearance. This possibility cannot be excluded; however, the very low frequency with which recent or recanalising thrombi were seen in renal vessels would count against it. Furthermore, it is not otherwise possible to account for the larger vessel changes.

Several explanations of the observed hypertension are possible. Alterations in pressure waveforms as a result of device insertion may affect baroreceptor function. Alternatively an increase in cardiac output may arise as a result of the LVAD working in tandem with a normally functioning left ventricle. Finally a reduction in left atrial and left ventricular end-diastolic pressures brought about by the LVAD may affect humoral factors which are concerned with the control of blood pressure. Until the cause of the observed hypertension is established, it is not possible to predict whether or not this will present a problem to long-term implantation in human adults with poor left ventricular function.

Pulmonary artery pressure rose immediately following device implantation, but by 2 weeks this had fallen to preoperative values. This accords with previous work which showed that circulating catecholamine levels and pulmonary vascular resistance return to normal 2 weeks postoperatively (Olsen et al. 1977). Pulmonary hypertension has been described following total artificial heart implantation in the calf (Weidermann et al. 1981). In our series there was neither haemodynamic nor histological evidence of this complication.

These renovascular changes may be a potential problem for long-term use of these devices. The incidence of systemic embolisation from the device's textured lining appears to be low but the calcification and infection of the prosthetic valves is a potential source of emboli, systemic infection and early device failure. For the various reasons already outlined, the calf model has significant limitations and these must be borne in mind when extrapolating to the clinical situation.

5 Pathological Complications in Clinical Application

A substantial world-wide experience in the clinical implantation of VADs and TAHs has now been accumulated. Most experience has been gained in temporary use of these devices as bridges to transplantation. Unfortunately the large majority of reports focus on the use of a single device and very few comparative studies have been undertaken. Nevertheless the pathological changes seen are broadly similar.

When considering the complications of device insertion it is important to consider the clinical status of the patient immediately prior to surgery and the nature of the surgery itself. A prolonged low-output state before pump implantation predisposes to the multiple system failure which may complicate short-term assistance.

5.1 Haemorrhage and Anticoagulation

In most studies uncontrollable haemorrhage is identified as a major cause of death after ventricular assistance. Bleeding necessitating operative exploration is also a common complication, occurring in 52% of patients in one large series (Kanter et al. 1988). This is considered to be largely a result of the haemostatic abnormalities induced by the extended duration of cardiopulmonary bypass before, during and after surgery (Harker 1986). Sustained activation of platelets and coagulation secondary to blood contact with artificial surfaces also results in a consumptive coagulopathy (AL-MONDHIRY and PIERCE 1989). Additional factors such as infection, hepatic impairment and acute pancreatitis have also been implicated in this process. Haemolysis has not been a clinically significant problem with temporary cardiac assistance although changes in erythrocyte deformability have been reported in patients during left ventricular assistance (FRATTINI et al. 1989; HUNG et al. 1989).

5.2 Thrombosis and Embolism

Clinical temporary ventricular assistance has been associated with a low degree of pump-related thromboembolic complications (SCHOEN et al. 1986). In contrast, patients who have undergone long-term TAH implantation have almost uniformly experienced serious thromboembolic sequelae (JOYCE et al. 1986).

The pathogenesis of thrombus formation in the artificial heart is undoubtedly multifactorial. Contributing factors may include the geometry and flow dynamics of the device, the anticoagulation regimen used and concomitant problems such as infection. Crevices and other surface discontinuities can serve as a nidus for thrombus formation. Flow studies indicate that thrombus formation tends to occur in areas associated with eddy currents and stagnant flow (WARD et al. 1987). Particularly vulnerable sites include junctions and seams, conduit connectors, prosthetic valves and the diaphragm-housing interface. Design modifications have gone some way to reduce sites of predilection for thrombus formation, but have not eliminated them (DEW et al. 1990).

A comparison of platelet activation and fibrin metabolism in recipients of TAH and heart transplants showed sustained elevations in the former group despite anticoagulation therapy (RING et al. 1989). Indeed, antiplatelet drugs and warfarin seem to be ineffective in preventing artificial heart-related thromboembolic complications long-term (AL-MONDHIRY and PIERCE 1989).

Calcification of bioprosthetic valves within conduits (FISHBEIN et al. 1982; NISTAL et al. 1988) acts as a focus for both thrombosis and infection. Embolisation of calcified fragments of neointima and underlying biomaterial have also been noted (VASKU 1989).

5.3 Infection

The surgical implantation of any foreign body predisposes the recipient to infection. Cardiac assist devices are especially prone to infection. Not only are the mediastinal tissues exposed to a foreign body, but the vascular compartment flows through the device. Furthermore, with the exception of the totally implantable devices currently being developed, transcutaneous conduits or drive lines are also present. Other indwelling devices such as vascular cannulae, tracheal tubes, urinary catheters and chest drains provide additional routes of infection and sites for colonisation.

In a series of TAH recipients, the commonest sites of infection were: mediastinum (36%), blood (29%), sputum (26%), drive lines (21%) and urine (12%) (Didishein et al. 1989). Infection of the artificial heart and native heart was seen in 7% and of valves and grafts in 5%. The cavities and voids which surround the device within the mediastinum provide a seed-bed for infection. In addition the biomaterials used in the construction of VADs have been shown significantly to impair the function of tissue neutrophils and so predispose to periprosthetic infection (Kaplan et al. 1990). The function of circulating neutrophils is not affected. Bacterial adhesion to biomaterial surfaces together with poor integration with surrounding host tissues is another exacerbating factor (Gristina et al. 1988).

Design modifications of percutaneous access devices have had some success in reducing infection (Holmberg et al. 1988; Allan et al. 1990). However, until a totally implantable system is available, these will remain a potential avenue for the introduction of infection.

Within devices thrombotic and infective complications appear to be interrelated. Examination of thrombi within explanted devices often shows them to be infective. Conversely, bacterial infection will promote thrombosis by numerous direct and indirect mechanisms.

Infection is particularly crucial in patients who are being bridged to transplantation and who will subsequently require immunosuppression to prevent rejection. Pretransplant mechanical support with a VAD or TAH has been shown significantly to increase the risk of infection-related mortality (Griffith et al. 1988; HSU et al. 1989).

5.4 Immunological Impairment

Infections associated with device implantation may be exacerbated by factors directly attributable to the device which impair the immune system. The generation of micro-thromboemboli within the device may result in blockade of the reticuloendothelial system and so impair the patient's ability to clear microorganisms from the circulation (Ward et al. 1987). Multiple blood transfusions and coagulopathy may contribute to this process. In long-term clinical implantation, lymphopenia has been demonstrated, although serum complement and polymorphonuclear leucocyte function remained intact (Wellhausen et al. 1988). Histological examination of lymphoid tissue at autopsy further revealed reduced numbers of germinal centres and atrophy of T-cell-dependent areas.

5.5 Renal Dysfunction

Postoperative renal function in patients who have undergone open heart surgery significantly depends on preoperative circulation, renal function and the duration of cardiopulmonary bypass (HILBERMAN et al. 1979). Experimentally ventricular assistance itself does not disturb renal function (WESTENFELDER et al. 1985). Although there may be a significant improvement in renal function after TAH implantation, there is no apparent correlation between the degree of pre-implant dysfunction and post-implant recovery (KAWAGUCHI et al. 1990).

5.6 Cardiac Complications

Theoretically it might be expected that prolonged ventricular assistance would result in atrophy of the myocardium of the native heart. In those cases in which recovery of native ventricular function is the goal of assistance, this could be a disastrous complication. Experimentally such atrophy has been demonstrated by morphometric techniques. It was shown to correlate with the duration of assistance and the bypass flow rate (KINOSHITA et al. 1988). The significance of this has to be interpreted with caution since the starting point experimentally is normal rather than diseased myocardium.

The use of the left ventricular apex as the point of anastomosis for the inlet conduit for implantable LVADs is hazardous in those patients with cardiogenic shock due to myocardial infarction. There is a risk that the initial infarct has involved this area, rendering the anastomosis insecure. Furthermore there is the ever-present danger that there may be subsequent reinfarction with extension to involve the apex. The outcome of this is catastrophic haemorrhage from the anastomosis and rapid demise (LEWIS et al. 1990).

5.7 Neurological Sequelae

Despite aggressive anticoagulation therapy, cerebral thromboembolic complications proved a very serious drawback in the early trials of permanent TAH implantation in man (LEVINSON et al. 1986). Embolic strokes were correlated with thrombus generation within the device. Design modifications have had only limited success in reducing these (OLSEN et al. 1975; KESSLER et al. 1978; LEVINSON et al. 1986). Furthermore, some patients have suffered secondary intracranial haemorrhage as a result of anticoagulation therapy. Elimination of this problem is dependent on the development of a totally inert biomaterial and this is discussed further later (see Sect. 6.1). The rate of thromboembolic phenomena is much lower with short-term use of TAH but remains unacceptable (GRIFFITH 1989).

Low cardiac output preoperatively can predispose to a range of acute cerebral ischaemic injuries in the absence of thromboemboli (Peters 1979). Careful assessment prior to surgery is needed to avoid the distressing situation in which a stroke patient is bridged toward a transplant for which the patient is no longer a suitable candidate.

Rheological changes such as erythrocyte rigidity related to device insertion have also been implicated in neurological changes (Hung et al. 1991).

6 Device Linings

The ideal biomaterial to provide the blood-contacting surface in a long-term mechanical circulatory support device must be non-toxic and non-thrombogenic and must not degrade over time. Biomer, an aromatic polyurethane with excellent flex life, has been the most widely used material for this application. Although it has excellent mechanical and non-toxic properties, it retains some thrombogenic properties.

Attempts have been made to reduce thrombus generation by making smooth surfaces within the blood-containing chamber of pumps. However, it is extremely difficult to manufacture a microscopically smooth polyurethane surface. Even minor surface imperfections measured in microns can serve as a nidus for platelet adhesion and thrombus accumulation. Although anticoagulation is routinely used, it is difficult to balance the propensity for thrombus formation in a given pump with effective anticoagulation therapy in each unique clinical setting.

6.1 Textured and Smooth Biomaterial Surfaces

An alternative approach for controlling thromboembolic events involves the use of textured biomaterials for the blood-contacting surfaces (Dasse et al. 1987). This approach has gained wide clinical acceptance when used in vascular grafts. Materials such as Dacron which are relatively thrombogenic, are used in porous woven grafts. These become lined by thrombus which becomes organised and is replaced by the formation of a neointima. This then functions as a permanent biocompatible blood-contacting surface (Fig. 25). The same principle has been applied in the construction of the ThermoCardioSystems VAD, which is unique among blood pumps in having textured blood-contacting surfaces. Sintered titanium microspheres consisting of small spheres of titanium fused together to provide the textured surface on the non-flexing components of the pump. Flexing surfaces consist of integrally textured polyurethane which is manufactured in such a way that fibrils of polyurethane are continuous with an underlying diaphragm. Earlier surfaces were made using adhesively bonded, flocked polyester fibrils on a polyurethane diaphragm. These were prone to become dislodged and this problem is eliminated with the integrally textured surfaces.

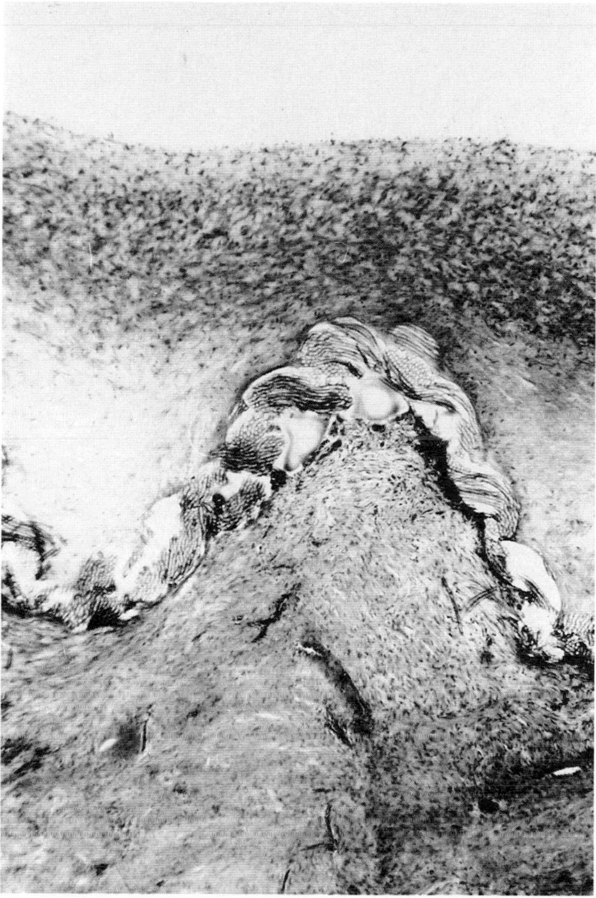

Fig. 25. Porous Dacron graft from a bovine LVAD implant. The graft lumen (*top*) is lined by a cellular neointima which is in contact with surrounding fibroblastic tissue through pores in the woven material. The neointima which develops in man is much less cellular than this. H&E, × 40

An important difference between the textured surfaces within blood pumps and those in vascular grafts is that the former are impermeable to surrounding tissue. Consequently, any contribution to the development of neointima from either in-growth or the release of exogenous tissue factors across a porous surface is eliminated. The typical neointima found on vascular grafts in man is largely acellular and formed of fibrin and collagen. In comparison with this the neointima on integrally textured polyurethane (ITP) and sintered titanium microspheres (STM) is cellular (Fig. 26). It is unlikely that cells migrate from the anastomosis, on the basis of the speed with which they appear and the distance of migration involved. The cell population lining textured surfaces must be assumed to be derived from circulating cells (GRAHAM et al. 1990).

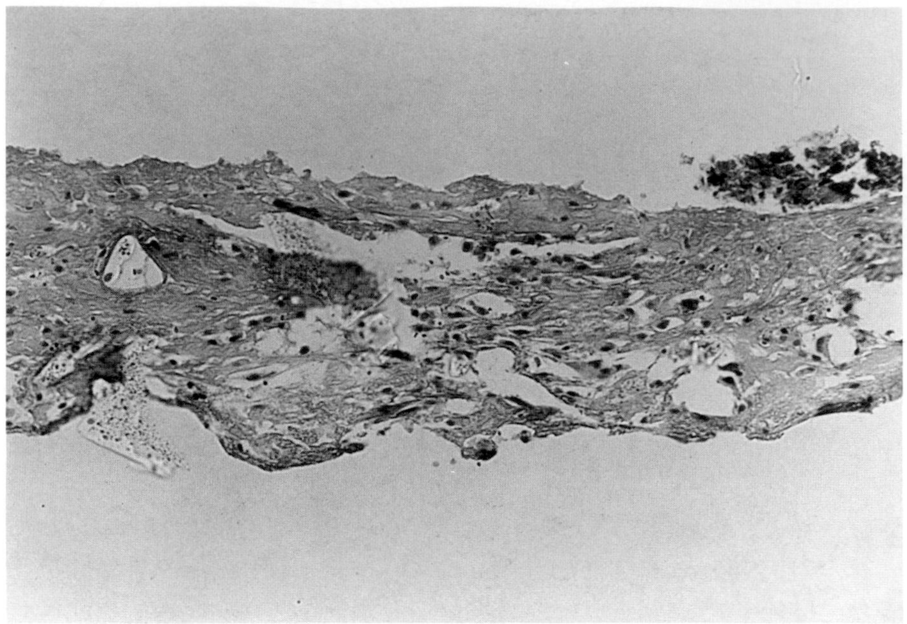

Fig. 26. Cellular neointima overlying integrally textured polyurethane. The outlines of fibrils can be seen surrounded by neointima on the deep surface (*lower*). H&E, × 40

6.2 Tissue Integration and Microbial Adhesion

The major impediments to the extended use of VADs and TAHs are associated with biomaterial–host interactions. In particular a lack of complete tissue integration, biomaterial-centered infection on the outer surfaces of devices and thrombosis within the blood-contacting chambers. These problems all relate to interactions between device surfaces and cells, be they prokaryotic or eukaryotic.

Foreign-body-centered infections are caused by adhesive bacterial colonisation of surfaces and are the result of the highly adaptive ability of bacteria to colonise inert biomaterials. Successful tissue integration depends on the ability of tissue cells similarly to adhere to biomaterial in an intimate and non-inflammatory manner.

Once attached to a substratum, bacteria produce a polysaccharide matrix within which propagation and spread can occur. An established infection cannot be adequately treated until the substratum is removed.

Tissue integration is the desired result of biomaterial implantation and has interesting parallels to microbial adhesion. The fate of a biomaterial implant may be seen to depend on a "race for the surface", a contest between tissue cell integration and bacterial adhesion to the same surface. If the race is won by the tissue then the surface is occupied and defended and is thus less available for bacterial colonisation (GRISTINA 1987). Perturbation of host defences by the biomaterial may be a vital factor tipping the balance in favour of microbial adhesion.

6.3 Cell Seeding

The early events in blood-biomaterial interaction are protein adsorption and platelet adhesion, activation and release leading to the formation of a platelet–fibrin coagulum. This process is limited within vascular grafts by a combination of flow, fibrinolysis and anticoagulation. The thin platelet - fibrin layer is relatively rapidly converted into a protein layer predominantly of fibrin. In smooth surface devices this is the ideal end-point. However, clinical experience has shown that surface imperfections and areas of stasis lead to propagation of thrombus and embolism.

In porous vascular grafts the platelet–fibrin layer becomes organised to from a neointima. The rationale behind the use of textured biomaterials in VADs is to promote a similar process on non-porous surfaces. Clinical studies have shown that these surfaces become populated by cells originating from the blood (GRAHAM et al. 1990). Attempts have been made to seed the biomaterial surface with fibroblasts prior to implantation (GRAHAM et al. 1987; BERNHARD 1989). Experimentally this has resulted in increased stability of neointima and reduced frequency of embolisation.

Since the antithrombotic properties of vessel walls depend on an intact lining of viable endothelial cells actively producing antithrombotic agents such as prostacyclin, the ideal cell type for seeding would be endothelial cells. Published reports of endothelial cell seeding of vascular prostheses have so far yielded poor results. Endothelial cell retention on grafts has been cited as a major problem (HERRING and LEGRAND 1989: HERRING 1991).

6.4 Surface Modifications

Physical and chemical manipulation of biomaterial surfaces to improve tissue integration is an active area of research at present. Examples of such surface modifications include the incorporation of antibiotics into biomaterials to impede bacterial adhesion and so promote tissue integration.

Components of the subendothelial cell matrix such as collagen type IV and fibronectin have been used to coat grafts to improve endothelial cell adhesion and retention (VOHRA et al. 1991). It remains to be seen whether or not such seeded endothelial cells will remain adherent when exposed to turbulent blood flow within a blood pump or whether they will produce anti-thrombotic prostacyclins.

The ultimate success or failure of long-term device implantation will depend on favourable interactions between biomaterials and host tissues at the cellular and subcellular level. Future research efforts in this field must focus on ways to optimise these interactions.

References

Allan A, Graham TR, Withington PS, Salih V, Dasse KA, Poirier VL, Lewis CT (1990) Development of a polyurethane percutaneous access device for long-term vascular access. ASAIO Trans 36: M349–351

Al-Mondhiry H, Pierce WS (1989) Hemostatic abnormalities in two patients implanted with total artificial hearts. Artif Organs 13: 464–469

Barcroft H (1933) Observations on the pumping action of the heart. J Physiol 78: 186–195

Baumgartner WA, Reitz BA, Oyer PE, et al. (1979) Cardiac homotransplantation. Curr Probl Surg 16:1

Bernhard WF (1989) A fibrillar blood-prosthetic interface for both temporary and permanent ventricular assist devices: experimental and clinical observations. Artif Organs 13: 255–271

Bernhard WF, LaFarge CG, Liss RH, Szycher M, Berger RL, Poirier V (1978) An appraisal of blood trauma and the prosthetic interface during left ventricular bypass in the calf and humans. Ann Thorac Surg 26: 427–437

Braunwald E, Kloner RA (1982) The stunned myocardium-prolonged, post-ischaemic ventricular dysfunction. Circulation 66: 1146–1149

Braunwald E, Kloner RA (1985) Myocardial reperfusion a double-edged sword? J Clin Invest 76: 1713–1719

Brodie TC (1903) The perfusion of surviving organs. J Physiol 29: 266–275

Carey C, Graham TR, Harrington D, Withingtom PS, Miles PG, Lewis CT (1991) Echocardiography during left ventricular assist. Artif Organs 14: 124–126

Chiang BY, Ye C-X, Gu Y-G, Gao X-D, Wang Y-S (1990) Limitation of myocardial infarct size by a right ventricular assist device. ASAIO Trans 36: M398–401

Copeland JG, Emery RW, Levinson MM, Copeland J, Maaleer JM, Riley JE (1985) The role of mechanical support and transplantation in treatment of patients with end stage cardiomyopathy. Circulation (Cardiovasc Suppl) 72(II): 7–12

Dasse KA, Chipman SD, Sherman CN, Levine AH, Frazier OH (1987) Clinical experience with textured blood contacting surfaces in ventricular assist devices. ASAIO Trans 10: 418–425

DeBakey ME (1934) A simple continuous-flow blood transfusion instrument. New Orleans Med Surg J 87: 386–389

DeBakey ME (1971) Left ventricular bypass pump for cardiac assistance. Am J Cardiol 27: 3–11

Dennis C, Hall DP, Moreno JR, Senning A (1962) Reduction of oxygen utilisation of the heart by left heart bypass. Circ Res 10: 298–305

DeVries WC, Anderson JL, Joyce LD, Anderson FL, Hammond EL, Jarvik RK, Kolff WJ (1984) Clinical use of the total artificial heart. N Engl J Med 310: 273–278

Dew PA, Pantalos GM, Holfert JW, Burns GL, Everett SD, Olsen DB (1990) Design mediated thrombus reduction in the Utah-100 total artificial heart. ASAIO Trans 36: M230–234

Didisheim P, Olsen DB, Farrar DJ, et al. (1989) Infection and thromboembolism with implantable cardiovascular devices. ASAIO Trans 35: 54–70

Embly EH, Martin CJ (1905) The action of anaesthetic quantities of chloroform upon the blood vessels of the bowel and kidney, with an account of an artificial circulation apparatus. J Physiol 32: 147–158

Emery RW, Eales F, Joyce LD, et al. (1991) Mechanical circulatory assistance after heart transplantation. Ann Thorac Surg 51: 43–47

Evans RW, Mannion DL, Garrison LP Jr, Maier AM (1986) Donor availability as the primary determinant of the future of heart transplantation. JAMA 255: 1892–1898

Fenoglio JJ, Ursell PC, Kellogg CF, Drusin RE, Weiss MB (1983) Diagnosis and classification of myocarditis by endomyocardial biopsy. N Engl J Med 308: 12–18

Fishbein MC, Levy RJ, Ferrans VJ, Dearden LC, Nashef A, Goodman AP, Capentier A (1982) Calcification of cardiac valve prostheses. J Thorac Cardiovasc Surg 83: 602–609

Frattini PL, Wachter C, Hung TC, Kormos RL, Griffith BP, Borovetz HS (1989) Erythrocyte deformability in patients on left ventricular assist systems. ASAIO Trans 35: 733–735
Ghosh PK (1989) Precedents and perspectives. In: Unger F (ed) Assisted circulation 3. Springer, Berlin Heidelberg New York, pp 8–48
Gibbs OS (1933) An artificial heart for dogs. J Pharmacol Exp Ther 49: 181–186
Graham TR, Chalmers JAC, Syndercombe-Court YD (1987) Initial experience with seeding of neointima in a rough surface left ventricular assist device. Artif Organs 11: 318–319
Graham TR, Dasse KA, Coumbe A, Salih V, Marrinan MT, Frazier OH, Lewis CT (1990) Neo-intimal development on textured biomaterial surfaces during clinical use of an implantable left ventricular assist device. Eur J Cardiothorac Surg 4: 182–190
Griffith BP (1989) Temporary use of the Jarvik-7 artificial heart – the Pittsburgh experience. In: Unger F (ed) Artificial circulation 3. Springer, Berlin Heidelberg New York, pp 269–281
Griffith BP, Kormos RL, Hardesty RL, Armitage JM, Dummer JS (1988) The artificial heart: Infection-related morbidity and its effect on transplantation. Ann Thorac Surg 45: 409–414
Gristina AG (1987) Biomaterial centered infection: microbial adhesion versus tissue integration. Science 237: 1588–1595
Gristina AG, Dobbins JJ, Giammara B, Lewis JC, DeVries WC (1988) Biomaterial centred sepsis and the total artificial heart. Microbial adhesion vs tissue integration. JAMA 259: 865–869
Harker LA (1986) Bleeding after cardiopulmonary bypass. N Engl J Med 314: 1446–1448
Hartmannova B, Vasku J, Dolezel S, et al. (1984) Mechanisms causing the death of 8 calves surviving with implanted artificial heart from 31 to 173 days. Exp Pathol 26: 221–225
Hastings WL, Aaron JL, Deneris TR, et al. (1981) A retrospective study of nine calves surviving five months on the pneumatic total artificial heart. ASAIO Trans 27: 71–76
Herring MB (1991) Endothelial cell seeding. J Vasc Surg 13: 731–732
Herring MB, LeGrand DR (1989) The history of seeded PTFE grafts in humans. Ann Vasc Surg 3: 96–103
Hilberman M, Myers BD, Carvie BJ, Derby G, Jamison RL, Stinson EB (1979) Acute renal failure following cardiac surgery. J Thorac Cardiovasc Surg 77: 880–888
Holmberg DL, Dew P, Crump C, Burns G, Taenaka Y, Olsen DB (1988) Percutaneous access devices in calves receiving an artificial heart. Artif Organs 12: 34–39
Hsu J, Griffith BP, Dowling RD, et al. (1989) Infections in mortally ill cardiac transplant recipients. J Thorac Cardiovasc Surg 98: 506–509
Hung TC, Butter DB, Kormos RL, Sun Z, Borovetz HS, Griffith BP, Yie CL (1989) Characteristics of blood rheology in patients during Novacor left ventricular assist system support. ASAIO Trans 35: 611–613
Hung TC, Butter DB, Yie CL, et al. (1991) Interim use of Jarvik-7 and Novacor artificial heart: blood rheology and transient ischaemic attacks (TIA's). Biorheology 28(1-2): 9–25
Jennings RB, Reimer KA (1983) Factors involved in salvaging ischaemic myocardium: effect of reperfusion of arterial blood. Circulation (Suppl 1): I-25–I-36
Joyce LD, Johnson KE, Pierce WS, et al.(1986) Summary of the world experience with clinical use of total artificial hearts as heart support devices. J Heart Transplant 5: 229–235
Kanter KR, Ruzevich SA, Pennington DG, McBride LR, Swartz MT, Willman VL (1988) Follow up of survivors of mechanical circulatory support. J Thorac Cardiovasc Surg 96: 72–80
Kaplan SS, Basford RE, Kormos RL, et al. (1990) Biomaterial associated impairment of local neutrophil function. ASAIO Trans 36: M172–175
Kawaguchi AT, Grandjbahch I, Pavie A, et al. (1990) Liver and kidney function in patients undergoing mechanical circulatory support with Jarvik-7 artificial heart as a bridge to transplantation. J Heart Transplant 1: 631–637
Kessler TR, Pons AB, Jarvik RK, Lawson JH, Razzeca KJ, Kolff WJ (1978) Elimination of predilection sites for thrombus formation in the total artificial heart – before and after. ASAIO Trans 24: 532–536
Kinoshota M, Takano H, Taenaka Y, et al. (1988) Cardiac disuse atrophy during LVAD pumping, ASAIO Trans 34: 208–212
Kloner RA, Ellis SG, Lange R, Braunwald E (1983) Studies of experimental coronary artery reperfusion. Effects on infarct size, myocardial function, biochemistry, ultrastructure and microvascular damage. Circulation 68 (Suppl 1): 8–15
Lefemine AA, Dunbar J, DeLucia A (1986) Concepts in assisted circulation. Tex Heart Inst J 13: 23–37
Levinson MM, Smith RG, Cork RC, et al. (1986) Thromboembolic complications of the Jarvik-7 total artificial heart: case report. Artif Organs 10: 236–244

Lewis CT, Graham TR, Marrinan MT, Chalmers JA, Colvin MP, Withington PS, Coumbe A (1990) The use of an implantable left ventricular assist device following irreversible ventricular fibrillation secondary to massive myocardial infarction. Eur J Cardiothorac Surg 4: 54–56

Loisance DY, Deleuze P, Kawasaki K, et al. (1987) Total artificial heart as a bridge to re-transplantation in acute cardiac rejection. J Heart Transplant 6: 281–285

Loisance DY, Deleuze P, Hillion ML, et al. (1990) The real impact of mechanical bridge strategy in patients with severe acute infarction. ASAIO Trans 36: M135–137

Marcus E, Wong SNT, Luisada AA (1951) Homologous heart grafts: transplantation of the heart in dogs. Surg Forum 2: 212–217

McEnany MT, Kay HR, Buckley MJ, et al. (1978) Clinical experience with intra-aortic balloon pump support in 728 patients. Circulation 58: 124

Mochizuki T, Lawson JH, Olsen DB, et al. (1981) A seven month survival of a calf with an artificial heart designed for human use. Artif Organs 5: 125–131

Nishi K, Mori F, Miyamoto M, Esato K (1989) Myocardial protection by a left ventricular assist device during reperfusion following acute coronary occlusion. Jpn J Surg 19: 536–569

Nistal F, Garcia-Martinez V, Fernandez D, Artuiano E, Mazona F, Gallo I (1988) Degenerative pathologic findings after long-term implantation of bovine pericardial bioprosthetic heart valves. J Thorac Cardiovasc Surg 96: 642–651

Noda H, Takano H, Taenaka Y, et al. (1989) Treatment of acute myocardial infarction with cardiogenic shock using left ventricular assist device. Int J Artif Organs 12: 175–179

O'Connell JB, Dec GW, Billingham ME, et al. (1989) Results of cardiac transplantation in active myocarditis (abstract). J Heart Transplant 8: 99

Olsen DB, Murray KD (1984) Artificial heart. In: Unger F (ed) Assisted circulation 2. Springer, Berlin Heidelberg New York, pp 205–206

Olsen DB, Unger F, Oster H, Lawson JH, Kessler TR, Kolff J, Kolff WJ (1975) Thrombus generation within the artificial heart. J Thorac Cardiovasc Surg 70: 248–255

Olsen DB, Fukumasu H, Peters JK, et al. (1977) Vascular and haemodynamic adaptions in the calf with a total artificial heart (abstract). 27th International Congress of Physiological Science 1682: 567

Pae WE Jr, Pierce WS (1980) Mechanical left ventricular assistance: current devices, future prospects. In: Moran JM, Michaels LL (eds) Surgery for the complications of myocardial infarction. Grune and Stratton, New York, pp 411–426

Pae WE Jr, Pierce WS (1981) Temporary left ventricular assistance in acute myocardial infarction and cardiogenic shock: rationale and criteria for utilisation. Chest 79: 692–695

Pae WE Jr, Gains WE, Pierce WS, Waldhausen JA (1985) Mechanical circulatory assistance for post-operative cardiogenic shock. Surgical Rounds (July): 49–63

Pennington DG, Merjavy JP, Codd JE, Swartz MT, Miller LL, Williams GA (1984) Extracorporeal membrane oxygenation for patients with cardiogenic shock. Circulation 70: 130–137

Pennington DG, Bernhard WF, Golding LR, Berger RL, Khuri SF, Watson JT (1985) Long-term follow-up of post-cardiotomy patients with profound cardiogenic shock treated with ventricular assist devices. Circulation 72 (Suppl 2): 216–226

Pennington DG, Golding LJ, Hill D, et al. (1986) Temporary mechanical support for cardiogenic shock. ASAIO Trans 32: 629–632

Pennock JL, Pae WE Jr, Pierce WS, Waldhausen JA (1979) Reduction of myocardial infarct size: comparison between left atrial and left ventricular bypass. Circulation 59: 275–297

Pennock JL, Pierce WS, Wisman CB, Bull AP, Waldhausen JA (1983) Survival and complications following ventricular assist pumping for cardiogenic shock. Ann Surg 198: 469–478

Peters G (1979) Spezielle Pathologie der Krankheiten des zentralen und peripheren Nervensystems, Kreislaufstörungen (2nd edn). Thieme, Stuffgart, pp 150–151

Pifarre R, Sullivan H, Montoya A, et al. (1990) Use of the total artificial heart and ventricular assist device as a bridge to transplantation. J Heart Transplant 9: 638–642

Portner PM, Green GF, Ramasamy N (1983) The blood interface at artificial surfaces within a left ventricular assist system. Ann NY Acad Sci 416: 471–503

Ramasamy N, Chen H, Miller PJ, Jassawalla JS, Oyer PE, Portner PM (1988) Bioprosthetic valve calcification and pseudoneointimal proliferation in bovine and ovine models. ASAIO Trans 34: 696–702

Ramasamy N, Chen H, Miller PJ, et al. (1989) Chronic ovine evaluation of a totally implantable electrical left ventricular assist system. ASAIO Trans 35: 402–404

Reichenbach D, Cowan MJ (1991) Healing of myocardial infarction with and without reperfusion. In: Virmani R, Atkinson JB, Fenoglio JJ (eds) Cardiovascular pathology. Major problems in pathology, Vol 23. W.B. Saunders, Philadelphia, pp 86–99

Reimer KA, Jennings RB, Tatum AH (1983) Pathobiology of acute myocardial ischaemia: metabolic, functional and ultrastructural studies. Am J Cardiol 52: 72A–81A

Richards AN, Drinker CK (1915) An apparatus for the perfusion of isolated organs. J Pharmacol Exp Ther 7: 467–483

Ring ME, Feinberg WM, Levinson MM, Bruck DC, Smith RG, Icenogle TM, Copeland JG (1989) Platelet and fibrin metabolism in recipients of the Jarvik-7 total artificial heart. J Heart Transplant 8: 225–232

Rockman HA, Adamson RM, Dembitsky WP, Bonar JW, Jaski BE (1991) Acute fulminant myocarditis: long-term follow up after circulatory support with left ventricular assist device. Am Heart J 121: 922–926

Sanfelippo PM, Baker NH, Ewy HG, et al. (1986) Experience with intra-aortic balloon counterpulsation. Ann Thorac Surg 41: 36–41

Schaper J, Schwarz F, Kittstein H, et al. (1982) The effects of global ischaemia and reperfusion on human myocardium: quantitative evaluation by electron microscopic morphometry. Ann Thorac Surg 33: 116–122

Schoen FJ, Bernhard WF, Khuri SF, Koster JK, Van De Vanter SJ, Weintraub RM (1982) Pathologic findings in post cardiotomy patients managed with a temporary left ventricular assist pump. Am J Surg 143: 508–513

Schoen FJ, LaFarge CG, Bernhard WF (1985a) Pathology and pathophysiology of temporary cardiac assist. Am Soc Artif Intern Organs 8: 174–181

Schoen FJ, Palmer DC, Haudenschild CC, Ratliff NB, Watson JT (1985b) Pathologic findings and their implications in patients managed with temporary ventricular assist. ASAIO Trans 31: 66–72

Schoen FJ, Palmer DC, Bernhard WE (1986) Clinical temporary ventricular assist. Pathologic findings and their implications in a multi-institutional study of 41 patients. J Thorac Cardiovasc Surg 92: 1071–1081

Tomioka N, Kishimoto C, Matsumori A, Kawai C (1986) Effects of prednisolone on acute viral myocarditis in mice. J Am Coll Cardiol 7: 868–872

Van Allen CM (1932) A pump for clinical and laboratory purposes which employs the milking principle. JAMA 98: 1805–1806

Vasku J (1989) A contribution to the assessment of pathophysiology in long-term total artificial heart recipients. In: Unger F (ed) Assisted circulation 3. Springer, Berlin Heidelberg New York, pp 340–376

Vasku J, Urbanek E, Vasku J, et al. (1981) Pathophysiological analysis of 3 experiments with the total artificial heart (TAH) with more than 100 days or survival. Proc Eur Soc Artif Organs 8: 17–22

Vohra R, Thomson GT, Carr HM, Sharma H, Walker MG (1991) Comparison of different vascular prostheses and matrices in relation to endothelial seeding. Br J Surg 78: 417–420

Waller BF (1988) The pathology of acute myocardial infarction: definition, location, pathogenesis, effects of reperfusion, complications and sequelae. Cardiol Clin 6:1

Ward RA, Wellhausen SR, Dobbins JJ, Johnson GS, DeVries WC (1987) Thromboembolic and infectious complications of total artificial heart implantation. Ann NY Acad Sci 516: 638–650

Weidermann H, Grosse-Siestrup C, Gerlach K, Kaufman A, Bucherl ES (1981) Pathological anatomical findings in calves after total artificial heart replacement. Proc Eur Artif Organs 8: 12–16

Weidermann H, Muller KM, Hennig E, Meissler M, Bucherl ES (1990) Experience with vascular grafts in total artificial heart replacement. Int J Artif Organs 13: 288–292

Wellhausen SR, Ward RA, Johnson GS, DeVries WC (1988) Immunologic complications of long-term implantation of a total heart. J Clin Immunol 8: 307–318

Westenfelder C, Haus RM, Border WA, Muniz H, Duffy D, Menlove RL, Bananovsky RL (1985) Renal function in calves with TAH. ASAIO trans 31: 383–387

Withington PS, Ooi LG, Graham TR, Coumbe A, White DG, Lewis CT (1991) Systemic hypertension with histological changes following prolonged left ventricular assist device insertion in calves. Artif Organs 14 (Suppl 1): 149–153

Working Group on Mechanical Circulatory Support of the National Heart, Lung and Blood Institute (1985) Artificial heart and assist devices: directions, needs, costs, societal and ethical issues. U.S. Dept of Health and Human Services, publication no. (NIH) 85–2723, Bethesda, Maryland

Pathology of Cardiac Pacemakers and Central Catheters

J.N. Cox

Current Topics in Pathology
Volume 86. Ed. C. Berry

1 Introduction

Cardiac pacing has become a major therapeutic tool in the treatment of a wide variety of conduction disturbances of the heart, many of which are life-threatening. The sophistication of modern designs, together with the introduction of the automatic implantable cardioverter defibrillator, has broadened the indications for the implantation of cardiac pacemakers, making them serious competitors to drug therapies for most of the aforementioned conditions. Both systems, alone or combined, are now widely used in various pathological heart conditions, and have also been adapted for use in infants and children.

Few deaths are directly related to the pacemaker or allied devices, but it is clear that certain complications or failures may lead to a fatal outcome indirectly and pathologists should be familiar with such problems. It is becoming more and more apparent that these devices (especially the automatic implantable cardioverter defibrillator) are acting as a bridge for patients awaiting cardiac transplantations and this affects pathological findings in this group.

Complications in patients carrying these devices may present as specific clinical symptoms, or there may be no clinically perceived effects.

2 Historical Background

Sutton et al. (1980) have reviewed the early physiological studies at the end of the last century and the beginning of this century which have allowed the human cardiac pacemaker to become a major therapeutic tool in the treatment of conduction disturbances. Lidwill of Australia appears to have been the first to have designed a machine for direct stimulation of the adynamic heart. In the 1920s he applied this technique to the hearts of several stillborn infants and in one case, when stimulation of the atrium had failed, he introduced the needle into the ventricular wall. This resulted in a response and after cessation of the current, a normal heart-beat was obtained; the patient survived (MOND et al. 1982a).

HYMAN (1930, 1932), who was familiar with some of the work done in Australia, later introduced a portable machine for delivering small repetitive impulses. When connected to needle electrodes and used to stimulate the asystolic dog's heart in the region of the sinus node, this produced contractions which spread to the entire organ. However, no significant progress was made until the important questions relating to major open heart surgery were defined. The use of total-body hypothermia required control of electrical activity (CALLAGHAN 1980; HOPPS 1981). Experiments in Bigelow's laboratory led CALLAGHAN and BIGELOW (1951) and BIGELOW et al. (1952) to develop transvenous catheter introduction in experiments with dogs, in the process of stimulating the sinoatrial node using a bipolar electrode. Zoll, who was familiar with the work of Bigelow's group, was able to use this technique for external pacing of the heart in a patient with Stokes-Adams attacks who was in complete heart block (ZOLL 1952; CALLAGHAN 1980).

In 1957 Weirich and associates showed that it was possible to improve the outcome in patients who developed heart block after cardiac surgery by using percutaneous epicardial wire electrodes fixed to an external pacemaker (WEIRICH et al. 1957). The following year, Senning's group at the Karolinska, Stockholm, introduced the first totally implantable pacemaker in a 43-year-old man with Stokes-Adams attacks. The electrodes were inserted into the left ventricular wall and connected to a nickel–cadmium rechargeable battery source which was placed in the abdominal wall. Although this first implantable generator lasted for only 3 h and had to be changed for a second which lasted for 8 days, this was a significant step forward (SENNING 1959; ELMQVIST et al. 1963; LAGERGREN 1978). In the meantime intensive work was carried out on improving electrodes, choosing the most suitable endovenous route for implantation, and finding ways and means of improving the pulse generators (FURMAN and SCHWEDEL 1959; FURMAN et al. 1961). Work on better pulse generators culminated in the successful implantation of the first totally implantable pacemaker (CHARDACK et al. 1960; CHARDACK 1981; GREATBATCH 1984). In the early part of the same year a similar feat was accomplished by another group in Uruguay (FIANDRA 1988). The era of the pacemaker as a mode of treatment of atrioventricular block with Stokes-Adams syndrome and related disorders had arrived.

3 The Cardiac Pacemaker

The cardiac pacemaker is made up of three essential components: the pulse generator, the insulated electrical conductor and the electrode (conductor and electrode forming the lead). Each of these has undergone tremendous improvements over the years and each continues to develop as new data and technology are acquired.

3.1 The Pulse Generator

The pulse generator is a power source with associated electrical circuitry for delivering the electrical stimulus and for regulating other important functions such as rate and mode of pacing.

The first totally implantable pacemakers were powered either by a rechargeable nickel–cadmium or a mercury–zinc battery, the latter with a calculated longevity of about 5 years. In fact, the longevity rarely exceeded 18 months, with 75% failure by 2 years due to a short shelf-life and a high current drain (Fig. 1). This type of generator was replaced by the hermetically sealed lithium anode battery, first used in 1968 and introduced into practice in 1972. The longevity of this type of source has gone well beyond 10 years in the majority of cases, with a prolonged shelf-life (Fig. 2). It has also been possible to reduce the size of the generators considerably to make them lighter and more flexible, and to develop a better performance (Furman 1979b, 1989; Hurzeler et al. 1980; Bilitch et al. 1981, 1985, 1988; Hanson and Grant 1984).

A nuclear power generator was also developed during the 1960s by the conversion of energy from plutonium-238. This alpha-emitter isotope with a half-life of 87.75 years was found to be ideal as a source of energy and has been used

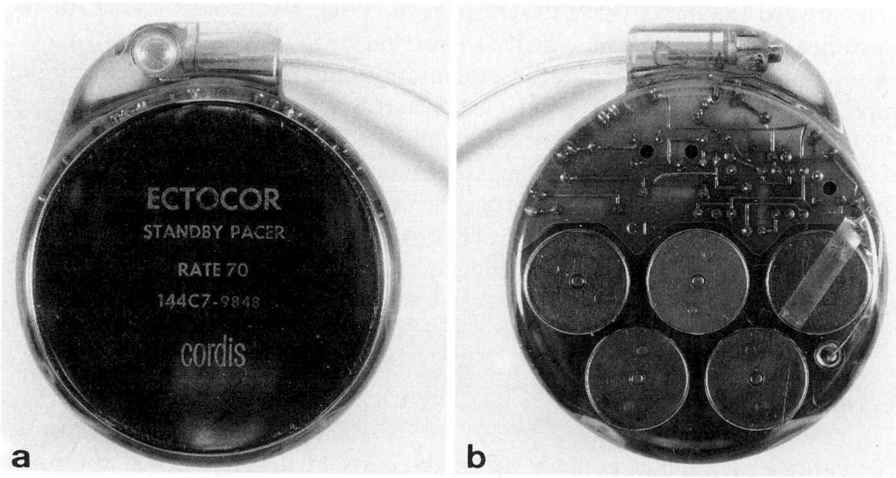

Fig. 1a,b. Pulse generator, early model. **a** Surface=anode; **b** component elements

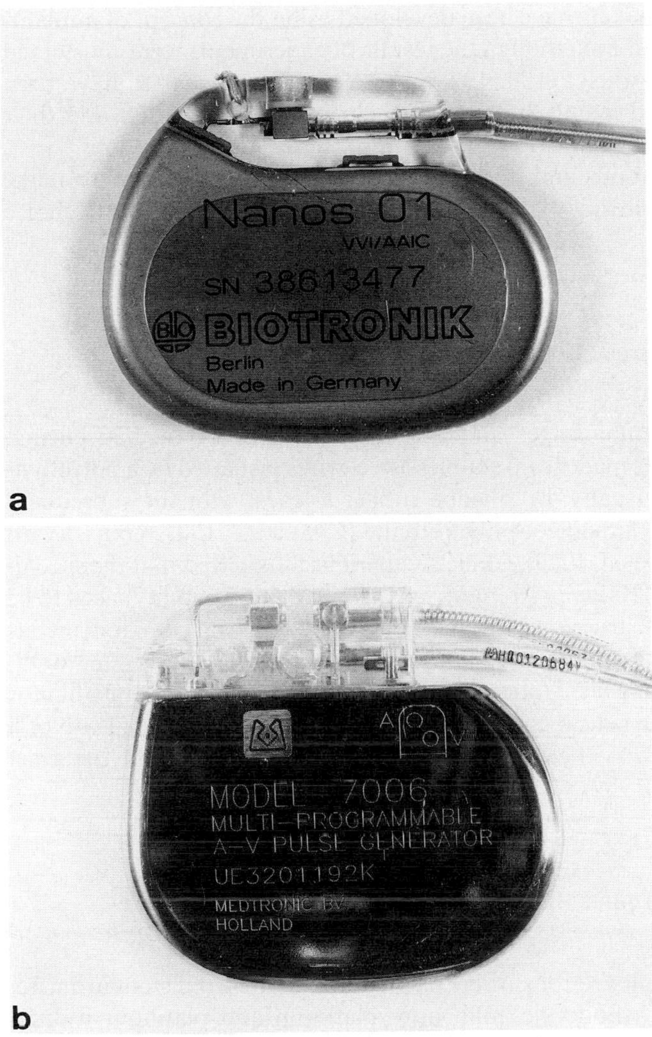

Fig. 2a,b. New lithium pulse generators: smaller, lighter, greater longevity and programmability

to manufacture a reliable thermoelectric generator with great longevity. The first implantation of this generator was in France in 1970, but with the cheaper, highly improved lithium varieties lasting for 10–20 years or more, isotopic generators have not met with much commercial success. There are still some thousands of patients who received these hermetically sealed generators when they were first introduced. They do not create a radiation hazard to themselves or to their surroundings (FURMAN 1979a, 1981a; JACOBSON 1979a, b; LAURENS 1979; PARSONNET et al. 1979, 1984; SMYTH et al. 1982). A new dual-chamber model, lighter, cheaper and efficient, has been introduced recently (PARSONNET et al. 1990).

Biogalvanic pacemakers have been developed using the concept of implantable bioelectric cells, but even though the results of experiments were considered to be encouraging (Cywinski et al. 1978), these projects appear to have been temporarily abandoned mainly because of their low energy density and their inconsistent performance (Greatbatch 1984).

Constant modifications and improvements of lithium generators to make them adaptable to most forms of pacing have made them the generators of choice for the present.

3.2 The Insulated Electrical Conductor

In the early experimental stages and first clinical trials of cardiac pacing, conductors were usually made from stainless steel wires insulated by a polyethylene coating or, more usually, by silicone rubber sleeves, with the subsequent development of a sheath made of polyurethane (Chardack 1981; Greatbatch 1984; Scheuer-Leeser et al. 1983). Clinical experience suggested that the specifications of the lead (variability in strength, extensibility and flexibility) need to be varied and led to the construction of the metallic coil system using different metals or their alloys, including multistrand platinum wires or nickel-alloy as uni- or bipolar coaxial units. These were followed by multifilar coils (bifilar, triple-filar or quadrifilar helix) or the helical coil of Elgiloy, most of which are made up of a mixture of alloys and carry their manufacturer's code name (Scheuer-Leeser et al. 1983; Bourke et al. 1989).

3.3 The Pacing Electrode

The first electrodes employed for cardiac pacing were made from standard wire, stainless steel, silver, orthodontic gold, pure platinum and platinum–iridium (10%) among others and were implanted into the myocardium either trans venously into the endomyocardium, subxiphoidial or transthoracically into the epimyocardium (Furman et al. 1979; Mond et al. 1982b; Mansour et al. 1973; Stewart et al. 1975).

3.3.1 Endocardial Ventricular Leads

The majority of the early electrodes were cylindrical with a flat or hemispherical tip and a surface area of approximately 45 mm^2 (Fig. 3). It soon became apparent clinically that their main functions (fixation, maintenance of a stable, low minimum stimulation threshold, and a maximum amplitude for sensing) were far from optimal, and in addition there was a high energy consumption leading to

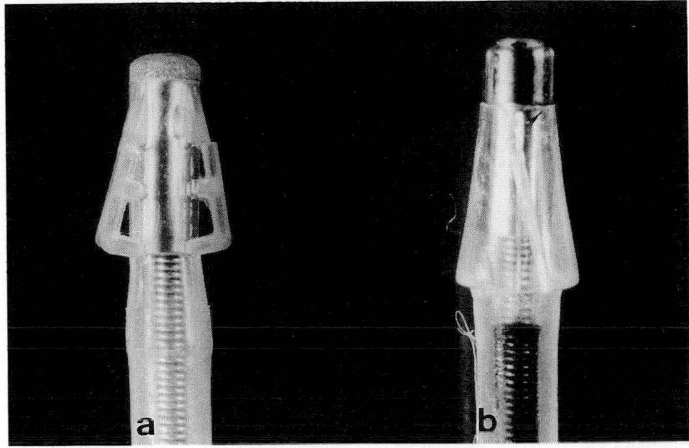

Fig. 3a,b. Earlier electrodes. **a** Conifix model; **b** cylindrical electrode with wedge-type fixation

accelerated battery depletion (EDHAG et al. 1978; SMYTH et al. 1976). Moreover, the incidence of the most common complications of these leads, i.e. dislodgement and displacement, ranged between 2% and 30% owing to their passive mode of fixation and anchorage, resulting in most cases in failure to pace (FURMAN et al. 1981).

When the lead was anchored, the fibrous tissue response at the site of fixation was responsible for an increase in stimulation threshold after long-term pacing, a decrease in sensing and an increase in energy consumption leading to premature generator decline (SLACK et al. 1982; RIPART and MUGICA 1983). In attempts to minimise these problems the size, shape and surface area (6–12 mm^2) of the electrodes were reduced. To ensure better anchorage, a conical shoulder or silicone rubber cuff was added proximally or a balloon-shaped tip was used – changes intended to serve as wedges between and beneath the trabeculae, for better stability and fixation. Short or long tines, bristles, hooks or metal cages were tried; all these fixations were considered to have a partially passive/partially active effects (Fig. 4) (BREDIKIS et al. 1978; FURMAN et al. 1979; SLOMAN et al. 1979; MOND and SLOMAN 1980; MOND et al. 1982b; IRNICH 1983; MOND and STOKES 1992). Other designs were introduced to "grasp" the myocardium, obtaining a true active fixation. They included corkscrew, screw-in, coil and Helifix designs, some of which were adapted for atrial pacing (EL GAMAL and VAN GELDER 1979; MORSE et al. 1983). Further progress was made with the introduction of the highly performing hemispherical totally porous platinum-iridium electrode and the porous-surfaced sintered treated electrode, both of which provided early, stable fixation as a result of fibrous tissue ingrowth into the electrode, with only a thin fibrous outer capsule on the surface. This resulted in a reduction in both the stimulation threshold and electrode polarisation (AMUNDSON et al. 1979; BERMAN et al. 1982; BEYERSDORF et al. 1988; BOBYN et al. 1981; MACCARTER et al. 1983; MUGICA et al. 1988).

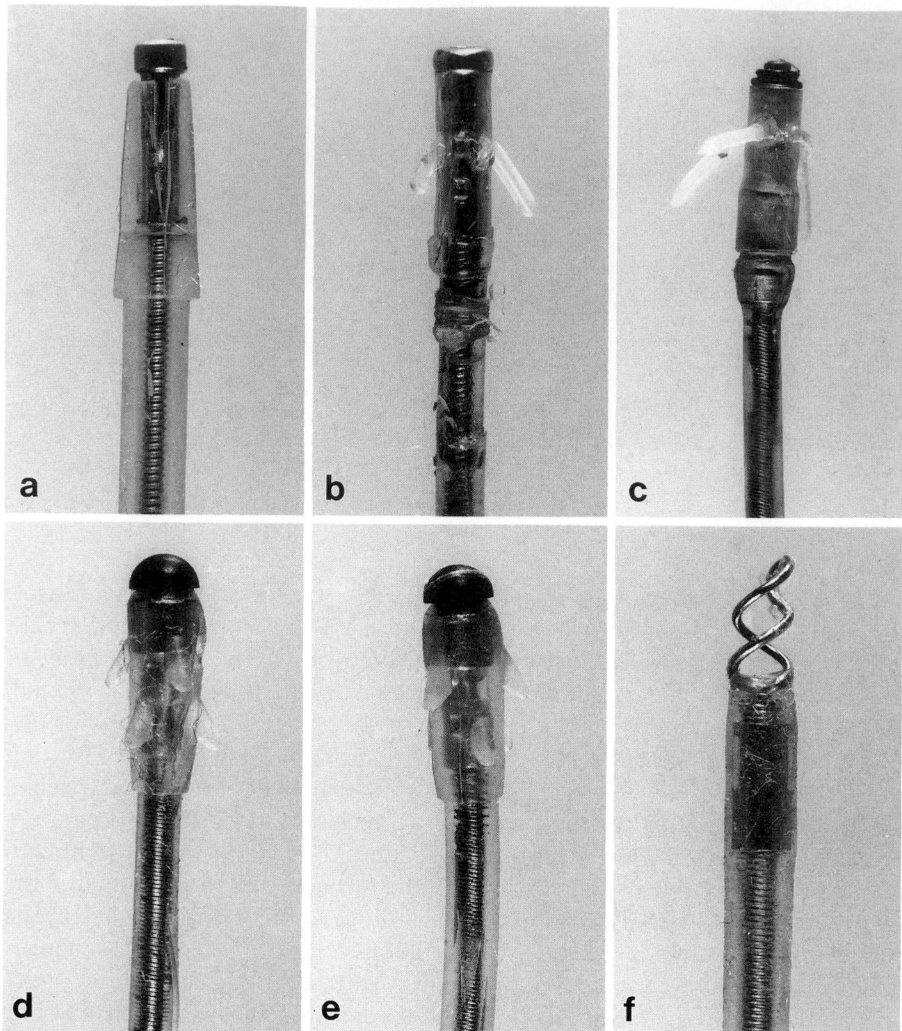

Fig. 4a-f. Six different recent electrode. **a** Shorter and smaller (blunt-tip) cylindrical platinum electrode with wedge-type fixation. **b** Ring-or dish-type platinum tip electrode. Long tined fixation. **c** Target-tipped electrode with long tines. **d** New hemispheric carbon-tipped electrode with smaller tines. **e** New hemispheric carbon-tipped electrode held in place by a platinum wire; small tines. **f** Helifix electrode (passive/active fixation). Fixation by rotation among the trabeculae

To obtain the "ideal electrode" producing little or no fibrotic tissue around its surface was now the major concern of designers and clinicians alike. To achieve this goal, it was necessary to obtain one with good biocompatibility. Experience had taught that carbon was the most suitable element and therefore many designs for carbon electrodes were proposed, produced either as activated pyrocarbon (a graphite core coated by a pyrocarbon layer) or as activated vitreous (glassy) carbon electrodes and presented in three main forms (hemispheric, annular, ring). The high biocompatibility of these electrodes has resulted in a marked reduction of the fibrotic tissue reaction, low stimulation thresholds and polarisation losses, with little energy consumption and good sensing behaviour (ELMQVIST et al. 1983; GARBEROGLIO et al. 1983; MUND et al. 1986; PIOGER and RIPART 1986; MUGICA et al. 1988; BOURKE et al. 1989).

The knowledge that glucocorticosteroids are able to lower stimulation thresholds and overcome post-implant exit block resulted in attempts to develop electrodes which delivered steroids directly at the electrode–endomyocardium interface. A number of delivery systems designed to deliver pharmacologically active agents (anticoagulants, non-steroidal anti-inflammatory drugs) at the site of electrode implantation were in use and these were adapted to deliver a corticosteroid [dexamethasone sodium phosphate (DSP)] in small quantities. In man, three systems are used: a minipump within a titanium tip electrode coated with a porous platinum layer, a polymeric matrix collar in silicon or porous ceramic and a polymeric matrix behind or within a porous electrode. Their small surface area, the little or no fibrous tissue reaction and the low stimulation threshold give these types of electrode a promising future, especially as they can be paced with little energy (2.5 V) (BREWER et al. 1988; KRUSE and TERPSTRA 1985; MATHIVANAR et al. 1990; MOND et al. 1988; MOND and STOKES 1992; RADOVSKY et al. 1988; SCHUCHERT et al. 1990; STOKES and BIRD 1990). Despite these variable results, the search for better performing electrodes continues and recently the sputter-deposited titanium-nitride electrode has made its appearance (SCHALDACH et al. 1990).

3.3.2 *Endocardial Atrial Leads*

As the sinus node is the physiological cardiac pacemaker it is evident that atrial pacing is the preferred mode in atrioventricular node dysfunction, bradyarrhythmia with sinus node intact and supraventricular tachycardias, in order to obtain optimal haemodynamic responses. Early attempts at atrial pacing with conventional electrodes saw a high percentage of displacements or dislodgements. It was not until the introduction of the curved "J" lead, which was made to be placed in the right atrial appendage, and its subsequent modifications (tines), that a sharp decline was observed in these complications. Now both unipolar and bipolar atrial pacing have become more common, especially as the more sophisticated electrodes together with active fixations are made adaptable and easier for implantation into the right atrial appendage or elsewhere (OGAWA et al. 1978; SMYTH 1978; LITTLEFORD and PEPINE 1981; MESSENGER et al. 1982; MORSE et al. 1983; MARKEWITZ et al. 1988; ORMEROD et al. 1988; PARSONNET et al. 1991). Atrial pacing has also been performed via the coronary sinus using special cylindrical electrodes (GREENBERG et al. 1978).

Atrial and ventricular pacing can also be accomplished by a non-invasive trans-oesophageal route. The technique is rapid and easily adapted to emergency situations and temporary pacing, especially in infants and children (Jenkins et al. 1985; Kerr et al. 1986; Blomstrom-Lundqvist and Edvardsson 1987; Alboni et al. 1989; Vrouchos and Vardas 1991).

3.3.3 Epicardial Leads

The epicardial sutured or sutureless electrode in its early design was in the form of a corkscrew with two or three turns insulated with silicone rubber except for the last three-quarters turn, which served as the stimulating surface with an area of approximately 12 mm^2 (Fig. 5). Introduction of these electrodes required general anaesthesia and thoracotomy, which were accompanied by many complications and high morbidity and mortality. Later a rapid, subxiphoid approach which may be performed under local anaesthesia was introduced, resulting in new interest in this mode of pacing. The electrode is screwed into the posterior or anterior wall of the right or left ventricle, and is very stable. Newer designs include the "fish-hook" type (also used for atrial pacing), and more recently a steroid-eluting system has been adapted with very favourable results. This mode of pacing is very useful in paediatrics (de Feyter et al. 1980; Bashore et al. 1982; Bognolo et al. 1983; Stokes 1988; Karpawich et al. 1988; Kugler et al. 1990).

4 Post-mortem Examination

To maximise the information obtained at autopsy, it is essential to have good collaboration between the cardiologists, surgeons and pathologists and, where

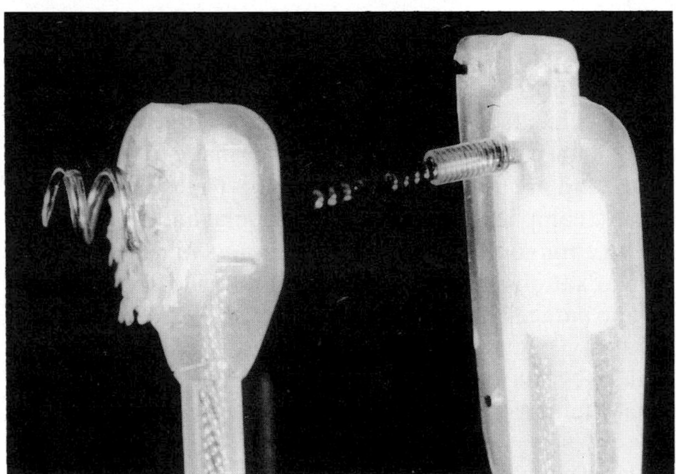

Fig. 5. Epicardial screw-on electrode *Left:* a two-turn electrode

possible, the manufacturers so that the main issues may be discussed and a consensus obtained.

In endocardial pacemaker carriers, chest x-rays (frontal and lateral views) are recommended before autopsy in order to obtain information as to be exact position of the pacing lead or eventual lead fractures. We find it preferable, once the sternum is removed, to dissect carefully the thoracic and neck organs with their accompanying vessels together with the pulse generator attached to the entire lead in one block. The lungs are then separated and an x-ray is taken of the specimen. In epicardial pacemaker carriers, the implanted subcutaneous generators are removed together with the lead loops in their fibrous tunnels and the heart and treated likewise. If infection of the generator pockets is suspected, material is taken immediately for culture before dissection.

With endocardial leads the right atrium is opened posteriorly so as to connect the superior and inferior vena cava, taking care to pass at some distance from the lead. The right ventricle is then opened anteriorly at about 1 cm from its right border. This allows a good view of the implantation site of the electrode and the route of the lead within the heart, as well as demonstrating the pathological lesions which may exist. Thereafter the superior vena cava and the tributary carrying the lead are then opened up to the point of lead entrance, avoiding all contact with the lead. From this point the latter is carefully dissected from the surrounding tissue or fibrous tunnel up to its connection with the pulse generator. Another x-ray of the specimen can be taken, but more importantly, appropriate photographs are strongly recommended.

The pulse generator is then examined in the search for seal defects at the point of connection with the lead. Once this has been done, the lead can be disconnected, and the generator (disinfected and maintained at room temperature - 37° C) is returned to the cardiologist or manufacturer for evaluation. The lead is then examined and compared with the x-rays. All defects are registered together with other pathological lesions that may exist along its course. Finally, the site of implantation is examined in the search for displacements, dislodgements or other lesions. All pulse generators must be removed since lithium generators may explode on cremation, causing damage to the ovens.

The heart and lead are fixed in formalin and after fixation the portion of the heart with the electrode and lead is separated from the rest. The specimen is then divided longitudinally to free the lead and electrode from the surrounding tissue capsule and the two halves are dehydrated, embedded in paraffin wax on their midsagittal surface, cut at 5 µm and stained with haematoxylin, and eosin, van Gieson-elastin and Masson's trichrome. Other sections are also taken from other pathological lesions observed along the lead or adjoining myocardium. Sections are taken from His bundle and sinus node in all cases, and from the atrioventricular node in special cases.

The base of the epicardial leads are freed from the fibrous tissue surrounding the Dacron sheath. The electrode is then unscrewed anti-clockwise to free it from the myocardium. The latter is sectioned perpendicular to the epicardium along the middle of the course of the electrode. The two halves are examined as above.

5 Morphological Lesions in Pacemaker Carriers

At post-mortem, morphological lesions of the heart are not always obvious and therefore it is impossible to over-emphasise the necessity for a close and constant collaboration between the cardiologist and pathologist.

Complications may be described as intraoperative when they occur on insertion, early when they occur in the first 2 months of use and late when they occur after this period. Although some anatomical lesions may occur at the time of implantation, clinical symptoms may appear months or years later, or never.

Complications associated with the pacemaker may derive from any one of the three components (pulse generator, conductor, electrode) or from more than one component (any combination is possible), and may be translated into functional disturbances of the myocardium.

5.1 Intraoperative Complications

Complications may occur at the time of pacemaker implantation and these depend on whether the lead inserted is an endocardial electrode through a transvenous route or an epicardial electrode by transthoracic thoracotomy or a subxiphoid approach.

5.1.1 Transvenous Approach

Transvenous access of the endocardial lead is generally by way of one of the neck or shoulder veins (principally on the right), by venous cutdown of one of the jugular veins (external or internal) or the cephalic vein, or by puncture of the jugular or subclavian veins. The latter route, although very popular, is still not accepted by all (Parsonnet 1978; Wirtzfeld 1980; Furman 1986; Lamas et al. 1988). Others have advocated the use of saphenous or external iliac veins as other entry points (Ellestad et al. 1980; Ellestad and French 1989).

5.1.1.1 Lesions During Implantation. Venous cutdown into jugular veins or the cephalic vein may be accompanied by vascular laceration with haemorrhage into the surrounding tissues. Such lesions may also occur during intraclavicular puncture of the subclavian vein and the accompanying artery may be damaged. When the injury occurs within the thorax, haemothorax ensues. The right recurrent laryngeal nerve may be damaged by this procedure, especially when the supraclavicular route is taken (Epstein et al. 1976; Copperman et al. 1982; Kevorkian 1982), and the brachial plexus may also be injured. Pneumothorax and/or haemothorax will occur if the apex of the lung is damaged. Air may be aspirated into the venous circulation during one of these procedures, leading to air embolism, acute right heart failure and death. Air may also escape into, and dissect, the surrounding tissues with the formation of subcutaneous emphysema. If the pulse generator is involved, pacemaker malfunction (especially with unipolar systems) follows (FURMAN 1986b; BYRD 1992; BASSAN and MERIN 1977; BERNARD and STAHL 1971; PARSONNET and MANHARDT 1977; LASALA et al. 1979; SMITH et al. 1985; GIROUD and GOY 1990). The frequencies of these complications are related to the experience and competence of the operators (FURMAN and BILITCH 1987; PARSONNET et al. 1989) but the lesions must be looked for by carefully dissecting the vessels of the region at post-mortem in any patient dying within 5 days after transvenous endocardial pacemaker implantation.

Perforation of the tricuspid valve leaflet may take place while manoeuvring the lead within the right ventricular cavity, for either temporary or permanent pacing. It is more likely to occur with the more rigid temporary pacing lead. Clinical symptoms appear to be extremely rare but the lesion is not altogether uncommon. Certain manoeuvres and manipulations of the catheter, especially withdrawing and repositioning, may result in entrapment of the electrode (especially those with tines) in the valve leaflets or chordae tendineae and attempts to retrieve the lead may result in partial avulsion of the leaflet and valvular insufficiency (PARSONNET and WERRES 1981; FURSTENBERG et al. 1984; CHRISTIE and KEELAN 1986; RES et al. 1989; OLD et al. 1989; FRANDSEN et al. 1990; RUBIO and AL-BASSAM 1991).

Perforation of the right ventricular wall may occur during manipulations to fix the electrode into the generally thin myocardium for either temporary or permanent pacing (Fig. 6). The tip of the electrode may remain embedded in the epicardial fat or lie within the pericardial space. The clinical symptoms may be immediate or may appear only weeks, months or years later or never. Pericardial friction rub may be the presenting symptom and haemopericardium leading to

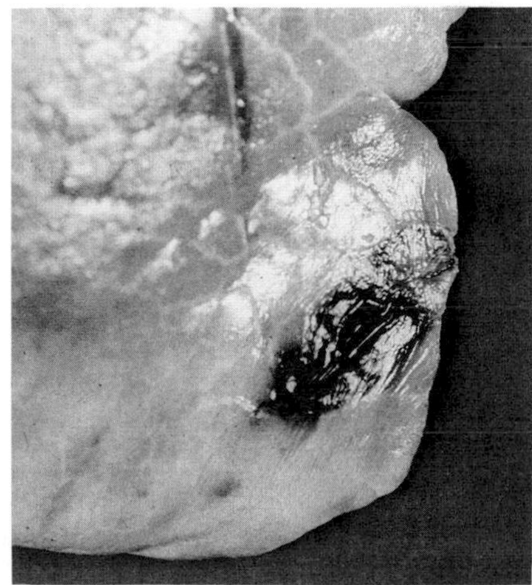

Fig. 6. Right ventricle posterior wall perforation leading to haemopericardium

tamponade, shock and even death may occur. Failure to capture is generally the alarm signal in most instances (Gibson et al. 1980; Mond et al. 1978; Chatelain et al. 1985; Sandler et al. 1989; Garcia-Jimenez et al. 1992; Snow et al. 1987).

Should the electrode attain the diaphragm by perforation of the posterior wall or stimulation of the phrenic nerve, twitching and diaphragmatic contractions may occur (Kevorkian et al. 1982; Gaidula and Barold 1974). For this reason some authors have resorted to implanting the electrode into the right ventricular outflow tract (Barin et al. 1991).

Right atrial pacing is becoming more and more fashionable, especially with the introduction of dual chamber pacemakers. Perforation of the atrial wall during manipulation of the lead to secure the electrode in the thin wall is not altogether uncommon (Irwin et al. 1987; Snow et al. 1987).

Acute myocardial infarction, although rare, has also been documented during introduction and stabilisation of pacemaker electrodes, and thoracic pain may be the only clinical indicator. A marked rise in diastolic pacing threshold with a shortened refractory period and ventricular fibrillation are suggestive of acute myocardial infarction (Mond and Sloman 1981b; Snow 1983; Manyari et al. 1983).

5.1.2 Transfemoral Approach

The femoral and iliac veins may be used to introduce temporary cardiac pacing in critically ill patients: This route of access has been chosen for permanent atrial and ventricular pacing but a number of complications have been recorded, including tearing of the wall of the vein and puncture of both artery and vein due to their close anatomical relationship and to anatomical variations. Double or triple punctures of the artery and vein may occur, and, like venous wall tears, may lead to massive haemorrhage and haematoma. Haemorrhages may extend into the retroperitoneal space and can be life threatening. Arteriovenous fistulae have also been documented. Subsequent venous thrombosis may lead to pulmonary thromboembolism. Other complications include phlebitis and sometimes thrombosis of the large thoracic veins. Atrial lead dislodgement is a major problem (Fig. 7) together with perforation of the right atrial appendage or right ventricular wall, and even phrenic nerve stimulation (Falkoff et al. 1978; El Gamal and van Gelder 1979; Ellestad et al. 1980; Ellestad and French 1989).

5.1.3 Epicardial Approach

Implantation of the epicardial leads in critically ill patients through thoracotomy under general anaesthesia was associated with a high morbidity and mortality, but the advent of the screw-on electrode and an approach by a subxiphoid incision has improved outcomes. An anterior axillary minithoracotomy under local anaesthesia

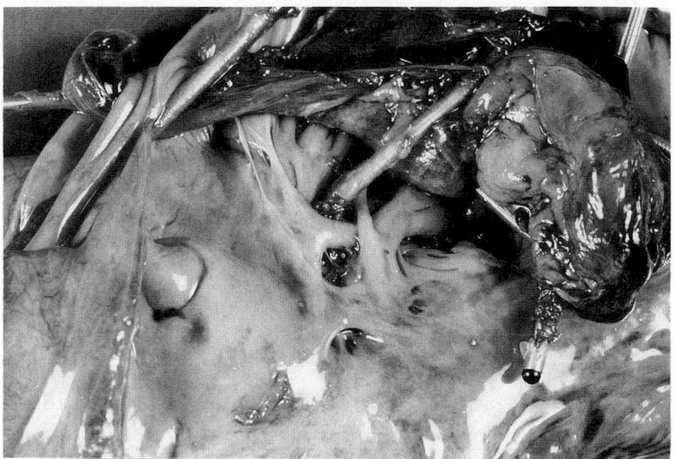

Fig. 7. Right atrial and auricular thrombosis with dislodgement of the atrial pacing lead partially enveloped by the thrombus

may be used. This approach gives improved electrode stability and decreased morbidity and mortality; nevertheless, complications are still encountered during implantation of the epicardial lead. These include pericardial adhesions, myocardial laceration, associated with a very thin right ventricular wall or a thin left ventricular apex. Perforations have also been described, accompanied by haemorrhage which may be fatal. This has led some authors to opt for implantation of the screw-on electrode into the thick anterolateral wall of the left ventricle (Vecht et al. 1976; Magilligan et al. 1976; de Feyter et al. 1980; Naclerio and Varriale 1980; Smith and Tatoulis 1990).

5.2 Complications Related to the Pulse Generator

Tremendous advances have been made within the last two decades in all aspects of implantable pacemakers and perhaps the most spectacular among them are the improvements and sophistication of the new designs of pulse generators.

5.2.1 Battery Failure

Power failure may occur prematurely and was a very common phenomenon with the earlier mercury–zinc oxide powered generators. Battery depletions may be expected or simply an accelerated event associated with shelf loss or internal self discharge, drainage due to pacing load or temperature increases or variations. The lithium power systems have markedly reduced the incidence of such failures. In cases of sudden death, control of pulse generator by qualified personnel is mandatory (Bilitch 1980; Hurzeler et al. 1980; Mond and Sloman 1981a; Abrahamsen and Aarsland 1981; Barold et al. 1988).

5.2.2 Pulse Generator Malfunctions

Although pulse generator malfunctions may go unnoticed, in many cases they can be life threatening. Many external or internal factors may be responsible for the deleterious effects which may occur on one or more of the components leading to failure.

5.2.2.1 Unipolar Electrocautery. Unipolar electrocautery may cause difficulties during implantation of a permanent pacemaker and destroy the circuitry of the pulse generator. Myocardial damage at the implantation site has also been reported after accidental large current bursts with this device (Furman and Parker 1978; Irnich 1984a; Heller 1990).

5.2.2.2 Phantom Programming. The term "phantom programming" describes programming errors (dysprogramming/misprogramming) of pulse generators which may be fatal. They may occur at the factory, during transport, at implantation or by electromagnetic interference (magnet, defibrillator paddles). At autopsy, the pathologist should determine the programme settings of the pacemaker to be able to compare them with those stipulated by the physician (Fieldman and Dobrow 1978; Mond and Sloman 1981a,b).

5.2.2.3 Runaway Pacemaker. The term "runaway pacemaker" refers to an increase in pacing rate to above 150 beats/min; the rate may even exceed 2000 beats/min. The condition is observed with battery failure, defects in pulse generator components, and influx of body fluids into the circuitry, and leads to a fatal outcome in around one-third of cases (Chudasama et al. 1978; Odabashian and Brown 1979; Inoue et al. 1979; Santini et al. 1980; Comer et al. 1981; Mond and Sloman 1981a, b; van Gelder and El Gamal 1981; Heller 1990).

5.2.2.4 Extracorporeal Electromagnetic Interference. Extracorporeal electromagnetic interference was a common event with the early unshielded pulse generators but has become less frequent with the new models protected by a metal shield. Household electrical equipment (e.g. electric razors, microwave ovens, electric toothbrushes) as well as devices used in the working environment and business surroundings (e.g. arc welding devices, escalators, automatic cash registers, radio and television transmitters) may exert electromagnetic interference on pulse generators leading to failure. In the hospital environment such interference has been documented in association with electrocoagulators, transurethral resections, electrical beds, physiotherapy short-wave apparatus and even static electricity produced by the surgeon's gloves during pacemaker implantation. Such interference may lead to shorter battery life or to permanent pulse generator damage (PANNIZZO and FURMAN 1980; MOND and SLOMAN 1981a,b; IRNICH et al. 1978; IRNICH 1984a. FURMAN 1982a).

Pacemaker failure due to damage of the circuitry may also occur following transthoracic countershock with an *external defibrillator* by applying the cardioverter paddles directly over, or in the vicinity of, the pulse generator. The effect may be immediate or occur several days later. Thus it is strongly recommended that the paddles be at least 10 cm away from the pulse generator. The newer pulse generators are now equipped with a zener diode or other suppressor diode which limits current entries and offers protection to the circuitry (PALAC et al. 1981; FURMAN 1981b; DAS and EATON 1981; GOULD et al. 1981; BUTROUS et al. 1983).

Although *extracorporeal shock wave lithotripsy* was shown to cause damage exceptionally to the circuitry of pulse generators (principally the dual-chamber models), it is generally recommended that such treatment be avoided when the pulse generator is implanted in the abdominal wall (LANGBERG et al. 1987; COOPER et al. 1988; FETTER et al. 1989; ECTOR et al. 1989).

With regard to *electromagnetic radiation,* therapeutic doses of x-rays (principally for breast and lung cancers) may cause damage to the circuitry of pacemakers. Since most modern pulse generators utilise complementary metal oxide semiconductors for their integrated circuits, which can be damaged when exposed to high doses of ionising radiation, and as the mode of failure cannot be predicted accurately, the resulting damage may be transient or permanent and is dose dependent. Thus all pulse generators, especially the programmable generators and the smaller newer devices with dense circuits, should be properly shielded from irradiation at therapeutic doses (FURMAN 1982b; ADAMEC et al. 1982; BLAMIRES and MYATT 1982; KATZENBERG et al. 1982; CALFEE 1982; SHEHATA et al. 1986; MULLER-RUNKEL et al. 1990; TESKEY et al. 1991).

Magnetic resonance imaging (MRI) was originally thought to have little or no effect on pulse generators in the model tested (FETTER et al. 1984); however, it has since been established that its high static and time-varying magnetic fields may provoke asynchronous pacing with no damage to the circuitry, while its high radiofrequency may trigger accelerated atrial pacing. In dual-chamber pacemakers it may cause complete inhibition of atrial and ventricular output (ERLEBACHER et al. 1986; HAYES et al. 1987; Holmes et al. 1986; Pavlicek et al. 1983).

5.2.2.5 Endogenous Myopotential Interference. Inhibition by myopotential arising from contraction artefacts of skeletål muscles surrounding or adjacent to the pulse generator creating myogenic bioelectric signals is not an uncommon phenomenon, especially with unipolar systems of pacing. The incidence varies between 30% and 90% depending on the model. The condition has also been described with bipolar demand systems but with a lower incidence; furthermore it appears to vary from one patient to another, as well as with the individual model, even from the same manufacturer. The inhibition and triggering of these endogenous signals can be provoked by muscle activation, electrode perforation or fracture, leakage in the generator, damage to the insulation with current leakage and variation in magnetic flux during testing over the pulse generator; the result is increases in muscle potential of variable intensities with oversensing or undersensing. The effect may be asymptomatic, but in most instances clinical symptoms occur, ranging from light-headedness, dizziness and syncope to Stokes-Adams attacks and even sudden death in about 20% of cases, the latter event being associated with cerebral or myocardial damage due to prolonged asystole or bradycardia-related ventricular tachyarrhythmias. Reduction in the anode surface area in the newer models, better metallic shielding or encapsulation of the pulse generators and adequate filtering measures have significantly reduced the incidence of this condition. Furthermore, the introduction of programmable systems capable of sensitivity adjustments has further helped to improve the outcome when this effect occurs. It has also been shown that the incidence can be reduced by subcutaneous rather than intramuscular implantation (Berger and Jacobs 1979; Breivik and Ohm 1980; Radcliffe et al. 1981; Furman 1982a; Secemsky et al. 1982; Iesaka et al. 1982; Hauser 1982; Sinnaeve et al. 1982; Gialafos et al. 1983; Quintal et al. 1984; van Gelder and El Gamal 1984; Irnich 1984a; Rosenqvist et al. 1986; Gabry et al. 1987; Lau et al. 1989).

5.2.2.6 Others. Acute myocardial infarction may cause a sudden increase in pacing threshold which can be lethal. Similar increases can also be observed in severe metabolic disturbances, in hyperkalemia in myxoedema and with certain drugs. A good and accurate clinical history is of value in determining the cause of death (Mond and Sloman 1981b; Walker et al. 1985; Salel et al. 1989).

5.3 Pathology Related to Surgery

5.3.1 Pacemaker Pocket Infection

Infection of the pacemaker pocket occurs in 1% – 10% of cases. It may occur within the first 8 weeks (Mayo Clinic classification: early, within 2 weeks; intermediate, 2 weeks to 6 months; late, above 6 months) at the site of implantation of the pulse generator. It may be preceded by a local haematoma within the pocket at or around the time of operation, which predisposes to infection. *Staphylococcus epidermidis* is the organism most often encountered. *Staphylococcus aureus, Enterobacter cloacae, Klebsiella, Escherichia coli, Proteus mirabilis, Corynebacterium* and *Candida* have also been reported. The infection is probably due to perioperative bacterial contamination introduced during the surgical procedure. In the case of transvenous permanent pacemakers, secondary progression of the infection along the lead may reach the endocardial electrode implantation site with subsequent endocarditis and eventually septicaemia. Mortality is relatively high in such cases. In all cases of infection the suture line is always involved with abscess formation.

Late infections (after 2 months or years post-implantation) are less frequent and are often associated with multiple surgical interventions at the site of the generator implantation or after replacements of pulse generators. Complete replacement of the entire system is the treatment of choice, with implantation of a new pulse generator at a different site (JARA et al. 1979; PETERS et al. 1982; WOHL et al. 1982; DE LEON et al. 1984; RUITER et al. 1985; GOLDMAN 1986; HURST et al. 1986; AMIN et al. 1991; COHEN et al. 1991).

Epicardial lead infection may result in recurrent pericarditis and even mediastinitis. Other lesions have also been described with this mode of pacing, including haemorrhage into the pericardial sac as a result of laceration of the myocardium, leading to tamponade and even pericardial constriction. Pleural effusion and secondary pulmonary infiltration may be consequences of the surgical procedure (PETERS et al. 1982; WANG and MOK 1983). Bronchocutaneous fistula has also been described in connection with epicardial leads (CHUA et al. 1973; TEGTMEYER et al. 1974), and cardiac strangulation or pulmonary arterial lasso resulting in pulmonary hypertension (BRENNER et al. 1988; PERRY et al. 1991) has been reported.

5.3.2 Gas Pocket

Gas retention in the pulse generator pocket may occur during surgery either at the time of preparation of the pocket or during revision or replacement of a pulse generator. The accumulated air between the pulse generator and the overlying distended skin separates the latter from the metallic casing which serves as the anode, thus leading to early interruption of pacemaker function. An unusual case has also been described in which an air pocket was formed after explosion of a pacemaker generator with secondary chemical cellulitis. Gas pocket must be distinguished from the subcutaneous emphysema described earlier (LASALA et al. 1979; KREIS et al. 1979; MCWILLIAMS et al. 1984).

5.3.3 Pocket Erosion

Pocket erosion is more frequently encountered with the larger, heavy pulse generators when used in children, the thin elderly, or debilitated patients and is due to pressure necrosis of the thin skin overlying the pulse generator. Adhesion of the latter to the sometimes markedly thickened and hard subcutaneous tissue is a sign of incipient erosion and may occur before the skin becomes dusky and dark red. Liponecrosis, a relatively early event, often precedes secondary bacterial infection. The lesion is very often situated over the prominent part of the pulse generator and rarely at the site of the surgical incision. Extrusion of the pulse generator has been described (SIDDONS and NOWAK 1975; GIBBONS et al. 1979; WANG and MOK 1983; KRATZ et al. 1984; BYRD et al. 1986).

5.3.4 Twiddler's Syndrome

Rotation or twisting (either spontaneous or by the patient) of the pulse generator in the subcutaneous pocket may lead to fracture of the pacing lead, dislodgement of the electrode tip or loosening of the terminal pin from its socket, each of which may result in cessation of pacing. The condition has been described with pulse generators in either the thoracic or abdominal sites and with unipolar or bipolar lead types. Twisting or twiddling of the pulse generator by the patient can be habitual or unconscious, with enlargement of the subcutaneous pacemaker pocket and accumulation of a serous (seroma) fluid. Repeated twiddling of the pulse generator in such a pocket may result in the coiling of a long pacing lead into several loops and finally cause one of the above abnormalities with loss of pacing. Lead retraction or dislodgement is associated principally with the transvenous mode of pacing, while lead breakage is commonly observed with the epicardial mode. The use of the Dacron-woven pouch seems to restrict the movements of the pulse generators in their pockets when manipulated by the patients, and furthermore, the introduction of smaller and lighter pulse generators has surely played a role in reducing this condition (Guharay et al. 1977; Weiss and Lorber 1987; Anderson and Nathan 1990; Shandling et al. 1991).

5.3.5 Pulse Generator Migration

Local displacement of the pulse generator is not an uncommon phenomenon, and is seen most often in very thin elderly patients irrespective of the implantation site (thoracic, abdominal). Pulse generator migration appears to be a rare event and Baumgartner et al. (1990) could find only ten recorded cases in the literature, adding one of their own. Four generators have been found in the peritoneal cavity, one in the retroperitoneum, two within the colon, one in the jejunum, one in the caecum, one in the small bowel and one in the urinary bladder. The clinical symptoms vary depending on the route taken by the pulse generator and its final location. Repeated infections, chronic diarrhoea, painful episodes and haematomas are frequently associated with such migrations.

5.3.6 Connector Socket/Connector Pin Incompatibility

The adaptability of the pulse generator socket and the connector pin is essential for the reliability of the pacemaker system. Should there be a loose fitting or connections are not properly sealed off, fluids and/or tissue ingrowths may enter the pulse generator socket, leading to failure to pace. In the cases that we have seen the sockets are cloudy or greyish-white or reddish when blood accompanies the fluid (Fig. 8a). Rust or corrosion may also appear on the screw stopper in some instances (Fig. 8b). Adhesive sealings, silicone oil or mineral jelly are being used in order to prevent these conditions, especially when there is need to change pulse

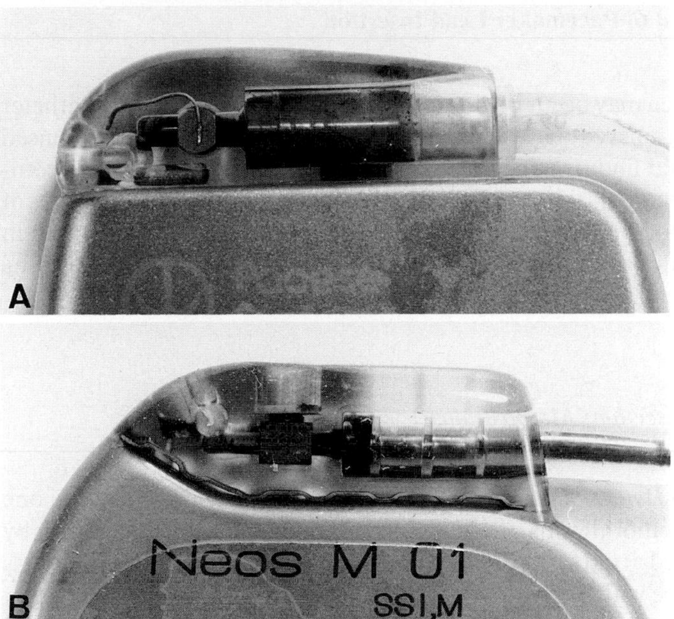

Fig. 8. Loose connector fittings:
a Fluids, including blood, have entered the pulse generator socket **b** The connector pin and the proximal end of the lead are rusty and corroded

generators and to be assured that there is sealing at the junction. Clinicians and manufacturers have been looking at this problem with the hope of arriving at some standardised designs or universal connector systems (FEREK et al. 1984; RAO 1984; CALFEE and SAULSON 1986; DORING and FLINK 1986; FURMAN 1990; COSTEAS and SCHOENFELD 1991).

5.3.7 *Pacemaker Pocket-Associated Neoplasia*

Neoplasms have been reported in association with pacemaker pockets. Carcinoma of the breast (three females, one male) is the most frequent tumour described, and a case of plasmacytoma has been reported in a male patient. Although there is debate over the role of the pulse generator in the genesis of the tumours, it is generally accepted that the association is most likely coincidental. Metastasis of a pulmonary histiocytoma to the pocket has also been documented (MAGILLIGAN and ISSHAK 1980; RASMUSSEN et al. 1985).

5.4 Problems Related to Pacemaker Lead Insertion

Most difficulties which may occur during implantation of the pacemaker catheter are associated with transvenous leads. The consequences may go unrecognised and may be incidental findings during radiological, echocardiographic or computed tomographic examinations or at autopsy. Major or minor abnormalities of the heart and/or blood vessels (principally the venous system) have resulted in some inadvertent malpositionings of the electrode, or in difficulties in attaining the right ventricle.

5.4.1 Transvenous insertion: Malpositions

5.4.1.1 Atrial Septal Defect. During introduction of the pacemaker lead via one of the neck veins or femoral veins, the lead may cross over into the left atrium by way of an unsuspected atrial septal defect or a patent foramen ovale. It may pass the mitral valve orifice with implantation of the electrode into the left ventricular wall. The malposition of the electrode in most cases does not produce clinical symptoms and is an incidental finding on radiology. Some patients have presented with amaurosis fugax as a result of thrombus formation at the site of implantation of the electrode. Partial or total perforation of the ventricular septum has also been documented (Nanda and Barold 1982; Ross et al. 1983; Tobin et al. 1983; Schiavone et al. 1984; Flicker et al. 1985; van Erckelens et al. 1991; Trohman et al. 1991; Shmuely et al. 1992; Iliceto et al. 1982).

5.4.1.2 Malformations of the Thoracic Veins. Persistence of the left superior vena cava occurs in approximately 0.5% of the general population and may be present in 3% - 10% or more of patients with associated congenital cardiac malformations. In such cases the right superior vena cava may be present, hypoplastic or absent (17%). The abnormality may go unrecognised unless suspected by echocardiography or discovered during cardiac catheterisation. When it is unsuspected, major difficulties may be encountered during implantation of a transvenous pacemaker lead via the subclavian or other vein on the right, while from the left it is possible to reach the right ventricular apex by way of the often dilated coronary sinus. Dislodgement of the electrode is the most common finding. The electrode may accidentally be implanted in the coronary sinus (intentional long-term atrial pacing is by a special type of electrode). The difficulties encountered with the persistent left superior vena cava are dependent on the extent of the abnormalities of the intrathoracic venous system, making it mandatory to dissect the venous system thoroughly at post-mortem (Greenberg et al. 1978; Gillmer et al. 1981; Hellestrand et al. 1982; Nanda and Barold 1982; Ronnevik et al. 1982; Flicker et al. 1985; Robbens and Ruiter 1986; Dirix et al. 1988; Riera et al. 1990; Dosios et al. 1991; Villani et al. 1991; Zerbe et al. 1992).

5.4.1.3 Middle Cardiac Vein Implantation. At the time of implantation the pacemaker lead may enter the middle cardiac vein by way of the coronary sinus, lodging in its lumen and thus stimulating the posterior interventricular septum. Right bundle branch block, a sign of left ventricular excitation, is suggestive of this malposition (Barold and Banner 1978; Waxman et al. 1979).

5.4.1.4 Hepatic Vein Implantation. The lead may cross the right atrium from the superior vena cava into the inferior vena cava to reach the hepatic vein (Nanda and Barold 1982).

5.4.1.5 Inadvertent Use of the Arterial System. Exceptionally, under certain conditions, an artery in the neck is mistaken for a cervical vein during lead implantation, with fatal outcome (Lapore et al. 1987).

5.4.2 Infection

Osteomyelitis of the clavicle and first rib associated with trauma at the time of subclavian catheterisation has been documented. Infection may occur during venepuncture or by haematological spread with symptoms appearing within days or weeks after the procedure or even months thereafter (Rosenfeld 1985).

5.4.3 Epicardial Insertion

The majority of lesions encountered with this type of pacing lead are surgical, as already described (de Feyter et al. 1980; Nanda and Barold 1982; Smith and Tatoulis 1990).

5.5 Pathology Related to Pacemaker Leads

A number of lesions of each element (insulator and conductor) of the insulated electrical conductor of the lead are known to produce certain clinical symptoms and/or electrical pacing abnormalities whose outcome may be fatal.

5.5.1 Insulator

The silicone elastomer (soft, thick) insulators have been replaced by a polyurethane, which has better physical, chemical and electrical characteristics. Lesions of the insulator may occur accidentally at the time of implantation by surgical instruments or improper handling of the material. Environmental stress cracking first presents as frosting and then as cracks in the insulator, and may finally involve the entire thickness of the wall. Blood or fluid may enter the sheath and reach the conductor with adverse effects. The insulator may be damaged by securing sutures at fixation (anchorage) points leading to pseudo-fracture. Compression of the lead between the first rib and clavicle or where the lead crosses the first rib may result in damage to the insulator. Atrial "J" leads may induce lesions in the "memory curve" of the lead. Mechanical wear and tear within or near remodelled thickened fibrous tissue sheaths in the vicinity of the tricuspid valve or chordae tendineae may do severe damage to the insulator, leaving the conductor bare. New current pathways are created, leading to high current flow and battery failure (van Gelder and El Gamal 1983; Timmis et al. 1983; Byrd et al. 1983; Raymond and Nanian 1984; Hanson 1984; Beyersdorf et al. 1985; Chatelain et al. 1985; Hubbell et al. 1986; Phillips et al. 1986; Fyke 1988; Arakawa et al. 1989).

5.5.2 Conductor

Transvenous conductor or lead fracture with an incidence between 1% and 7% was the main complication of the earlier rigid leads. The incidence is now estimated at below 2% with the introduction of the flexible multifilar coil leads. Lead fractures are encountered most frequently at points where there is sharp angulation or looping of the lead (between the clavicle and first rib) or compression in cases of abnormality of the thoracic cage (thoracic outlet syndrome). Some sites of predilection of fractures are: the site of venous access, between the venous entry and the pulse generator, a zone close to the insertion into the pulse generator socket and within the vessel lumen. Some cases have been described at the level of the tricuspid valve. Lead fracture may occur during implantation or later and leads to complete or incomplete loss of pacing and eventually to a fatal outcome. Retained, broken or sectioned unsecured portions of leads (with or without electrodes) have been reported to migrate to distant sites (iliac or femoral vein, pulmonary artery), resulting in vena caval thrombosis, iliofemoral phlebitis, venous perforation or pulmonary embolism (Kertes et al. 1983; Hill 1987; Suzuki et al. 1988; Clarke et al. 1989).

Epicardial lead fractures, although rarely reported, are not uncommon (Khair and Tristani 1979; Amin et al. 1991) although electrode failures have been described clinically with this system of pacing (De Feyter et al. 1980; Bashore et al. 1982).

5.6 Electrode–Endomyocardial Interface

5.6.1 Fibrosis

5.6.1.1 Transvenous Pacing Leads. At the time of implantation there is local trauma to the endocardium and surrounding myocardium at the point of contact, the extent of which depends on the difficulties encountered and manoeuvres

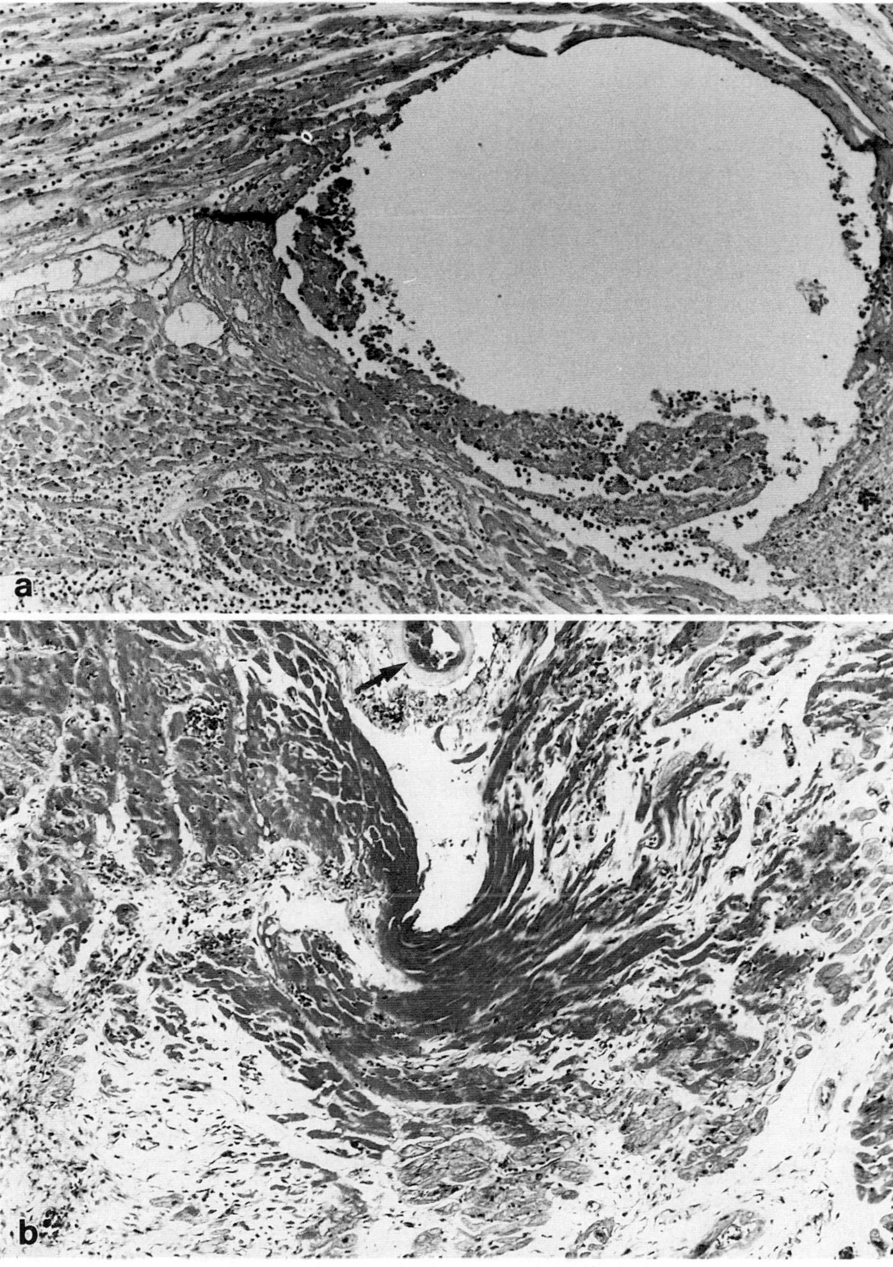

Fig. 9. a Necrosis, oedema and important polymorphonuclear infiltration of the surrounding myocardium at the implantation site at 26 h. Endovenous electrode implantation. H & E, × 16. **b** Acute necrosis, oedema, primarily mononuclear cell infiltration and thrombosis of small artery *(arrow)* at 11 days. Endovenous electrode implantation. H & E, × 16

necessary before stabilisation and fixation of the electrode are achieved. There is diffuse local interstitial oedema with myocardial necrosis. Within 12 h there is an acute inflammatory response, rich in polymorphonuclear cells, which is responsible for the early sharp rise in stimulation threshold (Fig. 9). The electrode surface is covered by an eosinophilic fibrinous layer which may persist for several months and extends along the surface of the lead. Granulation tissue appears within days and progressively transforms into fibrous scar tissue, fixing the electrode into its definite position with disorganisation of the surrounding myocardial fibres. The neighbouring endocardium is usually thickened and fibrous (Fig. 10). Occasionally, foci of chronic inflammatory cells are observed months or years after implantation within and/or around the scar tissue (Fig. 11). The latter is quite prominent with the larger, older electrodes, but is less abundant or negligible with the smaller, new-generation electrodes (Fig. 12). This fibrous tissue is responsible for the maintenance and plateau of the stimulation threshold observed clinically, which varies with the thickness of the tissue layer. During the manoeuvres in the attempt to secure the electrode, trabeculae and/or papillary muscles may be partially damaged or perforated, resulting in the accumulation of fibrin deposits around these areas and finally the formation of scar tissue which, in some cases, may fix the lead to these structures (Fig. 13). The electrode is sometimes lodged in one of the structures.

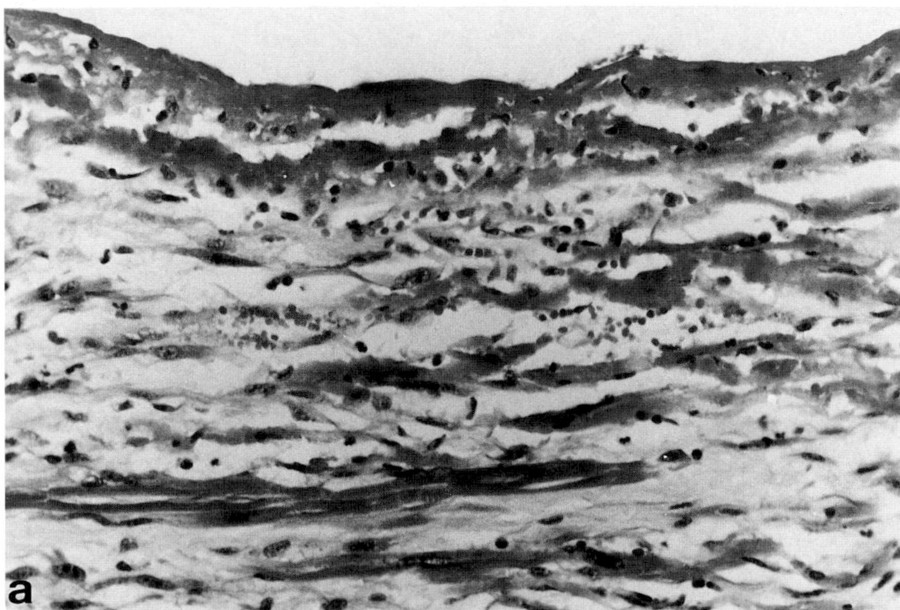

Fig. 10. a Eosinophilic, fibrinous layer which surrounds the electrode also extends along the lead. Notice adjacent myocardial fibre necrosis and inflammatory response. H & E, × 64.

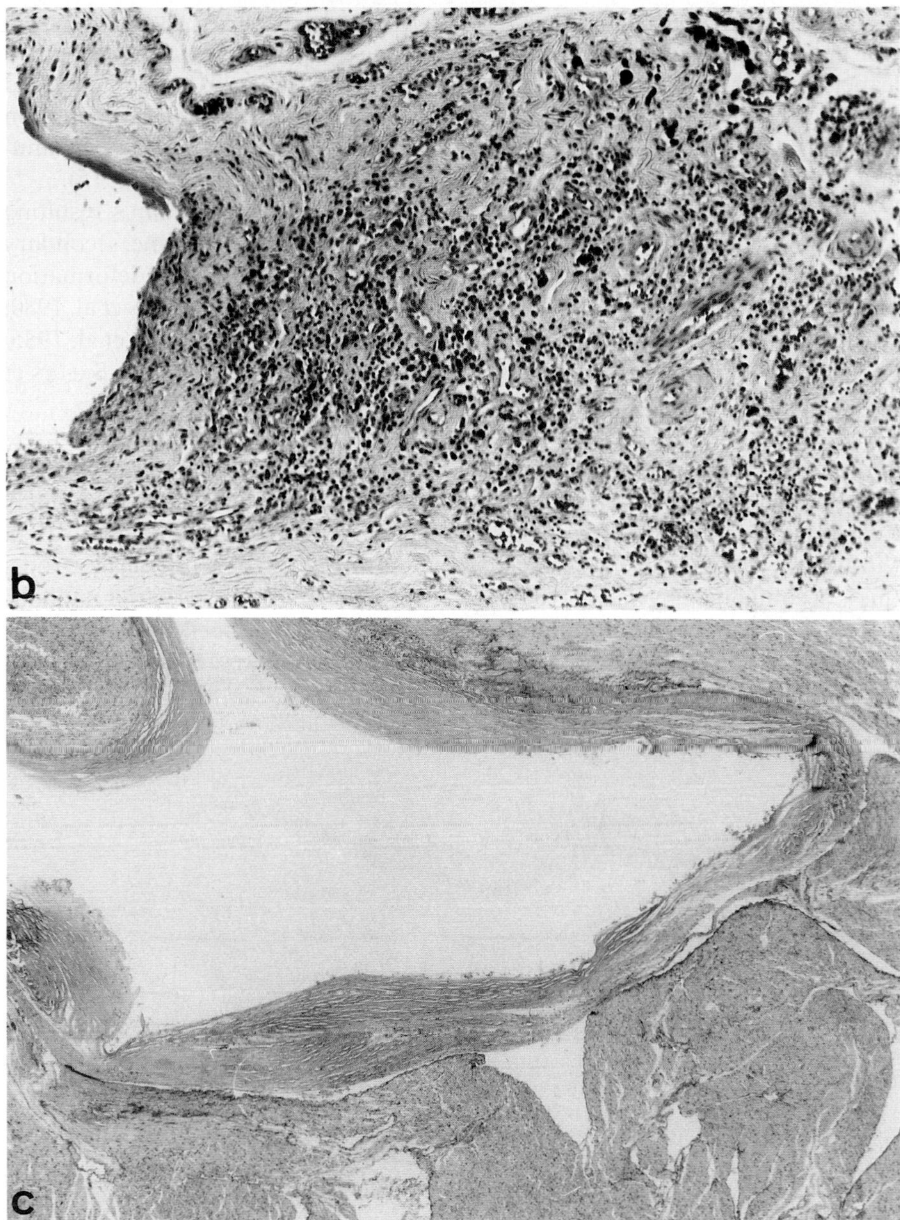

Fig. 10. b Important granulation tissue reaction of endocardial lead 2 weeks after implantation. H & E, × 25. **c** Endocardial fibrous thickening in the neighbourhood of the electrode implantation site 4 years later. van Gieson-elastin, × 10

Damage and/or perforation of the tricuspid valve leaflets (principally posterior and septal) and chordae tendineae may also occur. When perforated, the leaflet becomes fibrosed, thickened and often retracted (Fig. 14) and this may lead to valvular insufficiency. At this level, one may find fragmentation or disruption of the insulating material, sometimes accompanied by foreign body-type granulation tissue and even corrosion of the electrical conductor wires (Fig. 15).

The electrode may be inadvertently implanted in the coronary sinus, resulting in thrombosis of the vessel and its tributaries (Fig. 16) and, with time, secondary scarring, thickening of the vessel wall and ultimately constriction and deformation of its orifice. Coronary artery fistula may occur as a late event (Gibson et al. 1980; Robboy et al. 1969; Rajs 1983; Ripart and Mugica 1983; Chatelain et al. 1985; Old et al. 1989; Rubio and Al-Bassam 1991; Mond and Stokes 1992; Saeian et al. 1991).

5.6.1.2 Epicardial Pacing Leads. Trauma to the myocardium is more extensive with this mode of pacing, especially with the older electrode models. Immediately following implantation there is marked oedema and necrosis of the myocardium throughout the zone of the ventricular wall occupied by the screw-on electrode; this is accompanied by haemorrhage and within the first few hours after implantation a thick eosinophilic fibrinous deposit appears around the entire length of the electrode coil (Fig. 17). The myocardial fibres within the axis and around the coil

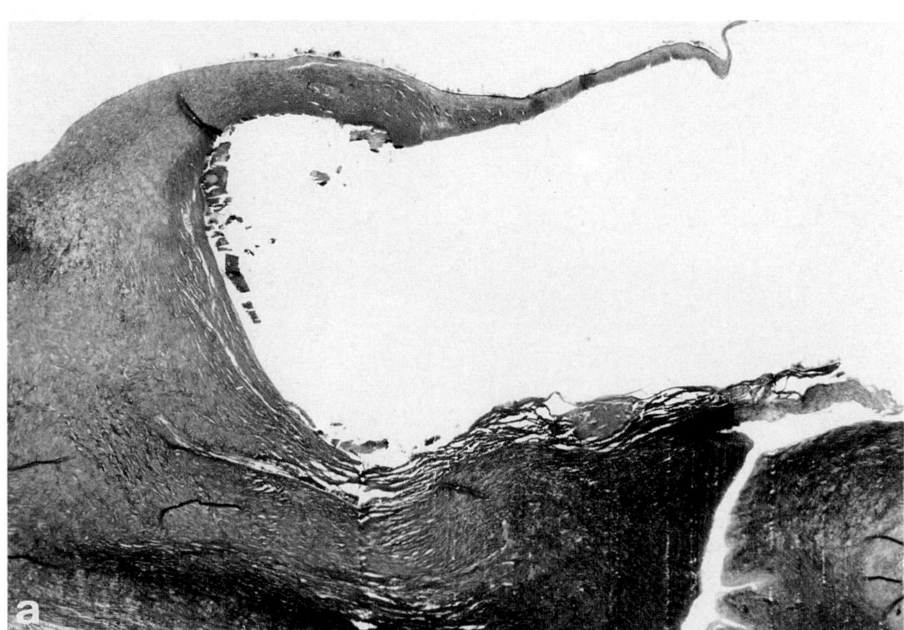

Fig. 11. a Important fibrotic tissue at the implantation site of endovenous lead 8 years after implantation. Note fragmented eosinophilic material covering the scarred tissue. van Gieson-elastin, × 10.

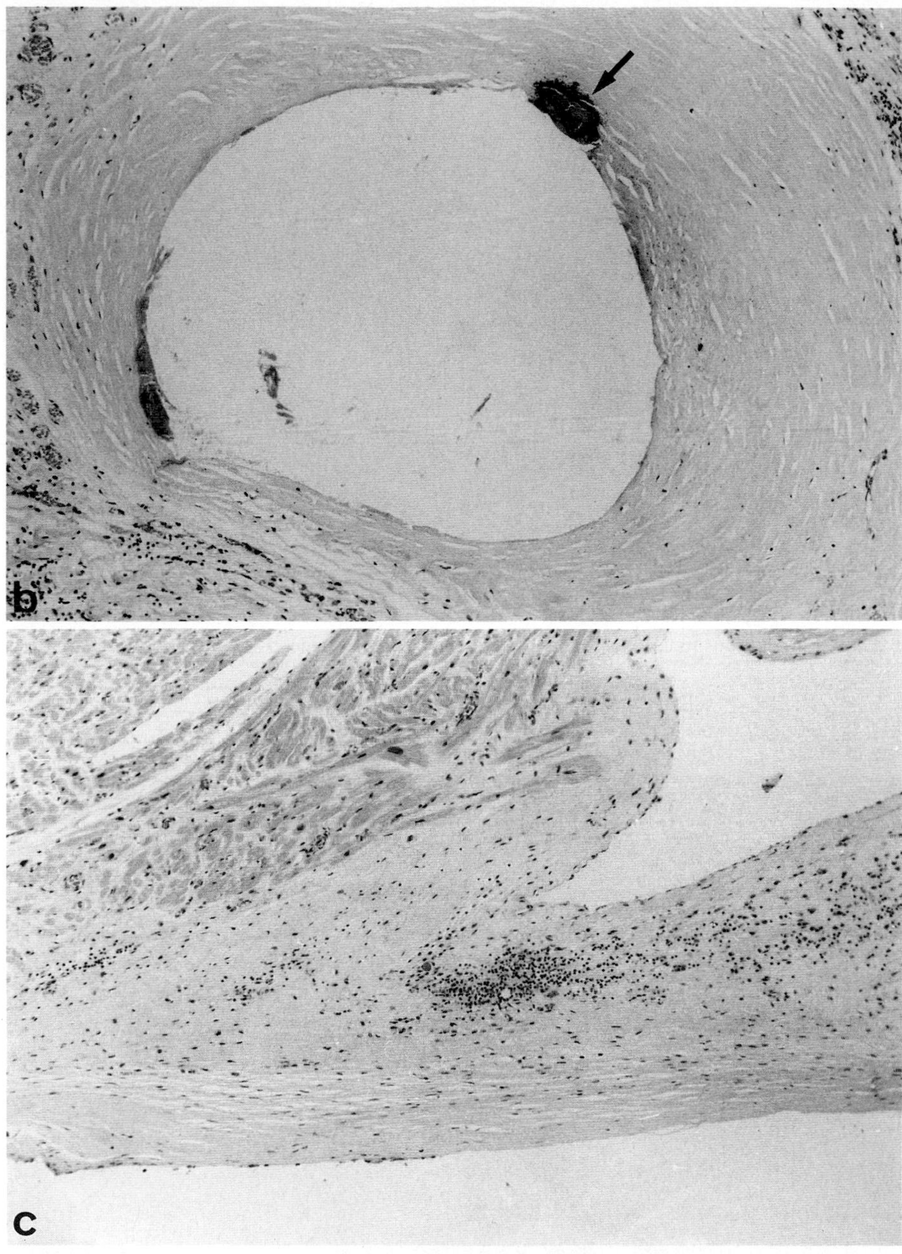

Fig. 11. b Extensive fibrotic tissue, partly hyalinised and calcified *(arrow)*, with moderate chronic inflammatory cells around the implantation site of endovenous electrode, 6 years after implantation. H & E, × 10. **c** Fibrosis and chronic inflammatory infiltration extending along the channel of the lead's trajectory. H & E, × 10

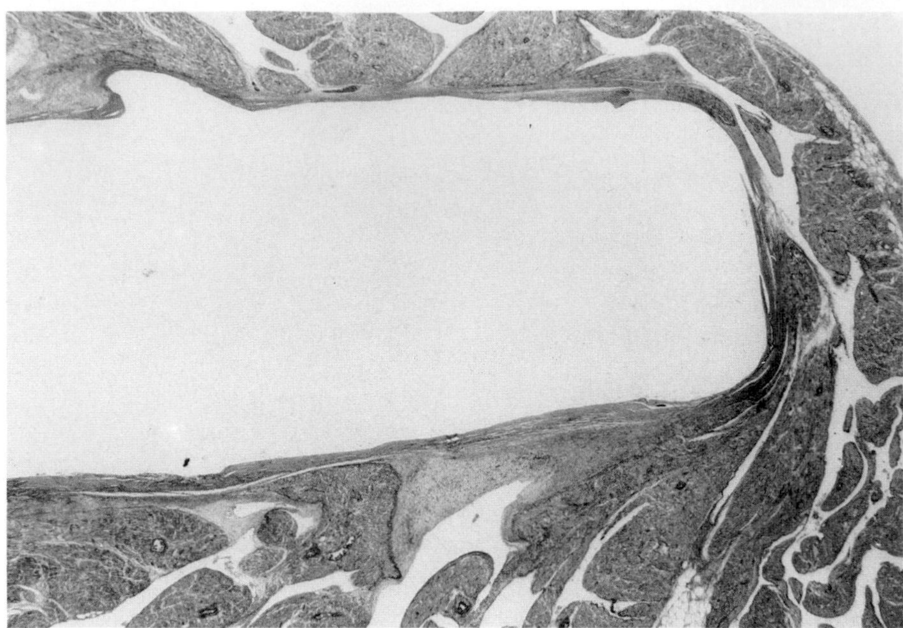

Fig. 12. Little fibrous tissue reaction with new carbon tip electrode, 5 1/2 years after implantation. H & E, × 6.3

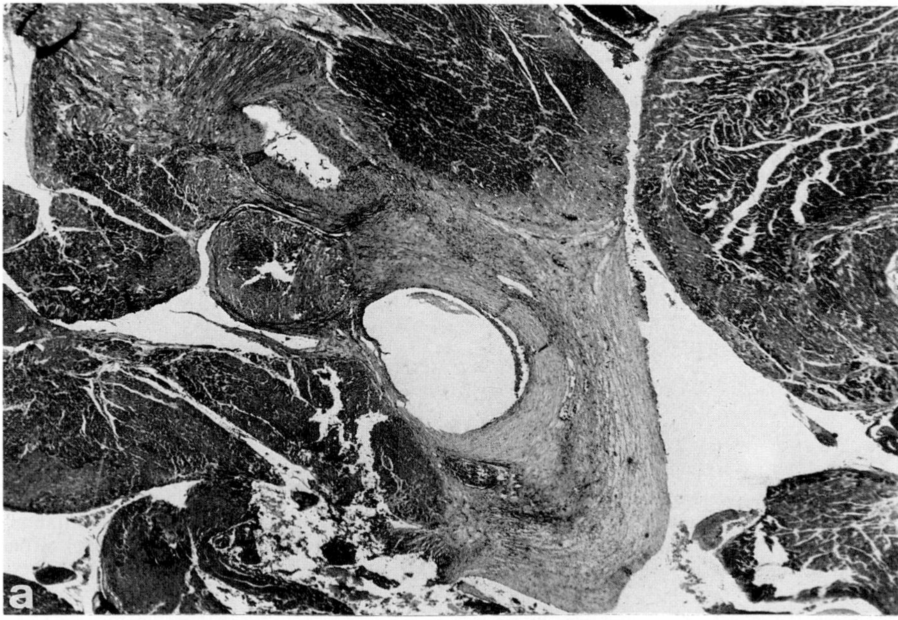

Fig. 13. a Extensive recent infarction proximal to the implantation site with organising thrombosis uniting the papillary muscle to the adjacent trabeculae, 10 days after endovenous implantation. H & E, × 6.3

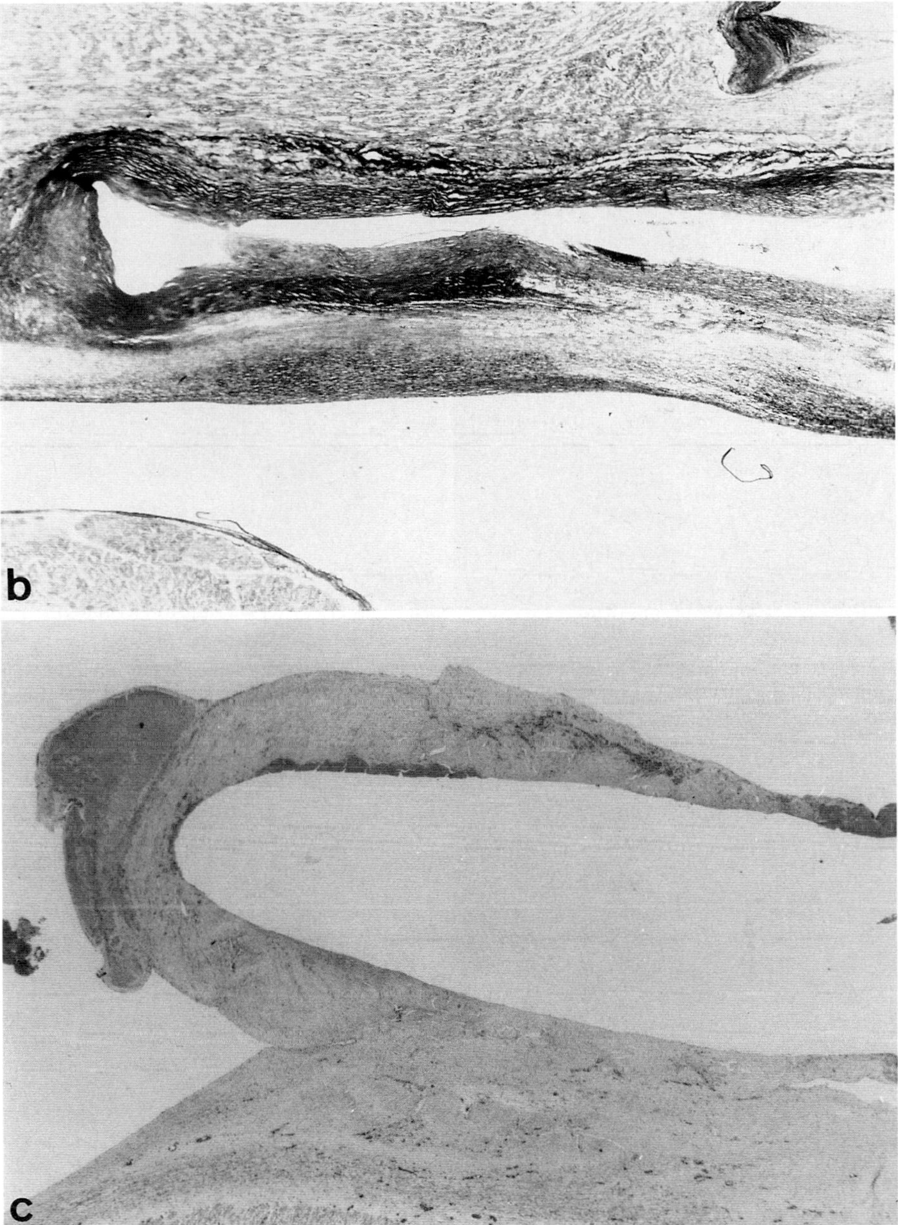

Fig. 13. b Implantation in papillary muscle with fibrosis and scarring. van Gieson-elastin, × 6.3. **c** Fibrous tissue fixing the electrode implantation site in a trabecular structure. H & E, × 10

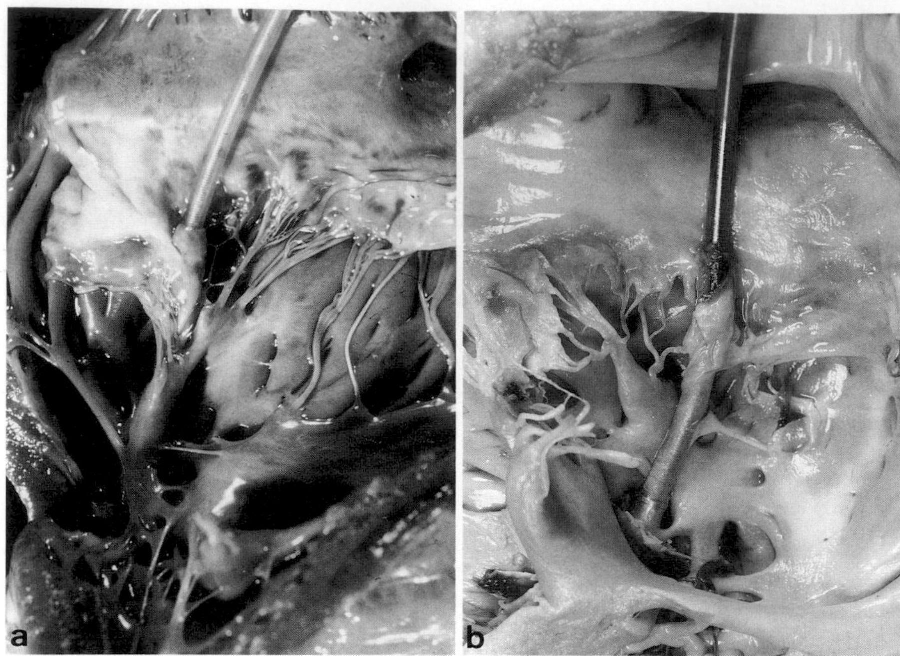

Fig. 14. a Perforation of the posterior tricuspid leaflet with marked fibrous thickening and retraction involving all the adjacent structures. **b** The septal leaflet, markedly thickened and fibrosed, is enrolled and retracted about the lead. The atrial endocardium is markedly thickened

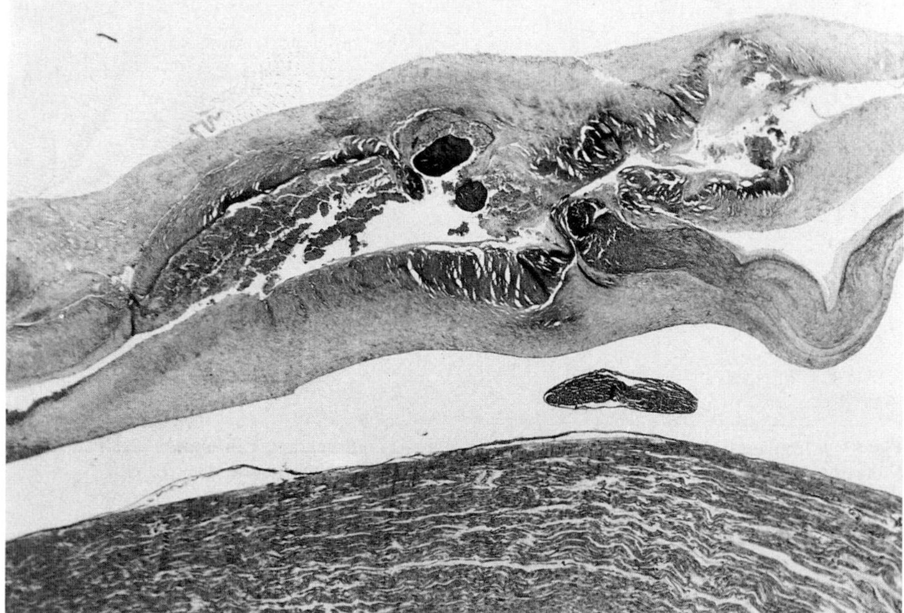

Fig. 15. Tricuspid valve leaflet perforation by endovenous lead. Note fragments of insulating material sometimes embedded within the fibrous tissue. H & E, ×4

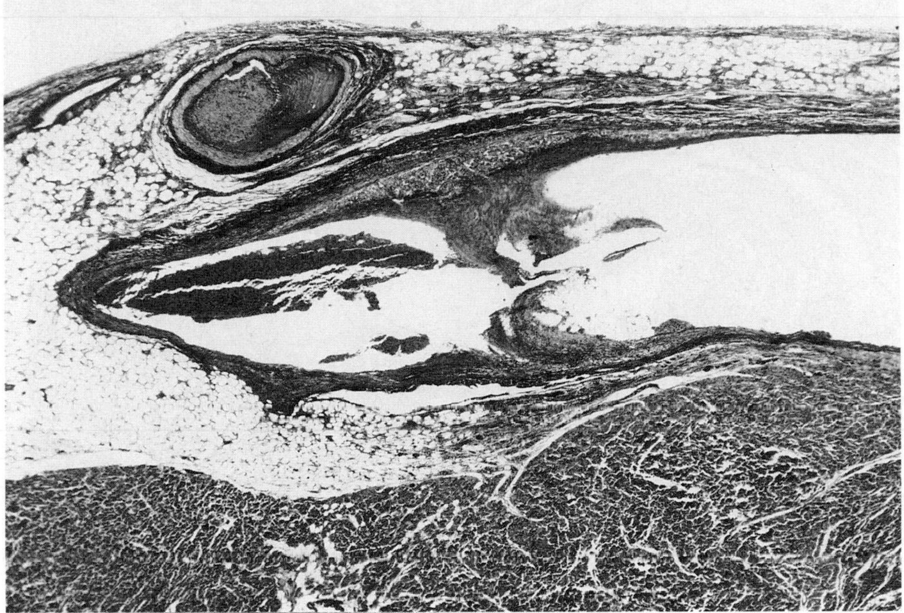

Fig. 16. Organising thrombus and fibrous thickening of coronary sinus at the site of implantation of endovenous electrode and thrombosis of tributary. van Gieson-elastin, × 4

are stretched, whorled or curved and show extensive coagulative necrosis and/or myocytolysis (Fig. 18). This is rapidly accompanied by an acute inflammatory reaction which progresses to granulation tissue (Fig. 19) by the third day and to fibrous scar tissue within 3 weeks. The scar tissue is generally extensive, which explains the higher pacing stimulation threshold observed with this type of electrode when compared with the endovenous electrode. The scar may also undergo hyalinisation and in many instances there are large collections of chronic inflammatory cells accompanied by numerous macrophages containing iron pigment (Fig. 20). Broken insulating material may be seen in the granulation tissue, sometimes with a foreign body giant cell reaction about the lumen of the unscrewed electrode coil (Fig. 21). There are two constant features with this mode of pacing lasting for months or even years: the presence of a granular fibrinous deposit along the course of the electrode and foci of myocytolysis and/or coagulative necrosis in the adjacent myocardium (Fig. 22). The fibrinous layer is continuously undergoing organisation.

Ventricular (reverse) perforation (myocardial penetration) or right atrial perforation may occur when the functional tip of the electrode protrudes into the ventricular or atrial cavity (Fig. 23). Cases of right ventricular rupture have also been documented with this mode of pacing.

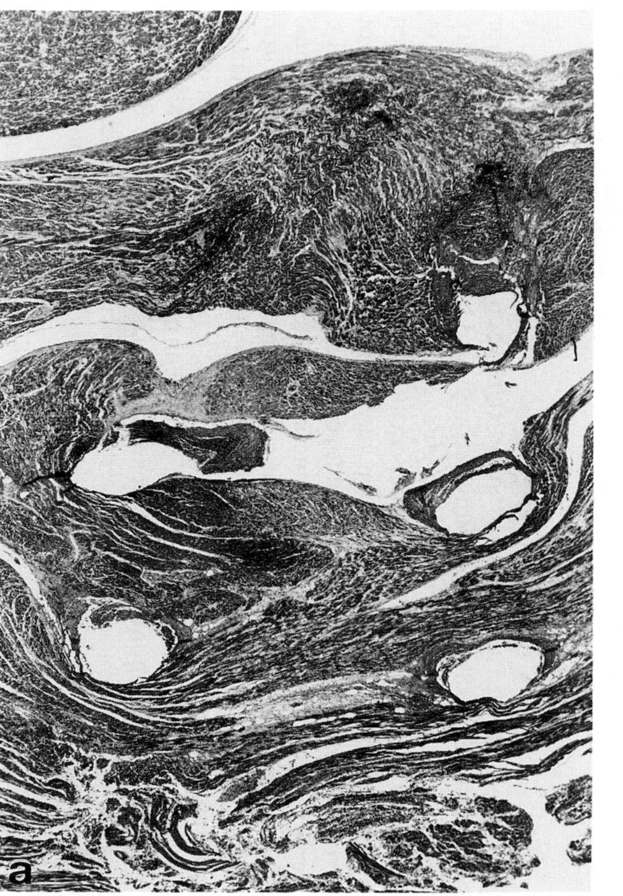

Fig. 17. a Important necrosis throughout the myocardial wall thickness at the site of the epicardial screw-on electrode, 23 h after implantation. H & E, ×4.

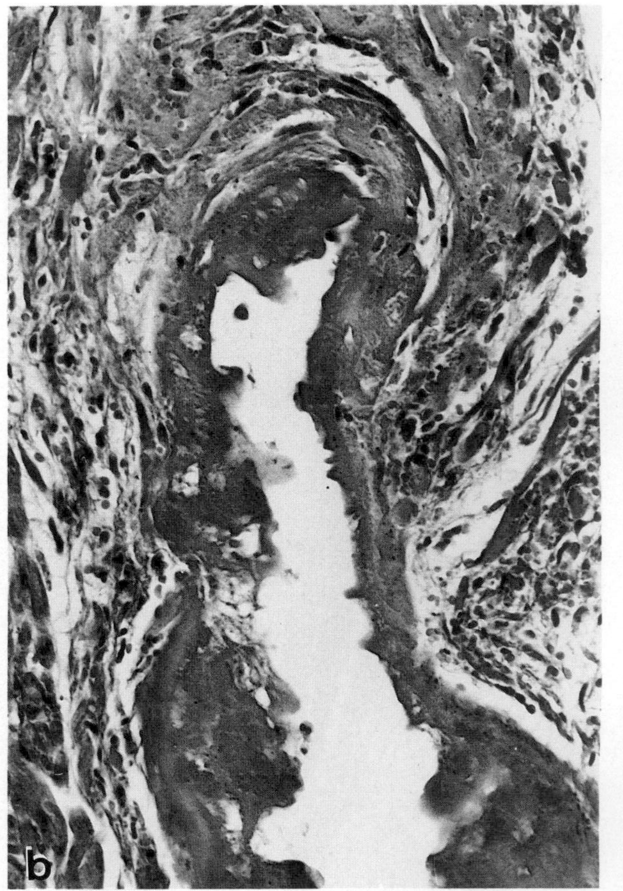

Fig. 17. b Abundant eosinophilic fibrinous deposit along the entire length of the channel of the epicardial screw-on electrode, 3 days after implantation. H & E, ×6

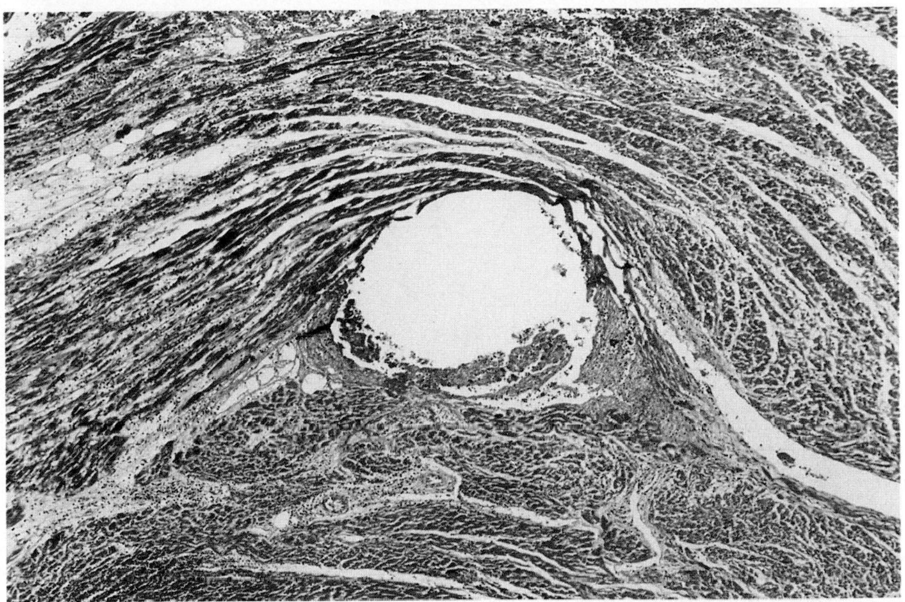

Fig. 18. Extensive myocardial necrosis with stretching, whorling and deformation of the myocardial fibres along the channel of the epicardial electrode, 3 days after implantation. H & E, × 10

Pericardial adhesions are common features of epicardial lead implantations, especially in the late stages post-implantation, while serosanguineous effusion and fibrinous pericarditis are observed within the first 2 weeks after implantation (BASHORE et al. 1982; CHATELAIN et al. 1985; KARPAWICH et al. 1988; KUGLER et al. 1990; SMITH and TATOULIS 1990).

5.6.2 Exit Block

Exit block is a relatively common and serious complication in pacemaker carriers (transvenous and epicardial electrodes), having an incidence of about 20%. It is characterised by failure to capture as a result of a markedly elevated stimulation threshold which exceeds the maximum output capacity of the pulse generator and can lead to pacemaker failure. High-threshold exit block may occur within the first 4-6 weeks or within the first year when fibrous tissue around the electrode is fully established. It is now generally accepted that the fibrous tissue around the electrode results in an increase in the distance between the electrode and excitable myocardial tissue (virtual electrode surface) and, as a result, increases the surface area of the electrically responsive electrode – endomyocardial interface, leading to the increase in stimulation threshold. The advent of the steroid-eluting leads which provoke a limited fibrous tissue response around the electrode site have eliminated

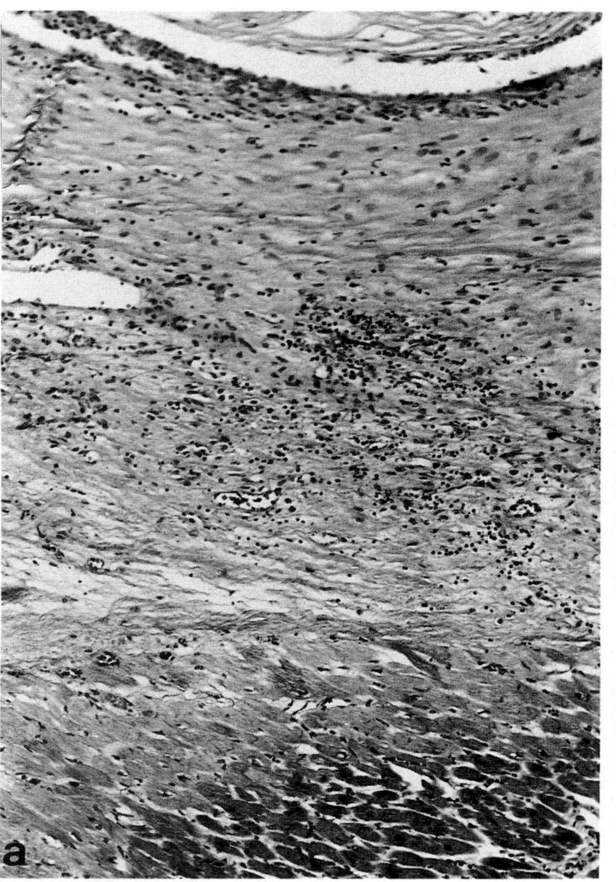

Fig. 19. a Thick zone of fibrous and granulation tissue along the channel of the screw-on electrode bordered by an area of necrotic myocardial fibres, 12 days after implantation. H & E, ×25.

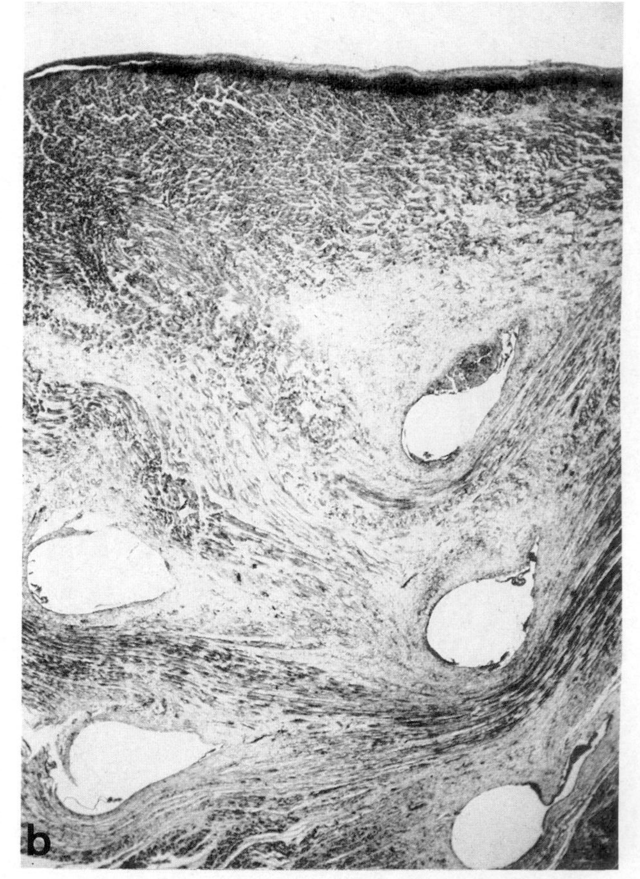

Fig. 19. b Diffuse fibrosis around and between the channel of the screw-on electrode at 18 months H & E, ×3

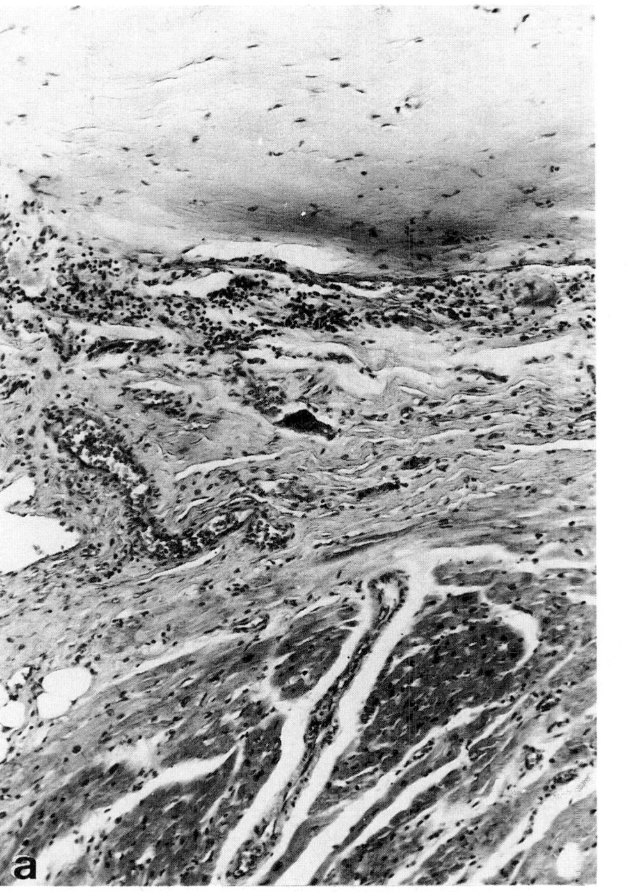

Fig. 20. a Hyalinisation of the fibrous tissue around the channel of the screw-on electrode with important granulation tissue at 5 years post-implantation. H & E, $\times 16$.

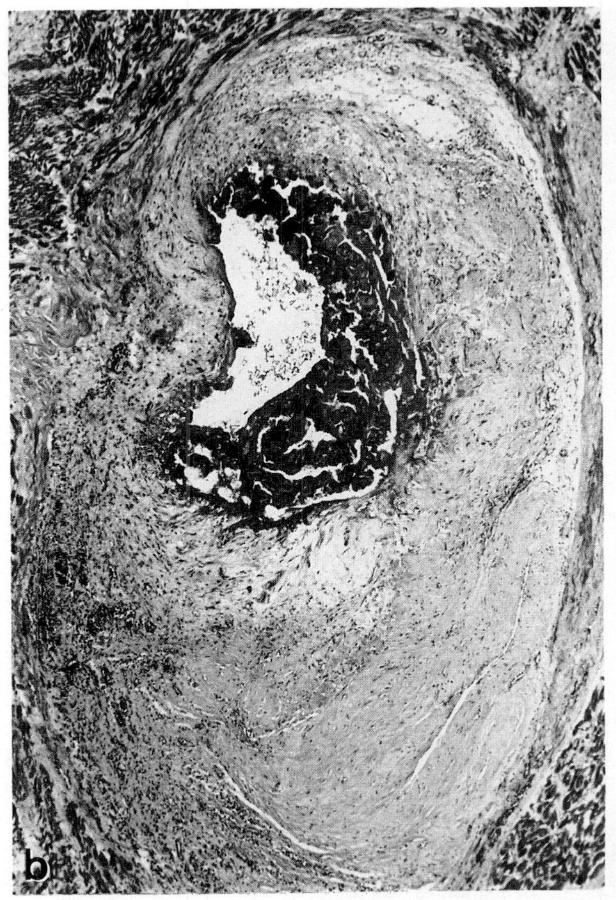

Fig. 20. b Thick fibrinoid layer around channel of screw-on electrode, 21 months after implantation. H & E, $\times 10$

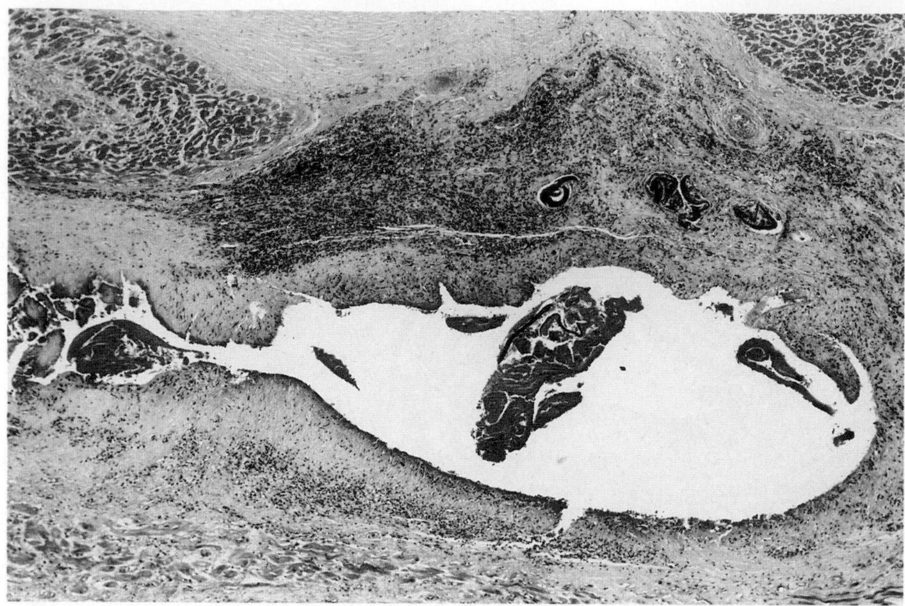

Fig. 21. Fragmented insulating material free or within the surrounding granulation tissue. It can also be seen in foreign body giant cells. Channel of screw-on electrode. van Gieson-elastin, × 4

the necessity of frequent reoperations and replacements of pacing systems and their components. Furthermore, their low stimulation threshold could eventually eliminate exit block.

Exit block is generally associated with certain other morphological lesions found at post-mortem, including myocardial infarction (recent or scarred tissue) in the neighbourhood of the electrode, ventricular perforation, increased distance between anode and cathode, variation in properties of materials (conductors and insulators), lead fractures (total or partial) and displacements or dislodgements of the electrode. The condition may also be observed in cases with severe metabolic imbalance, hyperkalemia, or drug overdose (anti-arrhythmics, antidepressants). As emphasised previously, a clinicopathological correlation is necessary in evaluating the results of autopsy (Hynes et al. 1981; Mond and Sloman 1981b; Ripart and Mugica 1983; Snow 1983; Stokes et al. 1987; Radovsky et al. 1988; Cameron et al. 1990).

5.6.3 Thrombosis

5.6.3.1 Transvenous Pacing Leads. Fibrin deposits cover the site of implantation shortly after positioning of the electrode and extend over the greater portion of the lead throughout its intracardiac and intravascular course. The fibrin layer is more prominent on silicone rubber leads than on polyurethane leads, and with time forms a translucent mantle around the leads. These deposits may undergo organisation with incorporation and integration with the surrounding fibrous tissue (Fig. 24) or local thrombus may develop immediately or weeks, months or even years following implantation.

Thrombosis along the lead is not altogether uncommon, especially in areas where the lead is in contact with a tricuspid valve leaflet or trabecula, the endocardium (mainly the right atrium) or the endothelium of the superior vena cava (where multiple thrombi are often observed). In most instances adherence to the wall develops at these

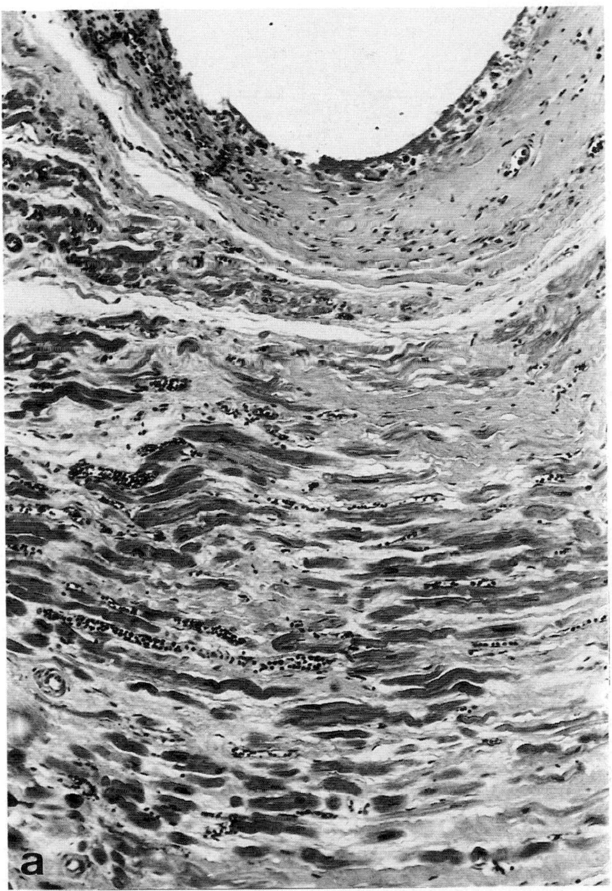

Fig. 22. a The fibrinous material along the channel is continuously undergoing organisation. Myocardial fibre necrosis can be present months or years later. Appearance 15 months after implantation of epicardial electrode. H & E, × 25.

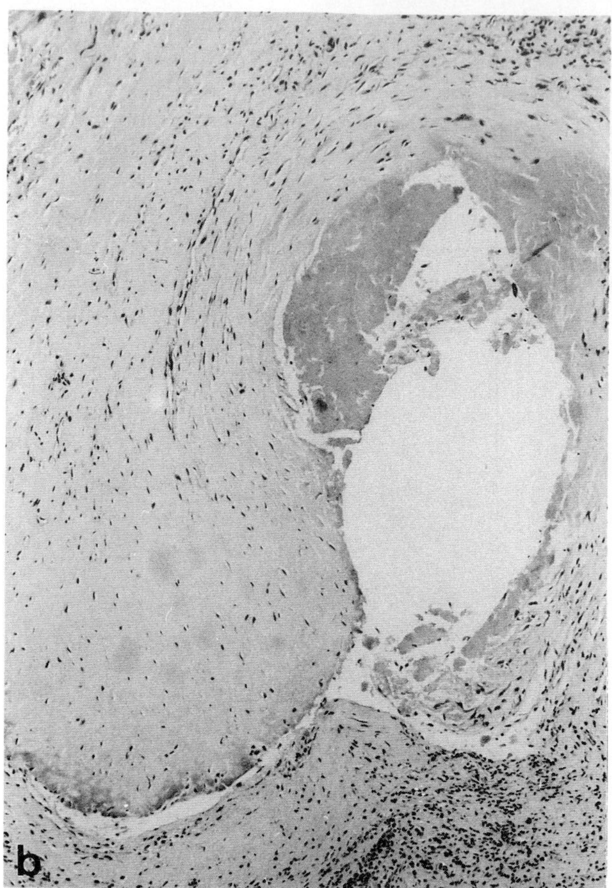

Fig. 22. b Granular eosinophilic, fibrinous material, 6 years after implantation with important foci of chronic inflammatory cells. H & E. × 10

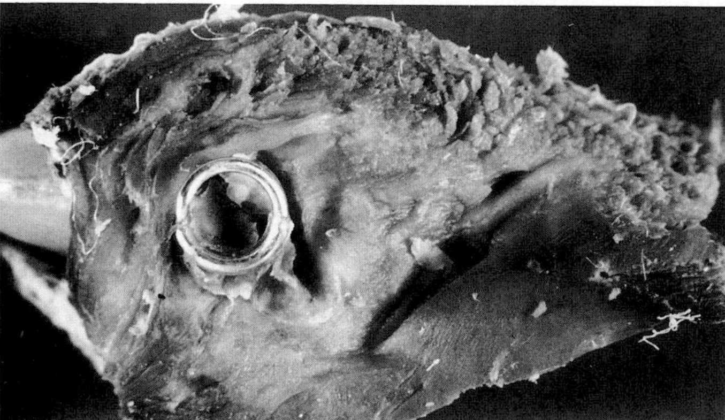

Fig. 23. Perforation (reverse) of epicardial screw-on electrode. A large portion of the coil is free in the right ventricular cavity

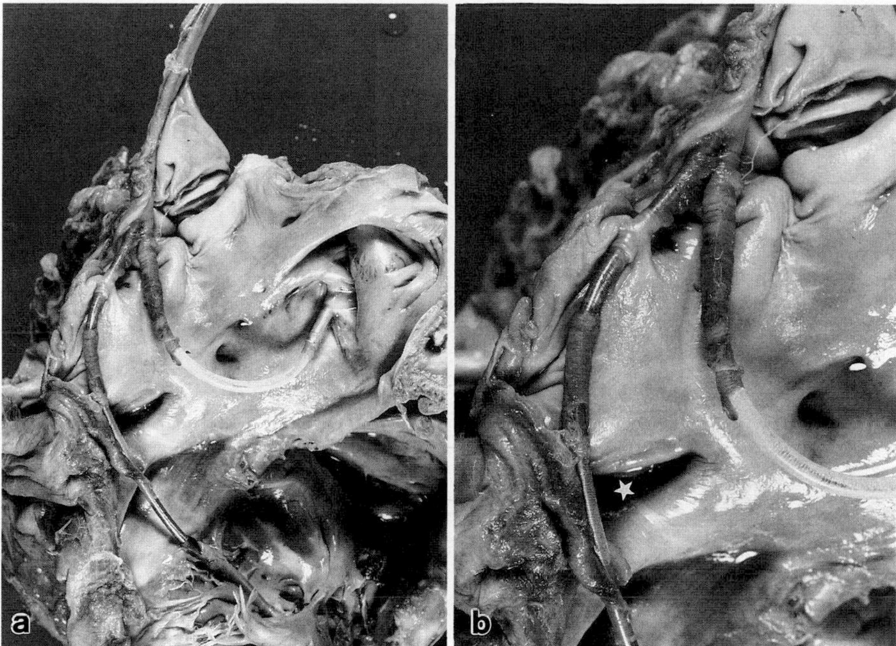

Fig. 24a,b. Thrombosis along both leads (ventricular, atrial) extending along the superior vena cava and fixing the leads at multiple points to the thickened endocardium. High-power view where the ventricular lead crosses the orifice of the coronary sinus (*); it is covered by a translucent material which may cover practically the entire lead at times

sites (Fig. 25). With time, such adherences become fibrotic and present histologically as successive thickened fibrous layers (Fig. 26) (Robboy et al. 1969; Rajs 1983; Chatelain et al. 1985).

5.6.3.2 Epicardial Pacing Leads. Local thrombosis is exceptional and may only occur if there is penetration of the right ventricular wall with the screw-on electrode.

5.6.4 Infection

5.6.4.1 Transvenous Pacing Leads. Infection remains one of the most important complications associated with long-term pacing. Its incidence was formerly estimated to be between 0.3% and 19% but is now below 4% due to the care taken before and after surgery and the use, in many institutions, of antibiotic prophylaxis. Most infections take their origin in the pulse generator pocket and travel along the lead to reach the implantation site. Abscess formation may occur locally in the ventricular wall; mural vegetations may be observed involving the

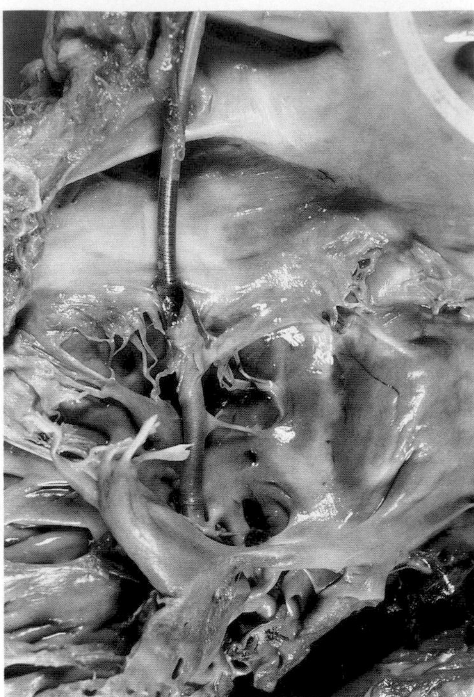

Fig. 25. Organising thrombus near the site of contact between the lead and the fibrosed, perforated and retracted tricuspid valve leaflet

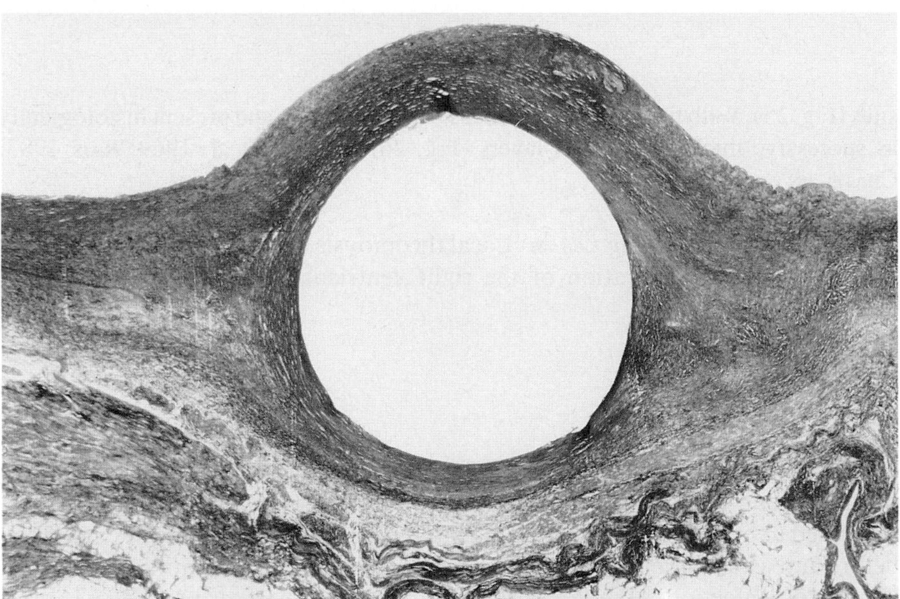

Fig. 26. Concentric rings of fibrous tissue rich in elastic fibres around the lead channel, merging with the thickened, fibrosed endocardium. Note marked thinning of the atrial wall. van Gieson-elastin, ×6.3

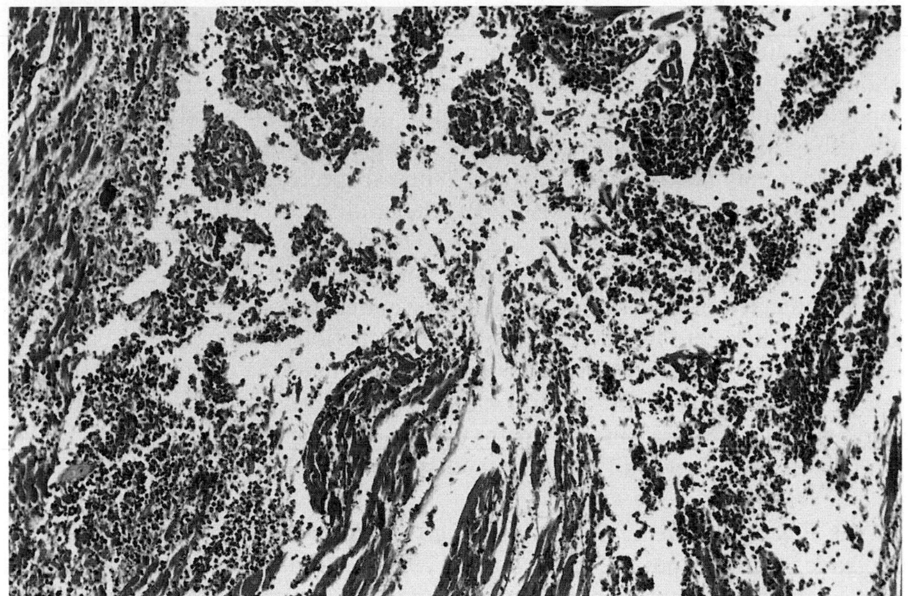

Fig. 27. Myocardial abscess, 3 days after implantation of epicardial screw-on electrode. H & E, × 25

endomyocardium at the multiple sites, including the tricuspid valve leaflets (sometimes with stenosis), and may even be disseminated along the lead. However, not all infections have their origin in the pacemaker system: some are of remote origin.

Infections may occur early or late and are often observed in patients (a) carrying multiple leads or retained sectioned leads, (b) at high risk or with intercurrent diseases including diabetes mellitus and malignancy. (c) under steroid, immunotherapy or anticoagulation therapy, (d) with postoperative haematoma or (e) subject to frequent pulse generator replacements or other manoeuvres. Clinical signs and symptoms may be absent and blood cultures may be unrevealing.

The organisms encountered are mostly those described with pulse generator infections. Mycotic infections (*Candida, Aspergillus* species, *Petriellidium boydii)* are extremely rare and may originate from distant sources. There may be widespread infection with generalised dissemination. These infections usually present with a very large thrombus filling and sometimes obliterating the right ventricular cavity and in some cases also the right atrial cavity. The wall of the ventricle and tricuspid valve may also be involved. Repeated pulmonary embolism is not uncommon and infarction or even death may result. Histologically, the organisms may go unrecognised if deep sections are not examined and the appropriate stains and cultures performed.

5.6.4.2 Septicaemia. Septicaemia occurs in about 1% of infections and carries a high mortality. It is often the consequence of infection at the implantation site; it is sometimes associated with endocarditis or an infected retained pacemaker lead. Septic pulmonary embolism is thus not infrequent. The clinical symptoms are often suggestive (chills, fever, rigors, a toxic confusional state with acute renal failure) but may be missing altogether. When suspected, blood culture at post-mortem is mandatory (BEELER 1982; BLUHM et al. 1984, 1986; MOORMAN et al. 1984; KRAMER et al. 1985; LEWIS et al. 1985; HONG-BARCO et al. 1988; COHEN et al. 1991; AMIN et al. 1991; ENIA et al. 1991; PARRY et al. 1991; MYERS et al. 1991).

The infected chronically implanted transvenous lead carries with it a very high mortality when left in place; thus, total extraction of the lead is strongly recommended. Due to the dense fibrous tissue around the electrode extraction can be extremely difficult. Several methods have been introduced, including cardiovascular bypass surgery, with variable results (MADIGAN et al. 1984; BYRD et al. 1991; STIRBYS 1991; GARCIA-JIMENEZ et al. 1992).

5.6.4.3 Epicardial Pacing Leads. Although infection of the epicardial screw-on electrode is rarely reported, it may occur. The infection, as with the transvenous leads, usually originates in the infected pacemaker pocket and reaches the implantation site by contiguous spread along the lead in the subcutaneous tissue, where abscess formation may occur (Fig. 27). Purulent pericarditis may be an associated feature. Treatment includes total extraction of the system, which may require major surgery to retrieve the pacing electrode (CHOO et al. 1981; BEELER 1982; CHATELAIN et al. 1985; AMIN et al. 1991).

5.7 Venous Lesions

5.7.1 Venous Thrombosis

Thrombosis of the catheterised veins (neck and/or lower extremities) and their recipient branches, as a consequence of transvenous pacing, is a very common phenomenon which may occur shortly after implantation or months or years there after. Its true incidence is not known since most patients remain asymptomatic; however, it remains a relatively common finding using the various new radiological techniques (venography, two-dimensional echocardiography, Doppler ultrasonography, CT scan, scintigraphy) now available, and a frequent accidental finding at post-mortem. Partial obstruction or complete occlusion has been reported in about 28% of patients with transvenous leads, sometimes associated with thickening and fibrosis of the venous wall and stenosis of the lumen. Prominent venous congestion of the tributaries and collaterals may follow. Thrombosis of the vessels is more prevalent at the ligation points of the veins at the time of entry and at the sites of free-lying ends of cut pacing leads which might be floating freely, and may occur where there are flipping or looped leads in the lumen and when several retained leads are left in the circulation. Thrombosis in the right atrium has also been documented in the absence of infection; in one case the patient was suffering from polycythaemia rubra vera. No cases have been described in patients with coagulation deficiency abnormalities (protein C, antithrombin III) but one case has occurred with a non-specific low-grade intravascular coagulation.

5.7.2 Caval Syndromes

The superior vena cava syndrome may occur with thrombosis of the jugular, axillary, subclavian and other veins of the region. There is marked distension of the many collateral systems with or without oedema. More than 30 cases of this condition have been described in the literature and many of these have been associated with fibrotic obliteration and stenosis of the vessels involved. Multiple leads, long leads with loops, retained leads and cut or broken leads are often associated findings.

The inferior vena cava syndrome has been described in association with looping of a pacing lead into the inferior vena cava with associated thrombosis of the vessel and the left renal vein. Combined superior and inferior vena cava syndrome has also been documented. Refractory congestive heart failure and cerebral oedema and haemorrhagic infarction of the brain have all been described (Lee and Chaux 1980; Pauletti et al. 1981; Schuster et al. 1982; Christopoulou-Cokkinou et al. 1982; Nanda and Barold 1982; Toumbouras et. al. 1982; Flaker et al. 1983; Yakirevich et al. 1983; Fritz et al. 1983; Antonelli et al. 1989; Goudevenos et al. 1989; Hendler et al. 1991; Sunder et al. 1992).

5.7.3 Pulmonary Thromboembolism

Pulmonary embolism in endovenous pacemaker carriers is known to occur but its incidence is not known. Estimates put it at about 30%. The condition is often misdiagnosed clinically although it is a relatively frequent finding at post-mortem. Recurrent pulmonary emboli in these patients may occur without symptoms. Some may lead to lung infarction, especially when massive. Thrombosis of the venous systems described above or infection of the pacemaker lead or both may be responsible for pulmonary thromboembolism (sometimes septic) and must be carefully and systematically looked for at post-mortem. It may not be easy to ascertain the origin of the embolus, as there may be other predisposing factors in these patients, such as cardiac fibrillation or the sick sinus syndrome, which might be responsible for the event. Pulmonary embolism is also known to be caused by the migration of a retained lead, resulting in sudden death (Kinney et al. 1979; Drizin et al. 1982; Davis et al. 1983; Pasquariello et al. 1984; Seeger and Scherer 1986; Langenfeld et al. 1988).

6 Cardiac Pacing in Infants and Children

Permanent pacemaker implantation in the paediatric age group is becoming more widespread due to the rapid advances in all areas of pacing technology and because of a better knowledge and understanding of the conditions in which the technique is applicable. The indications include congenital complete atrioventricular block (symptomatic or asymptomatic) or atrioventricular block related to neonatal systemic lupus erythematosus (SLE) (sometimes diagnosed in utero) in infants delivered by mothers with SLE or presenting with anti-Ro antibodies. Sudden death is not uncommon in this group. Congenital QT syndrome (torsades de pointes), sinus node dysfunctions (bradycardia–tachycardia) often related to complications of operative procedures for complex congenital cardiac defects and certain forms of hereditary neuromuscular disorders with cardiac involvement and rhythmic disturbances may also require pacing.

Detailed electrophysiological studies are necessary in most of these patients in order to localise the level of the conduction disturbances precisely (above, within or below the His bundle) so as to determine the exact mode (atrial, ventricular) of pacing required for the particular patient.

Because of the small size of the venous system in infancy, the epicardial mode of pacing has been accepted by most centres as the method of choice, especially among those patients below 4 years old or weighing less than 15 kg. The screw-on electrodes, as in the adult, always produce excessive fibrous tissue around the implantation site leading to high chronic stimulation thresholds, a major complication in these patients, with a high percentage (60%) of exit blocks and early battery exertion. Surprisingly, when the electrode is implanted in the right ventricle, the stimulation threshold is higher than if it were implanted into the left ventricle, this being the reason why many centres use the latter as the preferred implantation site. New electrode designs ("stab-in" or "fish-hook") have resulted in the lowering of the stimulation threshold, but the levels remain higher than in patients in this age group who have received transvenous pacing electrodes.

Transvenous endocardial pacing has been used in some institutions, but with the introduction of the smaller polyurethane leads together with the modifications in size and design of the electrodes, fitted with passive and active fixation devices, this mode of pacing has gained popularity and is rapidly replacing the epicardial mode in most centres. Furthermore, access to the venous system now poses little or no problem even in infancy, although, with time, retrieval of the lead could be hazardous. With this mode of pacing, chronic stimulation thresholds are much lower and the percentage of exit blocks is markedly reduced.

The markedly reduced size and weight, the high performance and the longevity of the modern pulse generators, have all contributed to a decrease in or elimination of many of the complications which were observed with the older pulse generators in childhood. The latter were often implanted directly under thin skin or in the abdominal wall. Twiddler's syndrome, pulse generator migration (to the dome of bladder), myopotential inhibition, wound dehiscence, skin erosions, pocket infections (sometimes associated with septicaemia) and adapter problems are among the complications described in association with the pulse generators in the paediatric age group, but they appear to be less common with the new generation of pulse generators.

Most complications encountered with cardiac pacemakers in infancy and childhood are similar to those observed with adult pacemaker carriers, but appear to occur at a higher rate clinically. Pericardial adhesion is a common finding with the epicardial electrode due to surgery. Pericarditis and infection with septicaemia have also been documented with this mode of pacing, as well as stimulation of the recurrent nerve and cardiac strangulation in relation to growth of the patient. The new steroid-eluting epicardial electrode will surely play an important role in reducing the percentage of exit blocks, at the same time lengthening pacemaker battery life significantly. Dislodgements and lead fractures have been documented with both types of leads. Thrombosis of the endocardial lead appears to be uncommon; only one case has been described in the literature, in which a large thrombus filled the right ventricle. Infections do occur but are rare and occasionally are accompanied by sepsis.

Two important problems are of concern to physicians dealing with cardiac pacemakers in the paediatric age group: growth and cosmetic factors. Recently, it has been calculated that an 80-mm loop of endocardial lead in the right atrium will allow 6–12 years of growth in infants and children without the need for reoperation, and some authors have adopted subpectoral implantation of the new-generation pulse generators for cosmetic purposes, especially in girls, with promising results. Myopotential inhibitions were not observed with the use of bipolar pulse generators (Young 1981; Simon et al. 1982; De Leon et al. 1984; Michalik et al. 1984; Bricker et al. 1985; Goldman et al. 1985; Bharati et al. 1987; McGrath et al. 1988; Gillette et al. 1988; 1991a,b; Walsh et al. 1988; Kugler and Danford 1989; Till et al. 1990; Perry et al. 1991; Gheissari et al. 1991; Hamilton et al. 1991).

7 Cardiac Pacing in Cardiac Surgery

Temporary pacemakers may be used during open heart surgery to prevent arrhythmias or to provide support for cardiac output in the postoperative period. The stimulation threshold may be very high due to myocardial damage resulting in exit block. Lead fracture may also occur. Permanent cardiac pacing may be necessary to treat conduction disturbances after surgical damage to the conduction system. Most cases are observed after surgery on a thickened, remodelled and calcified aortic valve and its annulus. Pacing is also often necessary after surgery on the tricuspid valve. Exit block with eventual loss of pacing is the main complication, especially when scar tissue is established (Ohm and Skagseth 1980; Goldman et al. 1984; Gaillard et al. 1988).

The orthotopic transplanted heart is anatomically and functionally denervated with a high incidence of arrhythmias and sinus node dysfunctions which may require temporary or permanent pacing. Atrial pacing of the new heart is the treatment of choice and the exact position of the electrode is essential for success (Bexton et al. 1986; Markewitz et al. 1987, 1988b; Marti et al. 1991; Kacet et al. 1991; Breedveld et al. 1992; Heinz et al. 1992).

8 Suicide Among Pacemaker Carriers

Permanent pacemaker carriers may attempt suicide by manipulation of the pulse generator (Twiddler's syndrome). This is difficult or impossible to prove. External examination of the body may reveal self-inflicted wounds over the site of the pulse generator or along the lead, which may be sectioned in places. The pulse generator was found to be missing in one such case (Simon et al. 1980; Rosenthal et al. 1980; Harthorne 1980).

9 The Automatic Implantable Cardioverter Defibrillator

The use of the automatic implantable cardioverter defibrillator (AICD) is rapidly expanding as a modality for the treatment of life-threatening medically refractory ventricular tachyarrhythmias. During the early part of the century and especially during the 1960s and 1970s numerous animal experiments and technical designs made it possible to produce and operate the implantable Cardioverter defibrillator efficiently. This device was first implanted clinically in 1980 in patients with ventricular tachycardia and those with ventricular fibrillation were soon included.

The original system (first generation) was composed of a pulse generator (292 g/162 cc) connected to two pairs of electrodes: a transvenous pair (anode) was placed with one in the superior vena cava and the other in the right ventricular apex, while the second pair (cathode) was present in the form of a cup covering the epicardial surface of the apex. The cup was soon replaced by a rectangular titanium patch. The system was designed to monitor cardiac rhythm continuously, to identify ventricular fibrillation and to deliver corrective defibrillatory discharges to restore normal contraction.

Further modifications in the lead system were soon introduced (second generation) which led to encouraging results. It soon became apparent that many other clinical entities could be adequately treated with the device. Programmability was introduced into the system (third generation), making it possible to extend its utilisation. Newer devices (fourth generation) made it possible to include bradycardia pacing, antitachycardia pacing and even information storage among other features. These added possibilities and better electrophysiological evaluations have helped to open the way to new applications in a large number of clinicopathological conditions, including dilated and hypertrophic cardiomyopathies, idiopathic "primary" electrical disturbances and cardiac surgery (valvular prostheses, coronary bypass, cardiac transplants), all of which may present with life-threatening tachyarrhythmias (MIROWSKI et al. 1982, 1984b; ZIPES et al. 1984; MOWER et al. 1984; CANNOM and WINKLE 1986; GREVE et al. 1988; NISAM et al. 1988, 1991; MOWER and NISAM 1988; IDEKER et al. 1991; AHERN et al. 1991; EDEL et al. 1991; FAZIO et al. 1991; HAUSER and HEILMAN 1991; HEILMAN 1991; HOROWITZ 1992).

9.1 Surgical Implantation Technique

The mode of implantation varies with the type of device and the circumstances of implantation. Anterior thoracotomy was the first approach employed in human implants but is now largely employed in those patients who have had previous cardiac surgery. Median sternotomy is used in association with open heart surgery. The subcostal and subxiphoid approaches are rapid and less traumatic than the above approaches. By the subcostal route the entire system is implanted on the epicardial surface with the double patch defibrillatory system fixed over the left ventricle. The subxiphoid approach is ideal for isolated implantation with the percutaneous transvenous ventricular lead implanted in the right ventricular apex, while the two defibrillating patch electrodes are implanted over the ventricles. Sometimes the transvenous lead may be replaced by two screw-on epicardial electrodes fixed into the right ventricle free wall (FURMAN et al. 1984; WATKINS et al. 1984; BRODMAN et al. 1984; WATKINS and TAYLOR 1991).

New pulse generators are smaller and lighter (200 g) but despite this improvement, use in infants and children is still limited. The pulse generator is generally inserted in the abdominal wall, either subcutaneously, between the rectus muscle, or on the fascia. Attempts have been made to place it in the pectoral region, but this has resulted in discomfort (MOWER et al. 1984; TAKEUCHI et al. 1988; FRANK and LOWES 1992).

9.2 Pathology

Clinically, a number of potentially fatal complications have been recorded after implantation of the AICD. Two are of particular importance: (a) Spurious discharges with rapid supraventricular arrhythmias. These may exceed the device rate threshold and lead to undesirable shock and component failure. (b) Atrial acceleration may occur where the tachycardia is not terminated but is accelerated to a much faster rhythm, disorganised and polymorphic. This may even evolve into ventricular fibrillation and eventually to hypotension and shock.

9.2.1 Problems Related to Surgery

Massive subcutaneous bleeding during or after implantation may warrant numerous transfusions to keep the patient alive. Pericardial effusions after epicardial patch fixation are not uncommon (pericardial rub) and can lead to pericardial adhesion and eventually to restrictive pericarditis. Pleural effusions have also been documented. The transvenous leads present lesions similar to those presented by endovenous pacemaker leads.

9.2.2 *Problems Related to the Pulse Generator*

Fluid accumulation (seroma) in the pocket is a relatively frequent finding and often appears shortly after implantation. The collection is usually sterile, but must be checked for micro-organisms, including fungus. Pocket haematoma is a frequent finding and a source of pocket infection. Due to the size and weight of the pulse generator, erosions and abrasions occur more frequently than with the pacemaker generators. Battery failure (average life 18 months) is not an uncommon feature and is often associated with elevated defibrillation thresholds. This inconvenience calls for frequent pulse generator changes which increase the risk of pocket infection. Explantations and migration into the peritoneal cavity have been described, as well as Twiddler's syndrome and even turning of the pulse generator on its axis, leading to false magnetic signals.

9.2.3 *Lead-Related Problems*

Lead-related problems are similar to those described with transvenous pacemaker leads and include dislodgements, fractures, migration, erosions, insulation breaks and electrode/patch dislocation. Thick, dense fibrous tissue may surround the endocardial electrode tip.

9.2.4 *Patch-Related Problems*

Twisting of the patch can lead to malfunction of the device with a fatal outcome. Silastic erosions are infrequent findings, as is migration of the patch into the right ventricle. Elevated defibrillation thresholds could be the result of titanium fraying of the patch mesh. Coronary lacerations have also been described.

9.2.5 *Infection*

Infection remains one of the most serious problems of the device, with an incidence of 1%–7%. It may occur early or late as intraoperative contamination at implantation, at the time of pulse generator replacement or by haematogenous spread from a remote site. Pocket infection remains the main source and especially so after repeated pulse generator replacements, the quantity of pocket fibrous tissue apparently enhancing the infection rate. The entire system (leads and patches) may be involved, as often demonstrated by gallium scans. Patch infection is a serious problem and can lead to pericarditis and secondary pulmonary infection. Transvenous lead infections and sepsis present like those of endocardial pacemaker leads, though with a somewhat lower incidence.

9.2.6 Thrombosis

Thrombosis is related entirely to the transvenous leads, like the endovenous pacemaker leads, and involves not only the implantation site but the entire lead focally, at multiple zones or throughout its course. Total or partial venous thrombosis, including the superior vena cava, may occur and may give rise to pulmonary embolism.

9.2.7 Others

Cerebrovascular accidents as well as acute myocardial infarctions have been reported in the immediate postoperative period. One case of suicide, by a gunshot wound, has been reported, and as many AICD patients do have serious psychological problems, evidence of suicidal attempts must be excluded at post-mortem.

The problems outlined within Sect. 9.2 have been widely discussed within the literature (Zipes et al. 1984; Veltri et al. 1984; Mirowski et al. 1984b; Perkins et al. 1987; Singer et al. 1987; Kelly et al. 1988; Luceri et al. 1988; McDaniel et al. 1988; Thomas et al. 1988; Mercando et al. 1988; Gering et al. 1989; Ruder et al. 1990; Taylor et al. 1990; Siclari et al. 1990; Wunderly et al. 1990; Keren et al. 1991; Mittleman et al. 1991; Singer et al. 1991; Underhill et al. 1991; Meesmann 1992; Bakker et al. 1992).

9.3 Recent Developments

The implantable devices are rapidly changing as new technologies and refinements are introduced into the various components so as to improve their performance and eliminate complications. Several new designs of transvenous lead systems (non-thoracotomy approach) have been implanted with encouraging results. The lead is inserted by the subclavian route, with the entire system implanted in the heart but in some instances a thoracic patch is also associated. Thrombosis remains the main pathological lesion encountered with these new devices. New electrode systems have also been introduced in order to decrease the amount of fibrous tissue around the electrodes (Singer et al. 1987; Perkins et al. 1987; Alt et al. 1991; Moore et al. 1991; Block et al. 1992; Hauser et al. 1992; Hammel et al. 1992; Epstein et al. 1992).

10 Non-pharmacological Therapy for Ventricular Arrhythmias

Although pharmacological therapy is used in most centres as the treatment of choice for ventricular arrhythmias, other treatment modalities are rapidly replacing it in many specific clinicopathological conditions. Furthermore, many of the drugs currently employed are either unsuitable for use in pregnancy (possible teratogens) or may have adverse effects including cardiac, extracardiac toxicity or a proarrhythmogenic effect.

Besides the implantable devices discussed above, various surgical approaches have been envisaged to treat intractable ventricular arrhythmias with variable success rates. These can be grouped into the following categories:

1. *Non-specific:* (a) revascularisation, (b) left stellate ganglionectomy
2. *Isolation procedures:* (a) partial or complete endocardial encircling myotomy, (b) right ventricular isolation
3. *Arrhythmogenic tissue resection:* (a) surgical, (b) local catheter ablation

The arrhythmogenic tissue resection techniques are becoming extremely popular as selection of patient populations for a specific mode of therapy can be accomplished with greater accuracy, and the therapy can be directed to a specific arrhythmia at its site of origin. However, some of these procedures may involve a combination of cardiac pacing and resection, or when ablation is incomplete, the implantation of a permanent pacemaker or an AICD may be necessary.

Surgical resections are performed in patients with recurrent ventricular tachycardias, among others, in whom ventricular aneurysmectomy may eliminate the re-entry point. Guided electrophysiological mapping has improved our ability to target the specific area involved. Various techniques have been adapted in the resection or ablation of the zone involved, by electrode catheter delivery, including cryoablation, laser, partial endocardial myotomy and direct current shock.

Chemical ablation by intra-arterial injection of certain substances (antiarrhythmic drugs, iced saline, ethanol, collagen) has also been employed in some centres, especially in life threatening ventricular arrhythmics.

Catheter ablation is perhaps the most promising among the procedures although the first results were not very convincing. The damage to the zone involved is much less than that observed with surgical procedures, and furthermore with new electrophysiological techniques, including activation sequence mapping, it is now possible to identify the specific site of origin of the arrhythmic abnormality and thus to control the size of the lesion. Constant postoperative monitoring by detailed electrophysiological studies during the first several hours or days makes it possible to obtain a good assessment of the immediate results and to determine the efficacy of the procedure and eventually the need for additional supportive therapy.

Several catheter ablation techniques have been tested in various animal models and are now applied in man with variable results, but within recent years there has been significant progress due to the sophistication of the equipment in the various fields and the experience gained by physicians. The most common catheter ablation procedures include: (a) direct current shocks (pacemaker dependent), (b) electrode catheter ablation (closed chest, suction ablation) and (c) surgical catheter ablation by cryoablation (pacemaker dependent), critical positioned incisions, radiofrequency energy, laser and combinations thereof (in Wolff-Parkinson-White syndrome). Radiofrequency and lasers are now the methods of choice.

10.1 Pathological Aspects

Various complications and pathological lesions may be encountered with the above-mentioned procedures especially with direct current shocks. Sudden death shortly after the procedure is not uncommon and may even occur months later. Clinically new ventricular arrhythmias may appear. Pericardial effusion, cardiac tamponade, myocardial perforation and acute myocardial infarction may occur in the immediate postoperative period or days later. Cerebral haemorrhage, often associated with severe hypotension or acute pulmonary oedema, may also be observed in this period. Damage to the tricuspid valve or rupture of the aortic valve cuspids (with or without insufficiency) has also been documented, as have sepsis, subclavian thrombosis, pulmonary embolism, right atrial thrombosis, arterial

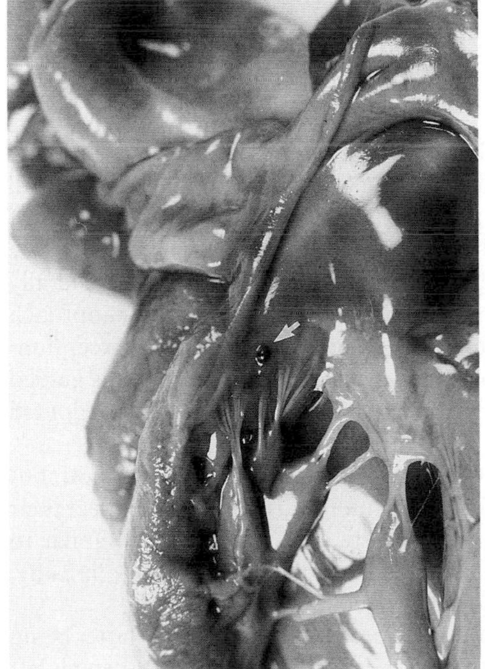

Fig. 28. Right atrial endocardial haemorrhage (*arrow*) near the insertion of the tricuspid valve

perforation and thrombosis. Patients with permanent pacemakers or AICDs may present lesions which are associated with those devices. Pathological examination is inconclusive unless a careful and detailed examination of the conduction system, the ablation site and adjacent areas is included.

Presently, there is active competition between the various pharmacological agents, the non-pharmacological procedures and the implantable devices as therapeutic approaches for patients with ventricular arrhythmias; however, the implantable devices may be more appropriate in many clinical settings, especially among those awaiting cardiac transplantation (Saksena and Gadhoke 1986; Marchlinski et al. 1987; Evans et al. 1988; Saksena 1988; Saksena et al. 1988; Curtis et al. 1989; DiMarco 1990; Singer and Kupersmith 1990a,b; Chin et al. 1991; Gillette et al. 1991c; Gindici et al. 1991; Huang 1991; Seifert et al. 1991; Sneddon et al. 1991; Breithardt et al. 1992; Gursoy et al. 1992; Scheinman et al. 1992; Trappe et al. 1992; Wang et al. 1992; Wietholt et al. 1992).

11 Pathology Related to Central Venous Catheters

Central venous catheters are widely used in the treatment of critically ill patients. They are considered to be an effective means of monitoring central venous pressure and of administering intravenous fluids, drugs and long-term parenteral nutrition.

11.1 Swan-Ganz Catheter

11.1.1 General Complications

The balloon-tipped flow-directed pulmonary indwelling catheter (Swan-Ganz catheter) is widely used for continuous haemodynamic monitoring of critically ill patients in various clinical settings and in the management of a variety of complicated medical and surgical conditions. It is used extensively in intensive care units, coronary care units, and during cardiac surgery. The catheter is generally inserted in the right subclavian vein by the percutaneous infraclavicular approach and in some instances by way of the cephalic or external jugular veins. Exceptionally, the left internal jugular vein is used. Under continuous pressure it is guided through the superior vena cava, right atrium and right ventricle and then floated into the pulmonary artery.

Complications with the Swan-Ganz catheter are not uncommon but their true incidence is unknown since there are many variables which affect their frequencies. Those which occur during or shortly after insertion are similar to those observed with endovenous pacemaker lead insertion (see p. 220). Clinically, minor atrial and ventricular contractions may occur during insertion.

Balloon rupture and/or perforations have been documented, the latter being associated with frequent reuse of the catheter or occurring when the catheter is left in place for long periods. Knotting, looping or curling of the catheter, a rare condition, is often associated with pulmonary hypertension, right ventricular dilatation and biventricular failure with low cardiac output. During insertion rupture or perforation of the pulmonary artery may lead to massive pulmonary haemorrhage with haemoptysis and even death, while a pseudo-aneurysm of the vessel wall may be the consequence of incomplete perforation.

Detailed post-mortem examination of Swan-Ganz catheter carriers have demonstrated many cardiac lesions related both to the catheter and to the length of time it has been in place. Many of the findings may have no clinical manifestations and thus may go unnoticed.

11.1.2 Endocardial Lesions

Endocardial lesions appear as superficial haemorrhages in the endocardium of both the right atrium and the right ventricle. They are more common in the atrium, although both cavities may be involved simultaneously. The lesions may be small or present as ecchymoses. They represent tears or ulcerations of the endothelial layer and are observed within hours or days after catheter insertion (Fig. 28). With time they are covered by fibrin. Although some attribute these lesions to haemodynamic disturbance, many associate them with local trauma, or with a combination of the two events.

11.1.3 Valvular lesions

Pulmonary valve petechial haemorrhages are not uncommon. They accompany abrasions due to trauma on the ventricular aspect of the valve along the line of closure and may involve one or more cusps. Fibrin deposits with thrombus formation and vegetations may occur with time. Single or multiple perforations have been described affecting one or more cusps below their free margins in patients who have been catheterised for long periods.

Tricuspid valve haemorrhages, mainly from the septal and anterior leaflets, are less prevalent, and are observed principally on the atrial aspect of the valve. Tears or ruptures of the leaflets, often associated with thrombi or vegetations, are relatively frequent findings. Rupture of the chordae tendineae has also been described.

11.1.4 Thrombosis

Thrombosis is a common feature with Swan-Ganz catheters. It begins as fine fibrinous deposits (fibrin and platelets) along the catheter within hours of insertion. These deposits may become adherent to the endocardial surface, especially in eroded areas, and fix the catheter to the surface in a continuous line or at multiple points. Thrombosis of the vein of insertion (subclavian, cephalic, jugular) is relatively frequent and is often accompanied by thrombosis of the superior vena cava with extension into the right atrium. The catheter is generally ensheathed by the thrombus; it may be fixed to the vessel wall and may undergo organisation. Like those on the pulmonary and tricuspid valves, these thrombi are variable in size and may be the source of isolated or repeated pulmonary embolism with pulmonary haemorrhage, infarction and death. Thrombus formation may take place around the tip of the catheter and/or within its lumen. These thrombi also may be a source of pulmonary embolism. When the thrombus is infected, septic pulmonary thromboembolitis ensues.

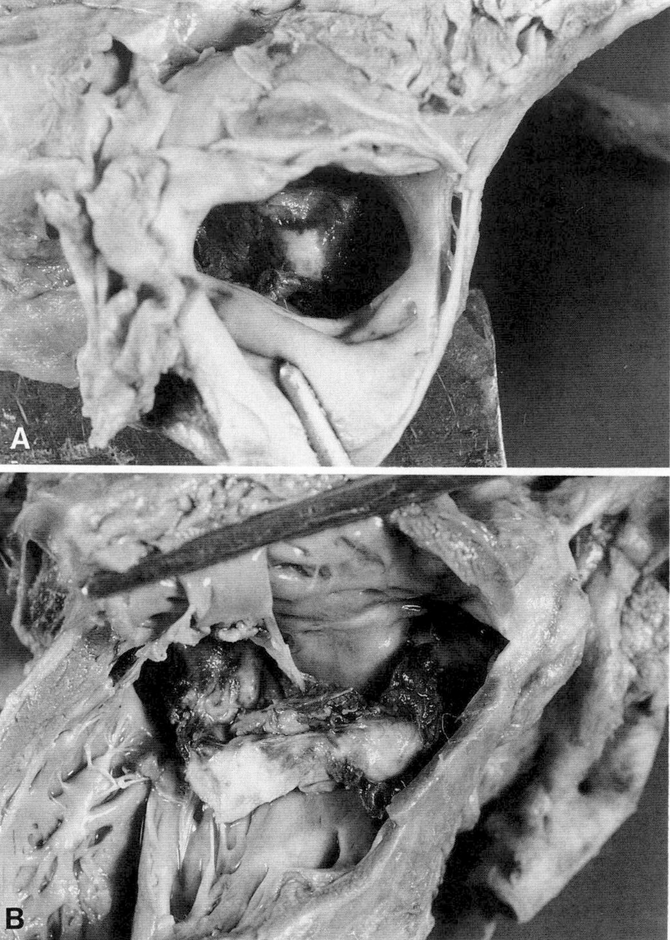

Fig. 29. a Right atrial and auricular thrombosis with partial obliteration of the superior vena cava after implantation of a central venous catheter in an infant. **b** Extension of the thrombus through the tricuspid orifice and into the right outflow track.

Pulmonary infarction may also result from vascular occlusion by migration of the catheter into a distal pulmonary artery, from unintentional catheter wedging, or secondary to entrapped air in a deflated balloon.

11.1.5 Infections

Although the incidence of infections with indwelling catheters is considered low, infections still remain a serious clinical problem. The Swan-Ganz catheter carries a higher incidence than is observed with other types of intracardiac catheter and this appears to be related to the duration of catheter insertion. Endocardial and valvular damage by the catheter with subsequent thrombus formation (bland thrombus) at those sites serves as the nidus for bacterial growth and the development of infective endocarditis. In this setting, endocarditis of the pulmonary valve is more frequent than that of the tricuspid valve. The pathogens are mostly commensals from the surrounding skin near the point of catheter insertion and occasionally from some remote site. The organisms most often cultured (from the catheter tip or haemocultures or both) include *Staphylococcus aureus, Staphylococcus epidermidis, Proteus species, Pseudomonas aeruginosa, Bacillus subtilis, Streptococcus viridans, Escherichia coli, Klebsiella* species and *Streptococcus faecalis*. Combinations have been recorded, as well as mycotic infections. Predisposing factors (age, host defence, underlying diseases, sepsis) may accelerate the process and lead to septicaemia. At post-mortem it is therefore imperative to obtain sterile blood from the heart for aerobic and anaerobic cultures, and when available, the catheter tip. All apparent pathological lesions including thrombus and vegetations should be controlled histologically for microorganisms, including fungus.

Sternoclavicular osteomyelitis has been described in association with subclavian catheterisation with the Swan-Ganz catheter (Swan et al. 1970; Foote et al. 1974; Elliott et al. 1979; Boscoe and DeLange 1981; Hunter et al. 1983; Lange et al. 1983; Rowley et al. 1984; Kaye and Smith 1988; Feng et al. 1990; Norwood et al. 1991).

11.2 Other Central Venous Catheters

Central venous catheters (single, double or triple lumen) other than the Swan-Ganz catheter are widely used in treating seriously ill patients. They are generally employed to measure right atrial pressure while monitoring treatment and to provide fluids, drugs and parenteral nutrition to those patients. Implantation is usually by one of the routes employed with the Swan-Ganz or intravenous pacemaker lead. Inadvertently, misplacement of the catheter may occur, especially when an internal jugular vein is catheterised, and this can lead to serious complications (Fig. 29). Perforation of the right atrium or right ventricle has also been described. Other pathological lesions observed with these catheters are similar to those seen with the Swan-Ganz catheter, but generally occur with a lower incidence. However, thrombosis and infections are much more common among those patients receiving hyperalimentation (Bernard and Stahl 1969; Bernard et al. 1971; Ford and Manley 1982; Van Haeften et al. 1988; Kaye and Smith 1988; Norwood et al. 1991).

Glossary

The intention is not to give an exhaustive list of the terms in the complex language of pacemakers and allied devices, but briefly to define some of the common terms frequently encountered or associated with those in the text. For a more comprehensive understanding of pacemaker language and coding systems the reader should refer to the list of references at the end of the glossary.

Asynchronous pacemaker: One which emits pulses at a fixed interval (fixed rate) and is not influenced by the spontaneous heart activity.

Bipolar lead configuration: Both electrodes (cathode and anode) are in contact with the heart.

Cross-talk: An alteration in pacemaker timing induced by the sensing in one chamber of a signal originating in the opposite cardiac chamber (also self-inhibition).

Delayed triggered: The cardiac signal triggers the pacemaker but the pulse is only released after a certain delay.

Dual (double chamber) pacing system: The sequential stimulation of the atrium and ventricle during slow atrial rates, and P wave synchronous ventricular pacing.

Electrostimulation: The alteration of the electrical potential across the cell membrane (myocardial fibre) by an electrical field to obtain a critical level resulting in cellular activity. In the heart a small local stimulus is sufficient to excite the entire organ.

Exit block: Failure to capture due to threshold elevation

Inhibitory pacing mode: The cardiac signal causes the pacemaker to reset its timing circuit and a new interval of surveillance begins.

Pacemaker pulse: An electrical signal of short duration when compared to its repetition time.

Pacing: Method for sustaining tolerable cardiac rhythmicity (by speeding it up or slowing it down).

Permanent cardiac pacing: Long-term pacing implantation as therapy for a defined condition, e.g. conduction disturbances.

Pulse amplitude: The height of the pacemaker pulse.

Pulse duration: The time interval between the first and last instants of the pulse at which the instantaneous amplitude reaches a stated fraction of the peak amplitude.

Pulse period: The time interval between selected identical points of consecutive pulses.

Refractory period: The pulse generator is designed to be *non-sensing* in order to prevent recycling of the generator by its own output or by the heart's response.

Sensing function: The ability to detect the cardiac activity and therefore to quicken or slow the heart's rate (pacing on demand). Many methods of determining cardiac activity are in use or under investigation (blood pH, venous blood temperature, stroke volume, O_2 saturation, respiration biosensor etc.).

Synchronous pacemaker: One which is not tied to a fixed rate and therefore co-ordinates its function with that of the heart (non-competitive) by the sensor electrode.

Temporary cardiac pacing: Usually pacing for a limited period, often in an acute situation, e.g. acute severe myocardial infarction, during or after cardiac surgery.

Threshold: The minimum quantity of electrical energy capable of producing a cellular (myocardial) response (current, voltage, energy thresholds); it is influenced by many factors.

Triggered: The cardiac signal causes an *immediate release* of an impulse which falls into the absolute refractory period.

Unipolar lead configuration: Only one electrode (cathode) is placed in the heart; the other (anode) is remote from the heart and is represented by the large surface plate of the pulse generator or its entire metal case.

References: BAROLD et al. 1980; BERNSTEIN et al. 1984, 1987; BREDIKIS and STIRBYS 1985; DALY 1980; IRNICH et al. 1979a,b, 1980; IRNICH 1980, 1984b; MOND 1991

References

Abrahamsen AM, Aarsland T (1981) Temperature dependent pulse generator dysfunction. PACE 4:523–524

Adamec R, Haefliger JM, Killisch JP, Niederer J, Jaquet P (1982) Damaging effect of therapeutic radiation on programmable pacemakers. PACE 5: 146–150

Ahern TS, Nydegger C, McCormick DJ, et al. (1991) Device interaction-antitachycardia pacemakers and defibrillators for sustained ventricular tachycardia. PACE 14 (II): 302–307

Alboni P, Paparella N, Cappato R, Pedroni P, Candini GC, Antonioli GE (1989) Reliability of transesophageal pacing in the assessment of sinus node function in patients with sick sinus syndrome. PACE 12: 294–300

Alt E, Volker R, Blomer H (1987) Lead fracture in pacemaker patients. J Thorac Cardiovasc Surg 85: 101–104

Alt E, Theres H, Heinz M, Albrecht K, Georg H, Bloemer H (1991) A new approach towards defibrillation electrodes: highly conductive isotropic carbon fibers. Pace 14 (II): 1923–1928

Amin M, Gross J, Andrews C, Furman S (1991) Pacemaker infection with Myobacterium avium complex. Pace 14 (I): 152–154

Amundson DC, McArthur W, Mosharrafa M (1979) The porous endocardial electrode. Pace 2: 40–50

Anderson MH, Nathan AW (1990) Ventricular pacing from the atrial channel of a DDD pacemaker: a consequence of pacemaker twiddling? Pace 13 (I): 1567–1570

Antonelli D, Turgeman Y, Kaveh Z, Artoul S, Rosenfeld T (1989) Short-term thrombosis after transvenous permanent pacemaker insertion. Pace 12: 280–282

Arakawa M, Kambara K, ITO H, Hirakawa S, Umeda S, Hirose H (1989) Intermittent oversensing due to internal insulation damage of temperature sensing rate responsive pacemaker lead in subclavian venipuncture method. Pace 12: 1312–1316

Bakker PFA, Hauer RNW, Wever EFD (1992) Infections involving implanted cardioverter defibrillator devices. Pace 15 (III): 654–658

Barin ES, Jones SM, Ward DE, Camm AJ, Nathan AW (1991) The right ventricular outflow tract as an alternative permanent pacing site. Longterm follow-up. Pace 14: 3–6

Barold SS, Banner R (1978) Unusual electrocardiographic pattern during transvenous pacing from the middle cardiac vein Pace 1: 31–34

Barold SS, Roehrich DR, Falkoff MD, Ong LS, Heinle RA (1980) Sources of error in the determination of output voltage of pulse generators by pacemaker system analyzers. Pace 3: 585–596

Barold SS, Falkoff MD, Ong LS, Heinle RA, Willis JE (1988) Resetting of DDD pulse generators due to cold exposure. Pace 11 (I): 736–743

Bashore TM, Barks JM, Wagner GS (1982) The epicardial screw-on electrode: an analysis of 114 consecutive patients with complete one-year follow-up. Pace 5: 59–66

Bassan MM, Merin G (1977) Pericardial tamponade due to perforation with a permanent endocardial pacing catheter. J Thorac Cardiovasc Surg 74: 51–54

Baumgartner G, Nesser HJ, Jurkovic K (1990) Ususual cause of dysuria: migration of a pacemaker generator into the urinary bladder. Pace 13: 703–704

Beeler BA (1982) Infections of permanent transvenous and epicardial pacemakers in adults. Heart Lung II: 152–156

Berger R, Jacobs W (1979) Myopotential inhibition of demand pacemakers: etiologic diagnostic, and therapeutic considerations. Pace 2: 596–602

Berman ND, Dickson SE, Lipton IH (1982) Acute and chronic clinical performance comparison of a porous and a solid electrode design. Pace 5: 67–71

Bernard RW, Stahl WM (1971) Subclavian vein catheterizations: a prospective study. I. Non-infectious complications. Ann Surg 173: 184–190
Bernard RW, Stahl WM, Chase RM, Jr (1971) Subclavian vein catheterizations: a prospective study. II. Infectious complications. Ann Surg 173: 191–200
Bernstein AD, Brownlee RR, Fletcher R, Gold RD, Smyth NPD, Spielman Sr (1984) Report of the Naspe mode code committee. Pace 7 (I): 395–402
Bernstein AD, Camm AJ, Fletcher RD et al. (1987) The NASPE/BPEG generic pacemaker code for antibradyarrhythmia and adaptive-rate pacing and antitachyarrhythmia devices. Pace 10 (I): 794–799
Bexton RS, Nathan AW, Camm AJ (1986) Ususual sinus mode response curves in two cardiac transplant recipients. Pace 9: 223–230
Beyersdorf F, Kreuzer J, Schmidts L, Satter P (1985) Examination of explanted polyurethane pacemaker leads using the scanning electron microscope. Pace 8: 562–568
Beyersdorf F, Schneider M, Kreuzer J, Falk S, Zegelman M, Satter P (1988) Studies of the tissue reaction induced by transvenous pacemaker electrodes. I. Microscopic examination of the extent of connective tissue around the electrode tip in the human right ventricle. Pace 11 (2): 1753–1759
Bharati S, Swerdlow MA, Vitullo D, Chiemmongkoltip P, Lev M (1987) Neonatal lupus with congenital atrioventricular block and myocarditis. Pace 10: 1058–1070
Bigelow WG, Hopps JA, Callaghan JC (1952) Radiofrequency rewarming in resuscitation from severe hypothermia. Can J Med Sci 30: 185–193
Bigger JT Jr (1991) Future studies with the implantable cardioverter defibrillator Pace 14 (II): 883–889
Bilitch M (1980) Performance of cardiac pacemaker pulse generators. Pace 3: 350–355
Bilitch M, Hauser RG, Goldman BS, Furman S, Parsonnet V (1981) Performance of cardiac pacemaker pulse generator. Pace 4: 607–612
Bilitch M, Hauser RG, Goldman BS, Furman S, Parsonnet V (1985) Performance of cardiac pacemaker pulse generator. Pace 8: 276–282
Bilitch M, Denes P, Goldman BS, et al. (1988) Performance of implantable cardiac rhythm management devices. Pace 11: 371–380
Blamires NG, Myatt J (1982) X-ray effects on pacemaker type circuits. Pace 5: 151–155
Block M, Hammel D, Isbruch F, et al. (1992) Results and realistic expectations with transvenous lead systems. Pace 15 (III): 665–670
Blomstrom-Lundqvist C, Edvardsson N (1987) Transoesophageal versus intracardiac atrial stimulation in assessing electrophysiologic parameters of the sinus and AV nodes and of the atrial myocardium. Pace 10: 1081–1095
Bluhm G, Jacobson B, Julander I, Levander-Lindgren, M, Olin C (1984) Antibiotic prophylaxis in pacemaker surgery – a prospective study. Scand J Thorac Cardiovasc Surg 18: 227–234
Bluhm G, Nordlander R, Ransjo U (1986) Antibiotic prophylaxis in pacemaker surgery: a prospective double blind trial with systemic administration of antibiotic versus placebo at implantation of cardiac pacemakers. Pace 9: 720–726
Bobyn JD, Wilson GJ, Mycyk TR, Klement P, Tait GA, Pillar RM, MacGregor DC (1981) Comparison of a porous-surfaced with a totally porous ventricular endocardial pacing electrode. Pace 4: 405–416
Bognolo D, Stokes K, Wiebush W, Vijayanagar R, Eckstein P, Jeffrey D (1983) Experimental and clinical study of a new permanent myocardial atrial sutureless pacing lead. Pace 6: 113–118
Boscoe MJ, de Lange S (1981) Damage to the tricuspid valve with a Swan-Ganz catheter, Br Med J 283: 346–347
Bourke JP, Howell L, Murray A, et al. (1989) Do electrode and lead design differences for permanent cardiac pacing translate into clinically demonstrable differences? (Comparison of sintered platinum and activated vitreous and porous carbon electrodes). Pace 12: 1419–1425
Bredikis J, Dumcius A, Stirbys P, Muckus K, Veteikis R, Koroliov V, Yarmilko P (1978) Permanent cardiac pacing with electrodes of a new type of fixation in the endocardium. PACE 1: 25–30
Bredikis JJ, Stirbys PP (1985) A suggested code for permanent cardiac pacing leads. Pace 8 (I): 320–321
Breedveld RW, Van Gelder LM, Mitchell AG, Peels CJ, Yacoub M, El Gamal MIH (1992) Optimized haemodynamics by implantation of a dual chamber pacemaker after heterotopic cardiac transplantation. Pace 15: 274–280
Breithardt G, Borggrefe M, Wietholt D, et al. (1992) Role of ventricular tachycardia surgery and catheter ablation as complements or alternatives to the implantable cardioverter defibrillator in the 1990s. Pace 15 (III): 681–689

Breivik K, Ohm O-J (1980) Myopotential inhibition of unipolar QRS-inhibited (VVI) pacemakers, assessed by ambulatory Holter monitoring of the electrocardiogram. Pace 3: 470–478

Brenner JI, Gaines S, Cordier J, Reiner BI, Hanney PJ, Gundry SR (1988) Cardiac strangulation: two dimensional echo recognition of a rare complication of epicardial pacemaker therapy. Am J, Cardiol 61: 654–656

Brewer G, Mathivanar R, Skalsky M, Anderson N (1988) Composite electrode tips containing externally placed drugs releasing collars Pace 11 (2): 1760–1769

Bricker JT, Garson A Jr, Traweek MS, Smith RT, Ward KA, Vargo TA, Gillette PC (1985) The use of exercise testing in children to evaluate abnormalities of pacemaker function not apparent at rest. Pace 8: 656–660

Brodman R, Fisher JD, Furman S, Johnston DR, Kim SG, Matos JA, Waspe LE (1984) Implantation of automatic cardioverter defibrillator via median sternotomy. Pace 7 (II): 1363–1369

Butrous GS, Male JC, Webber RS, Barton DG, Meldrum SJ, Bonnell JA, Camm AJ (1983) The effect of power frequency high intensity electric fields on implanted cardiac pacemakers. Pace 6: 1282–1292

Byrd, CL (1992) Safe introducer technique for pacemaker lead implantation. Pace 15: 262–267

Byrd CL, McArthur W, Stokes K, Sivina M, Yahr WZ, Greenberg J (1983) Implant experience with unipolar polyurethane pacing leads. Pace 6 (I): 868–882

Byrd CL, Schwartz SJ, Gonzales M, et al. (1986) Pacemaker clinic evaluations: key to early identification of surgical problems. Pace 9 (II): 1259–1264

Byrd CL, Schwartz SJ, Hedin N (1991) Intravascular techniques for extraction of permanent pacemaker leads. J Thorac Cardiovasc Surg 101 989–997

Calfee RV (1982) Therapeutic radiation and pacemakers. Pace 5: 160-161

Calfee RV, Saulson SH (1986) A voluntary standard for 3.2 mm unipolar and bipolar pacemaker leads and connectors. Pace 9 (II): 1181–1185

Callaghan JC (1980) Early experiences in the study and development of an artificial electrical pacemaker for standstill of the heart: view from 1949. Pace 3: 618–619

Callaghan JC, Bigelow WC (1951) An electrical artificial pacemaker for standstill of the heart. Ann Surg. 134: 8–17

Cameron J, Mond H, Ciddor G, Harper K, McKie J (1990) Stiffness of the distal tip of bipolar pacing leads. Pace 13 (II): 1915–1920

Cannom, DS, Winkle, RA (1986) Implantation of the automatic implantable cardioverter defibrillator (AICD): practical aspects. Pace 9 (I): 793–809

Chardack WM (1981) Recollections – 1958–1961. Pace 4: 592–596

Chardack WM, Gage AA, Greatbatch W (1960) A transistorized, self-contained, implantable pacemaker for the long-term correction of complete heart block. Surgery 48: 643–654

Chatelain P, Adamec R, Cox JN (1985) Morphological changes in human myocardium during permanent pacing. Virch Arch (Pathol Anat) 407: 43–57

Chin MC, Schuenemeyer T, Finkebeiner WE, Stern RA, Scheinman MM, Langberg JJ (1991) Histopathology of monopolar transcatheter radiofrequency ablation at the mitral valve annulus. Pace 14 (II): 1956: 1956-1960

Choo MH, Holmes DR Jr, Gersh BJ, Maloney JD, Merideth J, Pluth JR, Trusty J (1981a) Permanent pacemaker infections: Characterization and Management. Am J, Cardiol 48: 559-564

Choo MH, Holmes DR Jr, Gersh BJ, Maloney JD, Merideth J, Pluth JR, Trusty J (1981b) Infected epicardial pacemaker system. Partial versus total removal. J Thorac Cardiovasc Surg 82: 794 796

Christie JL, Keelan H Jr (1986) Tricuspid valve perforation by a permanent pacing lead in a patient with cardiac amyloidosis. Case report and brief literature review. Pace 9 (I): 124–126

Christopoulou-Cokkinou V, Kourepi-Logotheti, Kontaxis A, Mallios C, Vorides EM, Cokkinos DV (1982) Evidence of low-grade intravascular coagulation in patients with transvenous pacemakers. Pace 5: 341–344

Chua FS, Leininger BJ, Hanizda FA, Pifarre RF (1973) Bronchopleural cutaneous fistula from infected pacemaker electrodes. Chest 63: 284–286

Chudasama L, Ernest AC, Greif E, Nejat M (1978) Runaway temporary pacemaker: case report of a ``runaway temporary pacemaker" with a rate over 1500/min. Pace 1: 529–530

Clarke B, Jones S, Gray HH, Rowland E (1989) The tricuspid valve: an unusual site of endocardial pacemaker lead fracture. Pace 12 (I): 1077–1079

Cohen TJ, Pons VG, Schwartz J, Griffin JC (1991) *Candida albicans* pacemaker site infection. Pace 14 (I): 146–148

Comer TP, Saxena N, Salzman SH (1981) The case of two-timing pacemaker. Pace 4: 465–466

Cooper D, Wilkoff B, Masterson M, et al. (1988) Effects of extracorporeal shock wave lithotripsy on cardiac pacemakers and its safety in patients with implanted cardiac pacemakers Pace (I): 1607–1616

Copperman YJ, Beiser M, Samuel Y, Laniado S, Shanon E (1982) Recurrent laryngeal nerve paralysis following pacemaker introduction. Pace 5: 535–536
Costeas XF, Schoenfeld MH (1991) Undersensing as a consequence of lead incompatibility: case report and a plea for universality. Pace 14 (I): 1681–1683
Curtis AB, Abela GS, Griffin JC, Hill JA, Normann SJ (1989) Transvascular argon laser ablation of atrioventricular conduction in dogs: feasibility and morphological results. Pace 12: 347–357
Cywinski JK, Hahn AW, Nichols MF, Easley JR (1978) Performance of implanted Biogalvanic pacemakers. Pace 1: 117–125
Daly D (1980) Nondestructive determination of pacemaker sense amplifier passband. Pace 3: 687–694
Das G, Eaton J (1981) Pacemaker malfunction following transthoracic countershock. Pace 4: 487–490
Davis G, Kaplan K, Kwaan HC (1983) Pulmonary emboli from a platelet-rich thrombus attached to a pacemaker electrode. Pace 6 (I): 883–886
De Feyter JP, Majid PA, Hoitsma HFW, Stroes W, Roos JP (1980) Permanent cardiac pacing with sutureless myocardial electrodes: experience in first one hundred patients. Pace 3: 144–149
De Leon SY, Bojar R, Koster NK, Ilbawi MN, Munez, H, Idriss, FS (1984) Recurrent sepsis from retained endocardial electrode in children: successful removal with cardiopulmonary bypass. Pace 7: 166–168
Dimarco JP (1990) Nonpharmacological therapy of ventricular arrhythmias. Pace 13 (II): 1527–1532
Dirix LY, Kersschot IE, Fierens H, Goethals MA, Van Daele G, Claessen G (1988) Implantation of a dual chamber pacemaker in a patient with persistent left superior vena cava. Pace 11: 343–345
Doring J, Flink R (1986) The impact of pending technologies on a universal connector standard. Pace 9 (II): 1186–1190
Dosios T, Gorgogiannis D, Sakorafas G, Karampatsas K (1991) Persistent left superior vena cava: a problem in the transvenous pacing of the heart. Pace 14: 389–390
Drizin GS, Fein AM, Lippmann ML (1982) Clinical pulmonary embolism from migration of a retained transvenous permanent pacemaker electrode. Crit Care Med 10: 788–789
Ector H, Janssens L, Baert L, De Geest H (1989) Extracorporeal shock wave lithotripsy and cardiac arrhythmias. Pace 12: 1910–1917
Edel TB, Maloney JD, Moore S, et al. (1991) Six-year clinical experience with the automatic implantable cardioverter defibrillator. Pace 14 (II): 1850–1854
Edhag O, Lagergren H, Thorén A, Wahlberg I (1978) Influence of output capacitor, electrode and pulse width on power consumption in cardiac pacing. Pace I: 16–24
El Gamal M, Van Gelder B (1979) Preliminary experience with the Helifix electrode for transvenous atrial implantation. Pace 2: 444–454
Ellestad MH, Caso R, Greenberg PS (1980) Permanent pacemaker implantation using the femoral vein: a preliminary report. Pace 3: 418–423
Ellestad MH, French J (1989) Iliac vein approach to permanent pacemaker implantation. Pace 12: 1030–1033
Elliott CG, Zimmerman GA, Clemmer TP (1979) Complications of pulmonary artery catheterization in the case of critically ill patients. A prospective study. Chest 76: 647–652
Elmqvist R, Lagergren J, Pettersson SO, Senning A, William-Olsson G (1963) Artificial pacemaker for treatment of Adams-Stokes' syndrome and slow heart rate. Am Heart J 65: 731–748
Elmqvist H, Schueller H, Richter G (1983) The carbon tip electrode. Pace 6 (II): 436–439
Enia F, Mauro RL, Meschisi F, Sabella FP (1991) Right-sided infective endocarditis with acquired tricuspid valve stenosis associated with transvenous pacemaker: a case report. Pace 14: 1093–1097
Epstein AE, Anderson PG, Kay GN, Dailey SM, Plumb VJ, Shepard RB (1992) Gross and microscopic changes associated with a nonthoracotomy implantable cardioverter defibrillator. Pace 15 (I): 382–386
Epstein E, Quereshi MSA, Wright JS (1976) Diaphragmatic paralysis after supraclavicular puncture of subclavian vein. Br Med J I: 693–694
Erlebacher JA, Cahill PT, Pannizzo F, Knowlers RJ (1986) Effect of magnetic resonance imaging on DDD pacemakers. Am J Cardiol 57: 437 440
Evans GT Jr, Scheinman MM, Zipes DP, et al. (1988) The percutaneous cardiac mapping and ablation registry: final summary of results. Pace 11 (I): 1621–1626
Falkoff M, Heinle RA, Ong LS, Barold SS (1978) Inapparent double puncture of the femoral artery and vein. An important complication of temporary cardiac pacing by the transfemoral approach. Pace 1: 49–51
Fazio G, Veltri EP, Tomaselli G, Lewis R, Griffith LSC, Guarnieri, T (1991) Long-term follow-up of patients with non-ischemic dilated cardiomyopathy and ventricular tachyarrhythmias treated with implantable cardioverter defibrillators. Pace 14 (II): 1905–1910

Feng WC, Sing AK, Drew T, Donat W (1990) Swan-Ganz catheter-induced massive hemoptysis and pulmonary artery false aneurysm. Ann Thorac Surg 50: 644–646

Ferek B, Pasini M, Pustisek S, Jursic M, Tonkovic S (1984) Noninvasive detection of insulation break. Pace 7 (I): 1063–1068

Fetter J, Aram G, Holmes DR Jr, Gray JE, Hayes DL (1984) The effects of nuclear magnetic resonance imagers on external and implantable pulse generators. Pace 7: 720–727

Fetter J, Patterson D, Aram G, Hayes DL (1989) Effects of extracorporeal shock wave lithotripsy on single chamber rate response and dual chamber pacemakers. Pace 12: 1494–1501

Fiandra O (1988) The first pacemaker implant in America. Pace 11: 1234–1238

Fieldman A, Dobrow RJ (1978) Phantom pacemaker programming. Pace 1: 166–171

Flaker GC, Mueller KJ, Salazar JF, Madigan NP, Curtis JJ (1983) Total venous obstruction following atrioventricular sequential pacemaker implantation. Pace 6: 815–817

Flicker S, Eldredge WJ, Naidech HJ, Steiner RM, Clark DL (1985) Computed tomographic localization of malposition of pacing electrodes: the value of cardiovascular computed tomography. Pace 8: 589–599

Foote GA, Schabel SI, Hodges M (1974) Pulmonary complications of the flow-directed balloon-tipped catheter N Engl J Med 290: 927–931

Ford SE, Manley PN (1982) Indwelling cardiac catheters. An autopsy study of associated endocardial lesions. Arch Pathol Lab Med 106: 314–317

Frandsen F, Oxhoj H, Nielsen B (1990) Entrapment of a tined pacemaker electrode in the tricuspid valve. A case report. Pace 13: 1082–1083

Frank G, Lowes D (1992) Implantable cardioverter defibrillators: surgical considerations Pace 15 (III): 631–635

Fritz T, Richeson F, Fitzpatrick P, Wilson G (1983) Venous obstruction. A potential complication of transvenous pacemaker electrodes. Chest 83: 534–539

Furman S (1979a) Nuclear pacemakers. Pace 2: 135–136

Furman S (1979b) The sixth world symposium on cardiac pacing. Pace 2: 551–552

Furman S (1981a) Pacemaker longevity. Pace 4: 1–2

Furman S (1981b) External defibrillation and implanted cardiac pacemakers. Pace 4: 485–486

Furman S (1982a) Electromagnetic interference. Pace 5: 1–3

Furman S (1982b) Radiation effects on implanted pacemakers. Pace 5: 145

Furman S (1986a) Subclavian puncture for pacemaker lead placement. Pace 9: 467

Furman S (1986b) Venous cutdown for pacemaker implantation. Ann Thorac Surg 41: 438–439

Furman S (1989) Pacemaker longevity. Pace 12: 1437–1438

Furman S (1990) Connectors. Pace 13: 567

Furman S, Bilitch M (1987) Naspe x AM. Pace 10: 278–280

Furman S, Parker B (1978) Electrosurgical device interference with implanted pacemakers. JAMA 239: 1910

Furman S, Schwedel JB (1959) An intracardiac pacemaker for Stokes-Adams seizures. N Engl J Med 261: 943–948

Furman S, Schwedel JB, Robinson G, Hurwitt ES (1961) Use of an intracardiac pacemaker in control of heart block. Surgery 49: 98–108

Furman S, Pannizzo F, Campo I (1979) Comparison of active and passive adhering leads for endocardial pacing – I. Pace 2: 417–427

Furman S, Pannizzo F, Campo I (1981) Comparison of active and passive leads for endocardial pacing – II. Pace 4: 78–83

Furman S, Brodman R, Pannizzo F, Fisher JD (1984) Implantation techniques of antitachycardia devices. Pace 7 (II): 572–579

Furstenberg S, Bluhm G, Olin C (1984) Entrapment of an atrial tined pacemaker electrode in the tricuspid valve. A case report. Pace 7: 760–762

Fyke FE III (1988) Simultaneous insulation deterioration associated with side-by-side subclavian placement of two polyurethane leads. Pace 11: 1571-1574

Gabry MD, Behrens M, Andrews C, Wanliss M, Klementowicz PT, Furman, S (1987) Comparison of myopotential interference in unipolar-bipolar programmable DDD pacemakers. Pace 10: 1322–1330

Gaidula JJ, Barold SS (1974) Elimination of diaphragmetic contractions from chronic pacing, catheter perforation of the heart by conversion to a unipolar system. Chest 66: 86–88

Gaillard D, Lespinasse P, Vanetti A (1988) Cardiac pacing and valvular surgery. Pace11 (II): 2142–2148

Garberoglio B, Inguaggiato B, Chinaglia B, Cerise O (1983) Initial results with an activated pyrolytic carbon tip electrode. Pace 6 (II): 440–447
García Jiménez A, Albá CMB, Cortés JMG, Rodriguez CG, Diéguez IA, Pellejero FN (1992) Myocardial rupture after pulling out a tined atrial electrode with continuous traction. Pace 15: 5–8
Gering LE, Ruskin JN, Garan H (1989) Modified magnet test for a reversed automatic implantable cardioverter defibrillator. Pace 12: 1838–1840
Gheissari A, Hordof AJ, Spotnitz HM (1991) Transvenous pacemakers in children: relation of lead length to anticipated growth. Ann Thorac Surg 52: 118–121
Gialafos J, Maillis A, Basiakos L, Avgoustakis D (1983) Rectus abdominis as a source of myopotentials inhibiting demand pacemakers. Pace 6: 887–891
Gibbons JA, Devig PM, Aaron BL (1979) The recessed chest wall pacemaker pocket. Pace 2: 55–57
Gibson TC, Davidson RC, de Silvey DL (1980) Presumptive tricuspid valve malfunction induced by a pacemaker lead: a case report and review of the literature. Pace 3: 88–95
Gillette PC, Zeigler V, Bradham GB, Kinsella P (1988) Pediatric transvenous pacing: a concern for venous thrombosis? Pace 11 (II): 1935–1939
Gillette PC, Zeigler VL, Case CL, Harold M, Buckles DS (1991a) Atrial antitachycardia pacing in children and young adults. Am Heart J 122: 844–849
Gillette PC, Edgerton J, Kratz J, Zeigler V (1991b) The subpectoral pocket: the preferred implant site for pediatric pacemakers. Pace 14: 1089–1092
Gillette PC, Swindle MM, Thompson RP, Case CL, Armenia J, Harold M, Kerr C (1991c) Transvenous cryoablation of the bundle of His. Pace 14 (I): 504–510
Gillmer DJ, Vythilingum S, Mitha AS (1981) Problems encountered during insertion of permanent endocardial pacing electrode. Pace 4: 212–215
Giroud D, Goy JJ (1990) Pacemaker malfunction due to subcutaneous emphysema. Int J Cardiol 26: 234–236
Giudici MC, Flaker GC, Curtis JJ (1991) Intraoperative myocardial infarction during open-heart ablation of an atrioventricular accessory pathway. Pace 14: 399–403
Goldman BS (1986) Commentary for "salvage of infected cardiac pacemaker pockets using a closed irrigation system". Pace 9 (I): 915–916
Goldman BS, Hill TJ, Weisel RD, Scully HE, Mickleborough LL, Pym J, Baird RJ (1984) Permanent cardiac pacing after open-heart surgery: acquired heart disease. Pace 7: 367–371
Goldman BS, William WG, Hill T, Hesslein PS, McLaughlin PR, Trusler GA, Baird RJ (1985) Permanent cardiac pacing after open-heart surgery: congenital heart disease. Pace 8: 732-739
Goudevenos JA, Reid PG, Adams PC, Holden MP, Williams DO (1989) Pacemaker-induced superior vena cava syndrome: report of four cases and review of the literature. Pace 12: 1890–1895
Gould L, Patel S, Gomes GI, Chokshi AB (1981) Pacemaker failure following external defibrillation. Pace 4: 575–577
Greatbatch (1984) Twenty-five years of pacemaking. Pace 7: 143–147
Greenberg P, Castellanet M, Messenger J, Ellestad MH (1978) Coronary sinus pacing: clinical follow-up. Circulation 57: 98–103
Greve H, Koch TH, Gulker H, Heuer H (1988) Termination of malignant ventricular tachycardias by use of an automatical defibrillator (AICD) in combination with an antitachycardial pacemaker. Pace 11 (II): 2040–2044
Guharay BN, Ghose JC, Majumdar H, Basu AK (1977) The pacemaker-twiddler's syndrome: another disadvantage of abdominal implantation of pulse generators. Br J Surg 64: 655–660
Gursoy S, Brugada J, Souza O, Steurer G, Andries E, Grugada, P (1992) Radiofrequency ablation of symptomatic but benign ventricular arrhythmias. Pace 15: 738–747
Hamilton R, Gow R, Bahoric B, Griffiths J, Freedom R, Williams W (1991) Steroid-eluting epicardial leads in pediatrics: improved epicardial thresholds in the first year. Pace 14 (II): 2066–2092
Hammel D, Block M, Borggefe M, Konertz W, Breithardt G, Scheld HH (1992) Implantation of a cardioverter defibrillator in the subpectoral region combined with a nonthoracotomy lead system. Pace 15 (I): 367–372
Hanson JS (1984) Sixteen failures in a single model of bipolar polyurethane-insulated ventricular pacing lead: a 44-month experience. Pace 7 (I): 389–394
Hanson JS, Grant ME (1984) Nine-year experience during 1973-1982 with 1,060 pacemakers in 805 patients. Pace 7: 51–62
Harthorne JW (1980) Letter to the editor. Pace 3: 740–741
Hauser RG (1982) Bipolar leads for cardiac pacing in the 1980's: a reappraisal provoked by skeletal muscle interference. Pace 5: 35–37
Hauser RG, Heilman, MS (1991) The industrialization of the AICD. Pace 14 (II): 905–909

Hauser RG, Mower, MM, Mitchell M, Nisam S (1992) Current status of the Venlak (R) PRxpulse generator and Endotak-TM nonthoracotomy lead system. Pace 15 (III): 671–677
Hayes DL, Holmes DR Jr, Gray JE (1987) Effect of 1.5 tesla nuclear magnetic resonance imaging scanner on implanted permanent pacemakers. J Am Coll Cardiol 10: 782–786
Heilman MS (1991) Collaboration with Michel Mirowski on the development of the AICD. Pace 14 (II): 910–915
Heinz G, Hirschl M, Buxbaum P, Laufer G, Gasic S, Laczkovics A (1992) Sinus node dysfunction after orthotopic cardiac transplantation: Postoperative incidence and long-term implications. Pace 15: 731–737
Heller LI (1990) Surgical electrocautery and the runaway pacemaker syndrome. Pace 13: 1084–1085
Hellestrand KJ, Ward DE, Bexton RS, Camm AJ (1982) The use of active fixation electrodes for permanent endocardial pacing via a persistent left superior vena cava. Pace 5: 180–184
Hendler A, Krakover R, Stryjer D, Schlesinger Z (1991) A right atrial mass in the presence of a permanent pacemaker electrode in a patient with polycythemia vera. Pace 14: 2083–2085
Hill PE (1987) Complications of permanent transvenous cardiac pacing: a 14-year review of all transvenous pacemakers inserted at one community hospital. Pace 10 (I): 564–578
Holmes DR Jr, Hayes DL, Gray JE, Merideth J (1986) The effects of magnetic resonance imaging on implantable pulse generators. Pace 9: 360–370
Hong-Barco P, O'Toole J, Gerber ML, Domat I, Moquin M, Jackson SC (1988) Endocarditis due to six entrapped pacemaker leads and concomitant recurrent coronary arteriosclerosis. Ann Thorac. Surg. 46: 97–99
Hopps JA (1981) The development of the pacemaker. Pace 4: 106–108
Horowitz LN, (1992) The automatic implantable cardioverter defibrillator: review of clinical results 1980-1990. Pace 15 (III): 604–609
Huang SKS (1991) Advances in application of radiofrequency current to catheter ablation therapy. Pace 14: 28–42
Hubbell DS, Tyler GR Jr, Zoble RG (1986) Polyurethane sheath disintegration causing impaction of pacer lead and shock during attempted removal. Pace 9: 527–530
Hunter D, Moran JF, Venezio FR (1983) Osteomyelitis of the clavicle after Swan-Ganz catheterization. Arch Intern Med 143: 153–154
Hurst LN, Evans HB, Windle B, Klein GJ (1986) The salvage of infected cardiac pacemaker pockets using closed irrigation system. Pace 9 (I): 785–792
Hurzeler P, Morse D, Leach C, Sands MJ, Pennock R, Zinberg A (1980) Longevity comparisons among lithium anode power cells for cardiac pacemakers. Pace 3: 555–567
Hyman AS (1930) Resuscitation of the stopped heart by intracardiac therapy. Arch Intern Med 46: 553–568
Hyman AS (1932) Resuscitation of the stopped heart by intracardiac therapy. Experimental use of an artificial pacemaker. Arch Intern Med 50: 283-305
Hynes JK, Holmes DR Jr, Merideth J, Trusty JM (1981) An evaluation of long-term stimulation thresholds by measurement of chronic strength duration curves. Pace 4: 376–379
Ideker RE, Wolf PD, Alferness C, Krassowska W, Smith WM (1991) Current concepts for selecting the location, size and shape of defibrillation electrodes. Pace 14 (I): 227–240
Iesaka Y, Pinakatt T, Gosselin AJ, Lister JW (1982) Bradycardia dependent ventricular tachycardia facilitated by myopotential inhibition of a VVI pacemaker. Pace 5 (I): 23–29
Ilicetos S, DI Biase M, Antonelli G, Favales S, Rizzon P (1982) Two-dimensional echocardiographic recognition of a pacing catheter perforation of the interventricular septum. Pace 5: 934–936
Inoue H, Ueda K, Okhawa S-I, Mifune J-I, Sugiura M (1979) Runaway pacemaker. A case report with a runaway rate of 2100 ppm. Pace 2: 608–613
Irnich W (1980) The chronaxie time and its practical importance. Pace 3: 292–301
Irnich W (1983) Comparison of pacing electrodes of different shape and material – recommendations. Pace 6 (2): 422–426
Irnich W (1984a) Interference in pacemakers. Pace 7 (I): 1021–1048
Irnich W (1984b) Development of a coding system for pacemakers. Pace 7 (V): 882–901
Irnich W, de Bakker JMT, Bisping H-J (1978) Electromagnetic interference in implantable pacemakers. Pace 1: 52–61
Irnich W, Parsonnet V, Myers GH (1979a) Compendium of pacemaker technology. II. Definitions and glossary (part I). Pace 2: 88–93
Irnich W, Parsonnet V, Myers GH (1979b) Compendium of pacemaker technology. II. Definitions and glossary (part II). Pace 2: 634–640

Irnich, W, Parsonnet V, Myers GH (1980) Compendium of pacemaker technology. II. Definitions and glossary (part III). Pace 3: 68–72

Irwin JM, Greer GS, Lowe JE, German LD, Gilbert, MR (1987) Atrial lead perforation: a case report. Pace 10: 1378–1381

Jacobson PM (1979a) Radiation from implantable nuclear pacemakers. I. Dosimetry. Pace 2: 215–244

Jacobson PM (1979b) Radiation from implantable nuclear pacemaker. II. Analysis. Pace 2: 345–355

Jara FM, Toledo-Pereyra L, Lewis JW Jr, Magilligan DJ Jr (1979) The infected pacemaker pocket. J Thorac Cardiovasc Surg 78: 298–300

Jaye CG, Smith DR (1988) Complications of central venous cannulation. Br Med J 297: 572–573

Jenkins JM, Dick MD, Collins S, O'neill W, Campbell RM, Wilber DJ (1985) Use of the pill electrode for trans-esophageal atrial pacing. PACE 8: 512–527

Kacet S, Molin F, Lacroix D, Prat A, Pol A, Warembourg H, Lekieffre J (1991) Bipolar atrial triggered pacing to restore normal chronotropic responsiveness in an orthotopic cardiac transplant patient. Pace 14: 1444–1447

Karpawich PP, Stokes KB, Helland JR, Justice CD, Roskamp JO (1988) A new low threshold platinized epicardial pacing electrode: comparative evaluation in immature canines. Pace 11: 1139–1148

Katzenberg CA, Marcus FI, Heusinkveld RS, Mammana RB (1982) Pacemaker failure due to radiation therapy. Pace 5: 156–159

Kaye CG, Smith DR (1988) Complications of central venous cannulation. Trauma, infection and thrombosis. BMJ 297: 572–573

Kelly PA, Wallace S, Tucker B, Hurvitz RJ, Ilvento J, Mirabel GS, Cannom, DS (1988) Postoperative infection with the automatic implantable cardioverter defibrillator: clinical presentation and use of the gallium scan in diagnosis. Pace 11: 1220–1225

Keren R, Aarons D, Veltri EP (1991) Anxiety and depression in patients with life-threatening ventricular arrhythmias: impact of the implantable cardioverter-defibrillator. Pace 14 (I): 181–187

Kerr CR, Chung DC, Cooper J (1986) Improved transesophageal recording and stimulation utilizing a new quadripolar lead configuration. Pace 9: 644–651

Kertes P, Mond H, Sloman G, Vohra J, Hunt D (1983) Comparison of lead complications with polyurethane tined, silicone rubber tined, and wedge tip leads: clinical experience with 822 ventricular endocardial leads. Pace 6 (I): 957–962

Kevorkian M, Motte G, Kevorkian JP, Welti JJ (1982) Hiccup and electroventricular stimulation with a pervenous electrode. Pace 5: 440–441

Khair, GZ, Tristani, FE (1979) Pacing failure due to an unusual fracture of the sutureless myocardial electrode. Pace 2: 51–54

Kinney EL, Allen RP, Weidner WA, Pierce WS, Leaman DM, Zelis RF (1979) Recurrent pulmonary emboli secondary to right atrial thrombus around a permanent pacing catheter: a case report and review of the literature. Pace 2: 196–202

Kramer LK, Rojas-Corona RR, Sheff D, Eisenberg ES (1985) Disseminated aspergillosis and pacemaker endocarditis. Pace 8: 225–229

Kratz JM, Campbell WC, Leman RB, Harvin JS (1984) Steroid treatment of the painful pacemaker pocket. Pace 7: 71–73

Kreis DJ, LiCalzi L, Shaw RK (1979) Air entrapment as a cause of transient cardiac pacemaker malfunction. Pace 2: 641–644

Kruse Im, Terpstra B (1985) Acute and long-term atrial and ventricular stimulation thresholds with a steroid-eluting electrode. Pace 8: 45–49

Kugler JD, Fetter J, Flemming W, Kilzer K, Stoehr D, Felix G, Radio S (1990) A new steroid-eluting epicardial lead: experience with atrial and ventricular implantation in the immature swine. Pace 13: 976–981

Lagergren H (1978) How it happened: my recollection of early pacing. Pace 1: 140–143

Lamas GA, Fish RD, Braunwald NS (1988) Fluoroscopic technique of subclavian venous puncture for permanent pacing: a safer and easier approach. Pace 11: 1398–1401

Langberg J, Abber J, Thuroff JW, Griffin JC (1987) The effects of extracorporeal shock wave lithotripsy on pacemaker function. Pace 10: 1142–1146

Lange HW, Galliani CA, Edwards JE (1983) Local complications associated with indwelling Swan-Ganz catheters: autopsy study of 36 cases. Am J Cardiol 52: 1108–1111

Langenfeld H, Grimm W, Maisch B, Kochsiek K (1988) Atrial fibrillation and embolic complications in paced patients. Pace 11 (II): 1667–1672

Lasala AF, Fieldman A, Diana DJ, Humphrey CB (1979) Gas pocket causing pacemaker malfunction. Pace 2: 183–185

Lau C-P, Linker NJ, Butrous GS, Ward DE, Camm AJ (1989) Myopotential interference in unipolar rate responsive pacemakers. Pace 12: 1324–1330

Laurens P (1979) Nuclear-powered pacemakers: an eight-year clinical experience. Pace 2: 356–360

Lee ME, Chaux A (1980) Unusual complications of endocardial pacing. J Thorac Cardiovasc Surg 80: 934–940

Lepore V, Pizzarelli G, Dernevik L (1987) Inadvertent transarterial pacemaker insertion: an unusual complication. Pace 10 (I): 951–954

Lewis AB, Hayes DL, Holmes DR Jr, Vlietstra RE, Pluth JR, Osborn M (1985) Update on infections involving permanent pacemakers: Characterization and management. J Thorac Cardiovasc Surg 89: 758–763

Littleford PO, Pepine. CJ, (1981) A new temporary atrial pacing catheter inserted percutaneously into the subclavian vein without fluoroscopy: a preliminary report. Pace 4: 458–464

Luceri RM, Habal SM, Castellanos A, Thurer RJ, Waters RS, Brownstein SL (1988) Mechanism of death in patients with the automatic implantable cardioverter defibrillator. Pace 11 (II): 2015–2022

MacCarter DJ, Lundberg KM, Corstjens JPM (1983) Porous electrodes: concept, technology and results. Pace 6 (2): 427–435

Madigan NP, Curtis JJ, Sanfelippo JF, Murphy TJ (1984) Difficulty of extraction of chronically implanted tined ventricular endocardial leads. J Am Coll Cardiol 3: 724–731

Magilligan DJ Jr, Hakimi M, Davila JC (1976) The suturelss electrode: comparison with transvenous and sutured epicardial electrode placement for permanent pacing. Ann Thorac Surg 22: 80–86

Magilligan, DJ Jr, Isshak, G (1980) Carcinoma of the breast in a pacemaker pocket - simple recurrence or oncotaxis? Pace 3: 220–223

Mansour KA, Fleming WH, Hatcher CR (1973) Initial experience with a sutureless, screw-in electrode for cardiac pacing. Ann Thorac Surg 16: 127–135

Manyari DE, Klein GJ, Kostuk WJ (1983) Electrocardiographic recognition of variant angina during permanent pacing. Pace 6: 99–103

Marchlinski FE, Falcone R, Iozzo RV, Reichek N, Vassallo JA, Eysmann SB (1987) Experimental myocardial cryoinjury: local electromechanical changes, arrhythmogenicity, and methods for determining depth of injury. Pace 10 (I): 886–901

Markewitz A, Kemkes BM, Reble B, et al. (1987) Particularities of dual chamber pacemaker therapy in patients after orthotopic heart transplant. Pace 10: 326–332

Markewitz A, Wenke K, Weinhold C (1988a) Reliability of atrial screw-in leads. Pace 11 (2): 1777–1783

Markewitz A, Osterholzer G, Weinhold C, Kemkes BM, Feruglio GA (1988b) Recipient P wave synchronized pacing of the donor atrium in a heart-transplanted patient: a case study. Pace 11: 1402–1404

Marti V, Ballester M, Oter R, Obrador D, Bayés-de Luna, A (1991) Recovery of sinus node function after pacemaker implant for sinus node disease following cardiac transplant. Pace 14: 1205–1208

Mathivanar J, Anderson N, Harman D, Skalsky M, Ng M (1990) In vivo elution rate of drug eluting ceramic leads with a reduced dose of dexamethasone sodium phosphate. Pace 13 (II): 1883–1886

McDaniel CM, Berry VA, Haines DE, Dimarco JP (1988) Automatic external defibrillation of patients after myocardial infarction by family members: practical aspects and psychological impact of training. Pace 11 (II): 2029–2034

McGrath LB, Gonzalez-Lavin L, Morse DP, Levett JM (1988) Pacemaker system failure and other events in children with surgically induced heart block. Pace 11: 1182–1187

McWilliams ETM, Buchalter MB, O'Neill CA (1984) An unusual form of pacemaker failure. Pace 7: 765-776

Meesmann M (1992) Factors associated with implantation-related complications. Pace 15 (III): 649–653

Mercando AD, Furman S, Johnston D, Frame R, Brodman R, Kim SG, Fisher JD (1988) Survival of patients with the automatic implantable cardioverter defibrillator. Pace 11 (II): 2059–2063

Messenger JC, Castellanet MJ, Stephenson NL (1982) New permanent endocardial atrial J lead: implantation techniques and clinical performance: Pace 5: 767–772

Michalik RE, Williams WH, Zorn-Chelton S, Hatcher CR Jr (1984) Experience with a new epimyocardial pacing lead in children. Pace 7: 831–838

Mirowski M, Reid PR, Mower MM, Watkins L Jr, Platia EV, Griffith LSC, Juanteguy JM (1984a) The automatic implantable cardioverter-defibrillator. Pace 7 (II): 534–540

Mirowski M, Reid PR, Mower MM, Watkins L Jr, Platia EV, Griffith LSC, Guarnieri T, Thomas, A, Juanteguy JM (1984b) Clinical performance of the implantable cardioverter-defibrillator. Pace 7 (II): 1345–1350

Mirowski M, Mower MM, Reid PR, Watkins L, Langer A (1982) The automatic implantable defibrillator: new modality for treatment of life-threatening ventricular arrhythmias. Pace 5: 384–401

Mittleman RS, Mack K, Rastegar H, Manolis AS, Estes NAM III (1991) Inappropriate shocks and elevation of defibrillation thresholds in a patient with automatic defibrillator patch Silastic erosion and titanium mesh fraying. Pace 14: 1452–1455

Mond HG (1991) Unipolar versus bipolar pacing – poles apart. Pace 14: 1411–1424

Mond H, Sloman G (1980) The small-tined pacemaker lead – absence of dislodgement. Pace 3: 171–177

Mond HG, Sloman JG (1981a) The malfunctioning pacemaker system. Part I. Pace 4: 49–60

Mond HG, Sloman JG (1981b) The malfunctioning pacemaker system. Part II. Pace 4: 168–181

Mond HG, Stokes KB (1992) The electrode-tissue interface: the revolutionary role of steroid elution. Pace 15: 95–107

Mond HG, Stuckey JG, Sloman G (1978) The diagnosis of right ventricular perforation by an endocardial pacemaker electrode. Pace 1: 62–67

Mond HG, Sloman JG, Edwards RH (1982a) The first pacemaker. Pace 5: 278–282

Mond H, Holley L, Hirshorn M (1982b) The high impedance dish electrode-clinical experience with a new tined lead. Pace 5: 529–534

Mond H, Stokes K, Helland J, Grigg L, Kertes P, Pate B, Hunt D (1988) The porous titanium steroid eluting electrode: a double blind study assessing the stimulation threshold effects of steroid. Pace 11 (2): 214–219

Moore SL, Maloney JD, Edel TB, et al. (1991) Implantable cardioverter defibrillator implanted by nonthoracotomy approach: initial clinical experience with the redesigned transvenous lead system. Pace 14 (II): 1865–1869

Moorman JR, Steenbergen S, Durack DT (1984) Aspergillus infection of a permanent ventricular pacing lead. Pace 7 (I): 361–366

Morse D, Yankaskas M, Johnson B, Spagna P, Lemole GM, (1983) Transvenous pacemaker insertion with a zero dislodgement rate. Pace 6 (1): 283–290

Mower MM, Nisam S (1988) AICD indications (patient selection): past, present and future. Pace 11 (II): 2064–2070

Mower MM, Reid PR, Watkins L Jr, et al. (1984) Automatic implantable cardioverter-defibrillator structural characteristics. Pace 7 (II): 1331–1337

Mugica J, Duconge B, Henry L, Atchia B, Lazarus B (1988) Clinical experience with new leads. Pace 11 (II): 1745–1752

Muller-Runkel R, Orsolini G, Kalokhe UP (1990) Monitoring the radiation dose to a multiprogrammable pacemaker during radical radiation therapy: a case report. Pace 13 (I): 1466–1470

Mund K, Richter G, Weidlich E, Fahlstrom U (1986) Electrochemical properties of platinum, glassy carbon, and pyrographite as stimulating electrodes. Pace 9 (II): 1225–1229

Myers MR, Parsonnet V, Bernstein AD (1991) Extraction of implanted transvenous pacing leads: a review of a persistent clinical problem. Am Heart J 121: 881–888

Naclerio EA, Varriale P (1980) The sutureless electrode for cardiac pacing: problems, advantages and surgical technique. Pace 3: 232–235

Nanda NC, Barold SS (1982) Usefulness of echocardiography in cardiac pacing. Pace 5: 222–237

Nisam S, Thomas A, Moser S, Winkle R, Fisher J (1988) AICD: standardized reporting and appropriate categorization of complications. Pace 11 (II): 2045–2052

Nisam S, Mower M, Moser S (1991) ICD clinical update: first decade, initial 10000 patients. Pace 4 (II): 255–262

Norwood S, Ruby A, Civetta J, Cortes V (1991) Catheter-related infections associated septicemia. Chest 99: 968–975

Odabashian HC, Brown DF (1979) "Runaway" in a modern generation pacemaker. Pace 2: 152–155

Ogawa S, Dreifus LS, Shenoy PN, Brockman SK, Berkovits BV (1978) Haemodynamic consequences of atrioventricular and ventriculoatrial pacing. Pace 1: 8–15

Ohm O-J, Skagseth E (1980) Temporary pacemaker treatment in open-heart surgery: pre- to postoperative changes in the electrogram characteristics. Pace 3: 150-158

Old WD, Paulsen W, Lewis SA, Nixon JV (1989) Pacemaker lead-induced tricuspid stenosis: diagnosis by Doppler echocardiography. Am Heart J 117: 1165–1167

Ormerod D, Walgren S, Berglund J, Heil R Jr (1988) Design and evaluation of a low threshold, porous tip lead with a mannitol-coated screw-in tip ("Sweet Tip" Tm). Pace 11 (II): 1784–1790

Palac RT, Hwang MH, Klodnycky ML, Loeb HS (1981) Delayed pulse generator malfunction after D.C. countershock. Pace 4: 163–167

Pannizzo F, Furman S (1980) Pacemaker and patient response to the "point of sale" terminal as an actual and simulated electromagnetic interference source. Pace 3: 461–469

Parry G, Goudevenos J, Jameson S, Adams PC, Gold RG (1991) Complications associated with retained pacemaker leads. Pace 14: 1251–1257

Parsonnet V (1978) Permanent transvenous pacing in 1962. Pace 1: 265–268

Parsonnet V, Manhardt M (1977) Permanent pacing of the heart: 1952–1976. AM J Cardiol 39: 250–256

Parsonnet V, Werres R (1981) Entrapment of a temporary atrial loop pacing electrode. Am Heart J 101: 227–229

Parsonnet V, Myers GH, Manhardt M (1979) An appraisal of radioisotope fueled pacemakers after 5 years. Pace 2: 361–369

Parsonnet V, Gilbert L, Zucker IR, Werres R, Atherley T, Manhardt M, Cort J (1984) A decade of nuclear pacing. Pace 7: 90–95

Parsonnet V, Bernstein AD, Lindsay B (1989) Pacemaker-implantation complication rates: an analysis of some contributing factors. J Am Coll Cardiol 13: 917–921

Parsonnet V, Berstein AD, Perry GY (1990) The nuclear pacemaker: Is renewed interest warranted? Am J Cardiol 66: 837–842

Parsonnet V, Hesselson AB, Harari DC (1991) Long-term functional integrity of atrial leads. Pace 14 (I): 517–521

Pasquariello JL, Hariman RJ, Yudelman IM, Feit A, Gomes AC, El-Sherif, N, (1984) Recurrent pulmonary embolization following implantation of transvenous pacemaker. Pace 7: 790–793

Pauletti M, Di Ricco G, Solfanelli S, Marini C, Contini C, Giuntini C (1981) Venous obstruction in permanent pacemaker patients: an isotopic study. Pace 4: 36–42

Pavlicek W, Geisinger M, Castle L, Borkowski GP, Meaney TF, Bream BL, Gallagher JH (1983) The effects of nuclear magnetic resonance on patients with cardiac pacemakers. Radiology 147: 149–153

Perkins DG, Klein GJ, Silver MD, Yee R, Jones DL (1987) Cardioversion and defibrillation using a catheter electrode: myocardial damage assessed at autopsy. Pace 10 (I): 800–804

Perry JC, Nihill MR, Ludomirsky A, Ott DA, Garson A Jr (1991) The pulmonary artery lasso: epicardial pacing lead causing right ventricular outflow obstruction. Pace 14: 1018–1023

Peters R, Wohl B, Fisher M, Carliner N, Plotnick G (1982) Non-operative removal of a tined-tip endocardial pacemaker catheter. Pace 5: 129–132

Phillips R, Frey M, Martin RO (1986) Long-term performance of polyurethane pacing-leads: mechanisms of design-related failures. Pace 9 (II): 1166–1172

Pioger G, Ripart A (1986) Clinical results of low energy unipolar or bipolar activated carbon tip leads. Pace 9 (II): 1243–1248

Quintal R, Dhurandhar RW, Jain RK (1984) Myopotential interference with a DDD pacemaker-report of a case. Pace 7: 37–39

Radcliffe PJ, Jones S, Ward DE (1981) An unusual case of pacemaker current leakage causing muscle stimulation. Pace 4: 589–591

Radovsky AS, Van Vleet JF, Stokes KB, Tacker WA Jr, (1988) Paired comparisons of steroid-eluting and non-steroid endocardial pacemaker leads in dogs: electrical performance and morphologic alterations. Pace 11: 1085–1094

Rajs J (1983) Postmortem findings and possible causes of unexpected death in patients treated with intraventricular pacing. Pace 6: 751–760

Rao G (1984) Letter to the editor. Pace 7: 1086

Rasmussen K, Grimsgaard C, Vik-Mo H, Stalsberg H (1985) Male breast cancer from pacemaker pocket. Pace 8: 761–763

Raymond RD, Nanian KB (1984) Insulation failure with bipolar polyurethane pacing leads. Pace 7 (I): 378–380

Res JCJ, De Cock CC, Van Rossum AC, Schreuder J (1989) Entrapment of tined leads. Pace 12: 1583–1585

Riera JA S-I, Garcia JR, Samartin RC (1990) Anomalous placement of an endocardial pacing lead. Pace 13(I): 1475

Ripart A, Mugica J (1983) Electrode-heart interface:definition of the ideal electrode. Pace 6 (II): 410–421

Robbens EJ, Ruiter JH (1986) Atrial pacing via unilateral persistent left superior vena cava. Pace 9: 594–596

Robboy SJ, Harthorne JW, Leinbach RC, Sanders CA, Austen WG (1969) Autopsy findings with permanent pervenous pacemakers. Circulation 39: 495–501

Ronnevik PK, Abrahamsen AM, Tollefsen I (1982) Transvenous pacemaker implantation via a unilateral left superior vena cava. Pace 5: 808–813

Rosenfeld LE (1985) Osteomyelitis of the first rib presenting as a cold abscess nine months after subclavian venous catheterization . Pace 8: 897–899

Rosenqvist M, Nordlander R, Andersson M, Edhag O (1986) Reduced incidence of myopotential pacemaker inhibition by abdominal generator implantation. Pace 9: 417–421

Rosenthal R, Crisafi BR, Coomaraswamy RP (1980) Manual extraction of a permanent pacemaker: an attempted suicide. Pace 3: 229–231

Ross WB, Mohiuddin SM, Pagano T, Hughes D (1983) Malposition of a transvenous cardiac electrode associated with amaurosis fugax. Pace 6: 119–124

Rowley KM, Soni Clubb, Walker-Smith GJ, Cabin HS (1984) Right-sided infective endocarditis as a consequence of flow-directed pulmonary artery catheterization: a clinicopathological study of 55 autopsied patients. N Engl J Med 311: 1152–1156

Rubin L, Rosenberg D, Parsonnet V, Villaneuva A, Ferrara-Ryan M (1991) Comparison of titanium-mesh and porous disc electrodes for epicardial defibrillation. Pace 14(II): 1860–1864

Rubio PA, Al-Bassam MS (1991) Pacemaker-lead puncture of the tricuspid valve. Successful diagnosis and treatment. Chest 99: 1519–1520

Ruder MA, Mead RH, Smith NA, Winkle RA (1990) Defibrillator "Twiddler's" syndrome – letter to the editor. Pace 13: 1073–1074.

Ruiter JH, Degener JE, Van Mechelen R, Bos R (1985) Late purulent pacemaker pocket infection caused by *Staphylococcus epidermidis:* serious complications of in situ management. Pace 8: 903–907

Saeian K, Vellinga T, Troup P, Wetherbee J (1991) Coronary artery fistula formation secondary to permanent pacemaker placement. Chest 99: 780–781

Saksena S (1988) Nonpharmacologic therapy for tachyarrhythmias: the Tower of Babel revisited? Pace 11: 93–97

Saksena S, Gadhoke A (1986) Laser therapy for tachyarrhythmias: a new frontier. Pace 9: 531–550

Saksena S, Lindsay BD, Parsonnet V (1987) Developments for future implantable cardioverters and defibrillators. Pace 10: 1342–1358

Saksena S, Hussain SM, Gielchinsky I (1988) Surgical ablation of tachyarrhythmias: reflections for the third decade. Pace 10: 1342–1358

Salel AF, Seagren SC, Pool PE (1989) Effects of encainide on the function of implanted pacemakers. Pace 12: 1439–1444

Sandler MA, Wertheimer JH, Kotler MN (1989) Pericardial tamponade associated with pacemaker catheter manipulation. Pace 12(I): 1085–1088

Santini M, Messina G, Masini V (1980) Intermittent and arrhythmic "runaway" pacemaker. Pace 3: 730–732

Schaldach M, Hubmann M, Weikl A, Hardt R (1990) Sputter-deposited TiN electrode coatings for superior sensing and pacing performance. Pace 13: 1891–1895

Scheinman MM, Akhtar M, Dreifus L et al. (1992) Catheter ablation for cardiac arrhythmias, personnel and facilities. Pace 15: 715–721

Scheuer-Leeser M, Irnich W, Kreuzert J (1983) Polyurethane leads: facts and controversy. Pace 6: 454–458

Schiavone WA, Castle LW, Salcedo E, Graor R (1984) Amaurosis fugax in a patient with a left ventricular endocardial pacemaker. Pace 7: 288–292

Schuchert A, Hopf M, Kuck KH, Bleifeld W (1990) Chronic ventricular electrograms: Do steriod-eluting leads differ from conventional leads? Pace 13; 1879–1882

Schuster AH, Zugibe F Jr, Nanda NC, Murphy GW (1982) Two-dimensional echocardiographic identification of pacing catheter-induced thrombosis. Pace 5: 124–128

Secemsky SI, Hauser RG, Denes P, Edwards LM (1982) Unipolar sensing abnormalities: incidence and clinical significance of skeletal muscle interference and undersensing in 228 patients. Pace 5: 10–19

Seeger W, Scherer K (1986) Asymptomatic pulmonary embolism following pacemaker implantation. Pacc 9: 196–199

Seifert MJ, Morady F, Calkins HG, Langberg JJ (1991) Aortic leaflet perforation during radiofrequency ablation. Pace 14(I): 1582–1585

Senning, A (1959) Discussion of a paper by Stephenson SE Jr, Physiologic P-wave cardiac stimulator. J Thorac Surg 38: 639

Shandling AH, Ellestad MH, Castellanet MJ, Messenger JC (1991) Dacron-woven pacemaker pouch. Influence on long-term pacemaker mobility. Chest 99: 660–662

Shehata WM, Daoud GL, Meyer RL (1986) Radiotherapy for patients with cardiac pacemakers: possible risks. Letter to the editors. Pace 9: 919

Shmuely H, Erdman S, Strasberg B, Rosenfeld JB (1992) Seven years of left ventricular pacing due to malposition of pacing electrode. Pace 15(I): 369–372
Siclari F, Klein H, Tröster J (1990) Intraventricular migration of an ICD patch. Pace 13(I): 1356–1359
Siddons H, Nowak K, (1975) Surgical complications of implanting pacemakers. Br J Surg 62: 929–935
Simon AB, Kleinman P, Janz N (1980) Suicide attempt by pacemaker system abuse: a case report with comments on the psychological adaptation of pacemaker patients. Pace 3: 224–228
Simon AB, Dick M II, Stern AM, Behrendt DM, Sloan H (1982) Ventricular pacing in children. Pace 5:836–844
Singer I, Kupersmith J (1990) Nonpharmacological therapy of superventricular arrhythmias. Surgery and catheter ablation techniques: I. Pace 13: 1045
Singer I, Hutchins GM, Mirowski M, et al. (1987) Pathological findings related to the lead system and repeated defibrillations in patients with the automatic implantable cardioverter defibrillator. J Am Coll Cardiol 10: 382–388
Singer I, Van Der Laken J, Edmonds HL Jr, Slater AD, Austin E, Shields, CB, Kupersmith J (1991) Is defibrillation testing safe? Pace 14(II): 1899–1904
Sinnaeve A, Willems R, Stroobandt R (1982) Inhibition of on demand pacemakers by magnetwaving. Pace 5: 878–890
Slack JP, Hurzeler P, Morse D (1982) Predication of battery depletion in the ARCO LI3D. Pace 5: 567–570
Sloman JG, Mond HG, Bailey B, Cole A, Duffield A (1979) The use of balloon-tipped electrodes for permanent cardiac pacing. Pace 2: 597–585
Smith JA, Tatoulis J (1990) Right atrial perforation by a temporary epicardial pacing wire. Ann Thorac Surg 50: 141–142
Smith SA, Weissberg PL, Tan, L-B (1985) Permanent pacemaker failure due to surgical emphysema. Br Heart J 54: 220–221
Smyth NPD (1978) Atrial programmed pacing. Pace 1: 104–113
Smyth NPD, Tarjan PP, Chernoff EBS, Baker, N (1976) The significance of electrode surface area and stimulating thresholds in permanent cardiac pacing. J Thorac Cardiovasc Surg 71: 559–565
Smyth NPD, Purdy DL, Sager D, Keshishian JM (1982) A new multiprogrammable isotopic powered cardiac pacemaker. Pace 5: 761–766
Sneddon JF, Linker NJ, O'Nunain S, Simpson IA, Camm AJ, Ward DE (1991) Transcoronary atrioventricular nodal modification using microvascular collagen. Pace 14(II): 1976–1980
Snow N (1983) Acute myocardial ischemia during pacemaker implantation: implication for threshold determinations and potential complications. Pace 6: 35–37
Snow ME, Agatston AS, Kramer HC, Samet P (1987) The postcardiotomy syndrome following transvenous pacemaker insertion. Pace 10(I): 934–936
Stewart S, Cohen J, Murphy G (1975) Sutureless epicardial pacemaker lead: a satisfactory preliminary experience. Chest 67: 564–567
Stirbys P (1991) Removable or nonremovable endocardial electrodes: do not accept erroneous conclusions. Pace 14(I): 858–859
Stokes KB (1988) Preliminary studies on a new steroid- eluting epicardial electrode. PACE 11: 1797–1803
Stokes K, Bird T (1990) A new efficient Nano Tip Lead. Pace 13(II): 1901–1905
Stokes K, Chem B, Church T (1987) The elimination of exit block as a pacing complication using a transvenous steroid eluting lead (abstract 475). Pace 10(II): 748
Sunder SK, Ekong EA, Sivalingam K, Kumar A (1992) Superior vena cava thrombosis due to pacing electrodes: successful treatment with combined thrombolysis and angioplasty. Am Heart J 123: 790–792
Sutton R, Perrins J, Citron P (1980) Physiological cardiac pacing. Pace 3: 207–219
Suzuki Y, Fujimori S, Sakai M, Ohkawa S-I, Ueda K (1988) A case of pacemaker lead fracture associated with thoracic outlet syndrome. Pace 11: 326–330
Swan HJC, Ganz W, Forrester J, Marcus H, Diamond G, Chonette D (1970) Catheterization of the heart in man with use of a flow-directed balloon-tipped catheter. N Engl J Med 283: 447–451
Takeuchi ES, Qattrini PJ, Greatbatch W (1988) Lithium/silver vanadium oxide batteries for implantable defibrillators. Pace. 11(II): 2035–2039
Taylor RL, Cohen DJ, Widman LE, Chilton RJ, O'Rourke RA (1990) Infection of an implantable cardioverter defibrillator: management without removal of the device in selected cases. Pace 13(I): 1352–1355
Tegtmeyer CJ, Hunter JG Jr, Keats TE (1974) Bronchocutaneous fistula as late complication of permanent epicardial pacing. AJR 121: 614–676

Teskey RJ, Whelan I, Akyurekli Y, Eapen L, Green MS (1991) Therapeutic irradiation over a permanent cardiac pacemaker. Pace 14: 143–145

Thomas AC, Moser SA, Smutka ML, Wilson PA (1988) Implantable defibrillation: eight years clinical experience Pace. 11(II): 2053–2058

Till JA, Jones S, Rowland E, Shinebourne EA, Ward DE (1990) Endocardial pacing in infants and children 15 kg or less in weight: medium-term follow-up. Pace 13(I): 1385–1392

Timmis GC, Westveer DC, Martin R, Gordons S (1983) The significance of surface changes on explanted polyurethane pacemaker leads. Pace 6: 845–857

Tobin AM, Grodman RS, Fisherkeller M, Nicolosi R (1983) Two-dimensional echocardiographic localization of a malpositioned pacing catheter. Pace 6: 291–299

Toumbouras M, Spanos P, Konstantaras C, Lazarides DP (1982) Inferior vena cava thrombosis due to migration of retained functionless pacemaker electrode. Chest 82: 785–786

Trappe H-J, Klein H, Auricchio A, Wenzlaff P, Lichtlen PR, (1992) Catheter ablation of ventricular tachycardia: role of the underlying etiology and the site of energy delivery. Pace 15(I): 411–424

Trohman RG, Wilkoff BL, Byrne T, Cook S (1991) Successful percutaneous extraction of a chronic left ventricular pacing lead. Pace 14: 1448–1451

Uunderhill SJ, Sanders J, Davis C, Broudy D (1991) Letter to Editor – Twiddler's syndrome. Pace 14: 1555–1556

Van Erckelens F, Sigmund M, Lambertz H, Kreis A, Reupcke C, Hanrath, P (1991) Asymptomatic left ventricular malposition of a transvenous pacemaker lead through a sinus venosus defect: follow-up over 17 years. Pace 14: 989–993

Van Gelder LM, El Gamal HIH (1981) Externally induced irreversible runaway pacemaker. Pace 4: 578–581

Van Gelder L, El Gamal MIH (1983) False inhibition of an atrial demand pacemaker caused by an insulation defect in a polyurethane lead. Pace 6(I): 834–839

Van Gelder LM, El Gamal HIH (1984) Myopotential interference inducing pacemaker tachycardia in a DVI programmed pacemaker. Pace 7: 970–972

Van Haeften TW, Van Pampus ECM, Boot H, Strack-Van Schijndel RJM, Thijs LG (1988) Cardiac tamponade from misplaced central venous line in pericardophremic vein. Arch Intern Med 148: 1648–1650

Vecht RJ, Fontaine CJ, Bradfield JWB (1976) Fatal outcome arising from use of a sutureless "corkscrew" epicardial pacing electrode inserted into apex of left ventricle. Br Heart J 38: 1359–1362

Veltri EP, Mower MM, Reid PR (1984) Twiddler's syndrome: a new twist. Pace 7(I): 1004–1009

Villani GQ, Piepoli M, Quaretti P, Dieci G (1991) Cardiac pacing in unilateral left superior vena cava: evaluation by digital angiography. Pace 14(I): 1566–1567

Vrouchos GTh, Vardas PE, (1991) Sensing through the esophagus for temporary atrial synchronous ventricular VDD pacing. Pace 14(1): 511–516

Walker PR, Papouchado M, James MA, Clarke LM (1985) Pacing failure due to flecainide acetate. Pace 8: 900–902

Walsh CA, McAlister HF, Andrews CA, Steeg CN, Eisenberg R, Furman S (1988) Pacemaker implantation in children: A 21 year experience. Pace 11(II): 1940–1944

Wang RYC, Monk CK (1983) Erosion of an epicardial pacemaker secondary to postpericardiotomy syndrome. Pace 6: 33–34

Wang PJ, Ursell PC, Sosa-Suarez G, Okishige K, Friedman PL (1992) Permanent AV block or modification of AV nodal function by selective AV nodal artery ethanol infusion. Pace 15: 779–789

Watkins L Jr, Taylor E Jr (1991) The surgical aspects of automatic implantable cardioverter-defibrillator implantation. Pace 14(II): 953–960

Watkins L, Jr, Mower MM, Reid PR, Platia EV, Griffith LSC, Mirowski M (1984) Surgical techniques for implanting the automatic implantable defibrillator. Pace 7(II): 1357–1362

Waxman HL, Lazzara R, Castellanos A, El-Sherif N (1979) Ventricular pacing from the middle cardiac vein mimicking supraventricular morphology. Pace 2: 203–207

Weirich WL, Gott VL, Lillehei CW (1957) The treatment of complete heart block by the combined use of a myocardial electrode and an artificial pacemaker. Surg Forum 8: 360–363

Weiss D, Lorber A (1987) Pacemaker twiddler's syndrome. Int J Cardiol 15: 357–360

Widman WD, Edoga JK, Garfias D, McLean ER Jr (1984) Peripheral migration of pacemaker electrodes. Pace 7: 227–229

Wietholt D, Alberty J, Hindricks G, et al. (1992) Nd:YAG laser-photocoagulation:acute electrophysiological, hemodynamic, and morphological effects in large irradiated areas. Pace 15: 52–59

Wirtzfeld A (1980) The ideal site for pacemaker lead insertion? Pace 3: 485–486

Wohl B, Peters RW, Carliner N, Plotnick G, Fisher M (1982) Late unheralded pacemaker pocket infection due to *Staphylococcus epidermidis:* a new clinical entity. Pace 5: 191–195

Wunderly D, Maloney J, Edel T, McHenry M, McCarthy PM (1990) Infections in implantable cardioverter defibrillator patients. Pace 13(I): 1360–1364

Yakirevich V, Alagem D, Papo J, Vidne BA (1983) Fibrotic stenosis of the superior vena cava with widespread thrombotic occlusion of its major tributarties: an unusual complication of transvenous cardiac pacing. J Thorac Cardiovasc Surg 85: 632–638

Young D (1981) Permanent pacemaker implantation in children: current status and future considerations. Pace 4: 61–67

Zerbe F, Bornakowski J, Sarnowski W (1992) Pacemaker electrode implantation in patients with persistent left superior vena cava. Br Heart J 67: 65–66

Zipes DP, Heger JJ, Miles WM, Prystowsky EN (1984) Synchronous intracardiac cardioversion. Pace 7(II): 522–533

Zoll PM (1952) Resuscitation of the heart in ventricular standstill by electric stimulation. N Engl J Med 247: 768–771

The Pathology of Vascular Grafts

K.-M. Müller and G. Dasbach

1 Introduction

Due to a steadily growing number of patients and considerable diagnostic and therapeutic advances, vascular diseases are becoming more and more important in general and clinical practice. According to their type, localisation, severity, overall prognosis and associated illnesses, various conservative and surgical measurements are used (for survey studies see Vollmar 1982; Giessler 1987). Since the beginning of the 1950s reconstructive vascular surgery has established its position through the use of artificial prosthetic tubing.

Current Topics in Pathology
Volume 86. Ed. C. Berry

An important prerequisite for the development of synthetic vascular prostheses was the realisation that the prosthetic material must consist of porous walls made of a biologically indifferent material in order to be accepted by the organism. Numerous clinical and experimental studies have been conducted to investigate the suitability of synthetic materials such as Dacron, Ivalon, Moplen, nylon and Teflon for use in prostheses. At present, synthetic prostheses made of polyethylene terephthalate (Dacron, terylene) or expanded polytetrafluoroethylene (ePTFE is Teflon) are mainly used for prosthetic vascular replacement with alloplastic materials. Manufacturing processes for vascular prostheses have been altered in order to meet well-defined clinical requirements, and nowadays a great variety of seamless, knitted or woven tubes are available.

The key topic of this chapter is the reactive tissue alterations which follow implantation of porous, vascular prostheses into the arterial system, as assessed during different phases of incorporation. Morphological and immunohistochemical findings for Dacron and Teflon prostheses are evaluated with regard to transprosthetic organisation, degradation of synthetic material by macrophages and origin of the organisation of the developing "inner" and "outer" coats of vascular prostheses.

2 Materials and Methods

In order to analyse the pattern of incorporation of synthetic vascular prostheses into the high-pressure arterial system, 21 prostheses removed surgically and seven prostheses obtained during autopsy were examined immediately after removal. The material to be tested was removed after varying implantation periods ranging from 30 min to 10 years. Non-implanted (native) Teflon and Dacron prostheses were also studied.

The prostheses were cut transversely to the lumen. Apart from the usual fixation and staining with Haemalum and Eosin-stained paraffin sections, sections were stained with elastica–van Gieson and Goldner. Native preparations of Teflon and Dacron prostheses were not stained. Birefringent structures were well demonstrated by polarising microscopy.

Indirect avidin-biotin methods (HSU et al. 1981) were applied to demonstrate the presence of cell-bound markers. The following antigens were detected using polyclonal or monoclonal antibodies: (a) factor VIII-associated antibody (found in vascular endothelial cells in neo-angiogenic tissue); (b) LCA (monoclonal mouse anti-human leucocyte common antigen) for the differentiation of monocyte-macrophage infiltration through a reaction with surface-bound antigens located on lymphoid cells; (c) lysozyme reacting with lysozyme-positive macrophages and neutrophils and (d) α-1-antichymotrypsin, demonstrating histiocytes.

Indirect immunofluorescence microscopy was applied to paraffin sections to depict components of the extracellular matrix and to analyse their distribution pattern. Fluoro-chrome was provided by fluorescein isothiocyanate (FITC); predigestion with proteases made demonstration of antigen structures possible. We applied monospecific polyclonal antibodies against collagen type I, collagen type III, laminin and fibronectin.

Transmission polarising microscopy was applied to the demonstration of birefringent structures. Differential interference contrast microscopy was applied to further light microscopic differentiation. This permits an excellent and partly three-dimensional demonstration of the structural arrangement of synthetic fibres of the prosthetic fragments in the surrounding tissue during the process of incorporation.

Transmission polarising microscopy was used for the demonstration of birefringent structures. The application of special filter methods (red light filter, lambda filter) allowed further differentiation.

Differential-interference contrast microscopy was used for further light microscopic differentiation. In comparison with phase contrast microscopy, a much better and more representative demonstration of colourless or homogeneously stained objects is obtained. It permits an excellent and partly three-dimensional demonstration of the structural arrangement of the synthetic fibres of the prosthetic fragments in the surrounding tissue during the process of incorporation.

Scanning electron microscopy investigations were done using a DSM 940, Zeiss. The explanted prostheses were fixed with 2.5% glutaraldehyde and 1% osmium tetroxide, dehydrogenised and critical point treated. Native grafts and explanted grafts were treated by gold impregnation.

3 Survey of the Possibilities of Vascular Prostheses

The following gives a brief survey of the various types of prostheses and how they can be employed in vascular surgery. Biological prostheses include autogenic or allogenic veins or arteries and xenogenic prostheses as well as prostheses made of other biological materials, such as Lyodura. Alloplastic vascular prostheses can be classified according to the following criteria: shape, calibre, type of synthetic material, manufacturing and porosity. Furthermore, there are combined biological prostheses which are reinforced alloplastically, such as umbilical vein of Dardik or allo-autoplastic arterial prostheses, for instance the Sparks Mandril (Borchard and Loose 1980).

4 Teflon and Dacron Prostheses

The materials that may be used for arterial reconstruction are thermoplastic synthetics. Among the various types, only alloplastic synthetic prostheses made of Dacron and Teflon and autologous venous preparations have proved to be valuable, since these two synthetic materials are most suitable for arterial transplants. Alternative methods have failed for technical or biological reasons. Prostheses made of these two types of material (see Fig. 1) are nowadays regarded as the most important type of vascular replacement with regard to frequency and range of application (Borchard et al. 1980; Borchard and Loose 1980; Vollmar 1980, 1982; Giessler 1987; Sandmann and Kremer 1987).

The Teflon and Dacron prostheses examined differ fundamentally in wall structure and blood permeability. Impermeability for blood during implantation contrasts with the desire for better fibroblastic invasion, seen with highly porous prostheses. Generally speaking, it can be said that a porosity below 10 µm or above 45 µm shows adverse effects relative to blood density (10 µm) or incorporation (45µm). Dacron prostheses may be dense or woven and since structural density does not require preclotting, they are mainly used for aortic or iliac implants in patients with clotting disorders. More loosely structured, knitted prostheses made of Dacron are more suitable for implantation into the peripheral vascular system;

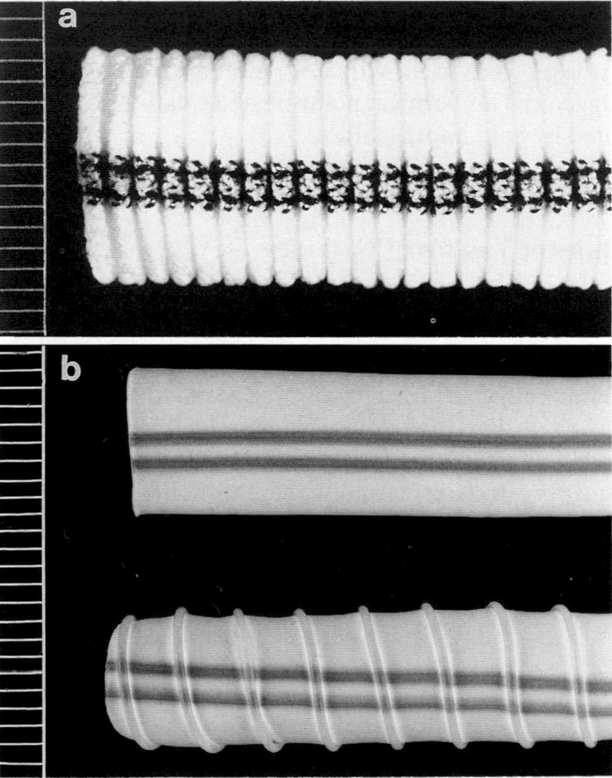

Fig. 1. Macrograph of **a** a knitted Dacron prosthesis marked with a black line. Crimping provides additional stability. **b** Two e-PTFE prostheses marked with double lines. The lower prosthesis in the picture is suitable for joint-crossing reconstructions; it possesses an outer spiral reinforcement

however, they require preliminary impregnation. Prostheses made of dense expanded polytetrafluoroethylene serve mainly as replacements for arteries with a smaller calibre (femoro-popliteal or crural), and for veins with a large calibre, and also as arteriovenous shunts (VOLLMAR 1982). To replace the horseshoe-shaped tracheal cartilages they are available with external ring or spiral reinforcements made of contrast-forming polypropylene (MÜLLER-WIEFEL 1986).

Inbuilt marking lines are designed to prevent torsion, and the prostheses are offered with calibres ranging from 0.4 to 3.5 cm, as either straight or Y-shaped synthetic tubes.

4.1 Teflon Prostheses (Expanded Polytetrafluoroethylene: e-PTFE)

Expanded polytetrafluoroethylene prostheses, which have been used since 1975 (BOYCE 1982), consist of an elongated fine-meshed PTFE tube forming a single- or double-layered structure. In some types the outer microporous part is surrounded by a very thin layer of highly porous material to prevent the formation of aneurysms. The basic molecular unit for e-PTFE is tetrafluoroethylene; this product of polymerisation has the trade name Teflon (Fluon; chemically: polytetrafluoroethylene) (VON FALKAI 1985). e (stretched)- PTFE consists of solid PTFE knots with fibrils radiating longitudinally in a herring bone pattern, forming a felt-like network. The internodal length of the fibrils ranges from 17μm to 90 μm (BOYCE 1982; VOLLMAR 1980, 1982) (see Figs. 2b and 3, parts 3 and 4).

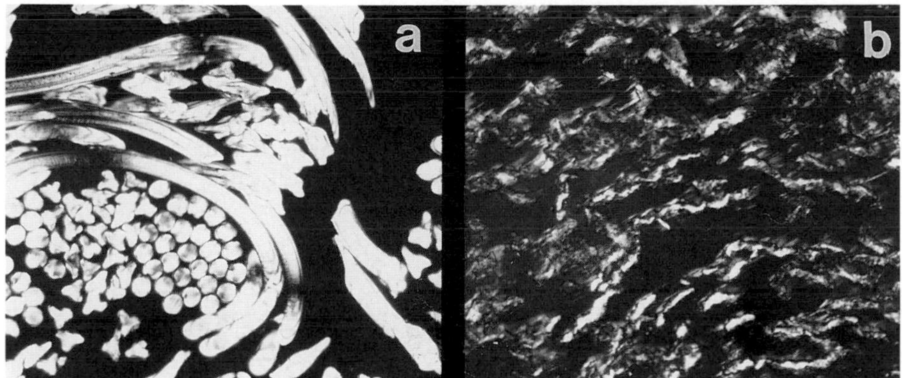

Fig. 2. Micrograph demonstrating the cross-section in plane-polarised light (native preparation, 200 ×) of **a** a woven Dacron prosthesis. Dacron fibrils and prosthetic gaps are seen. **b** Native Teflon vascular prosthesis. Demonstration of interfibrillary spaces

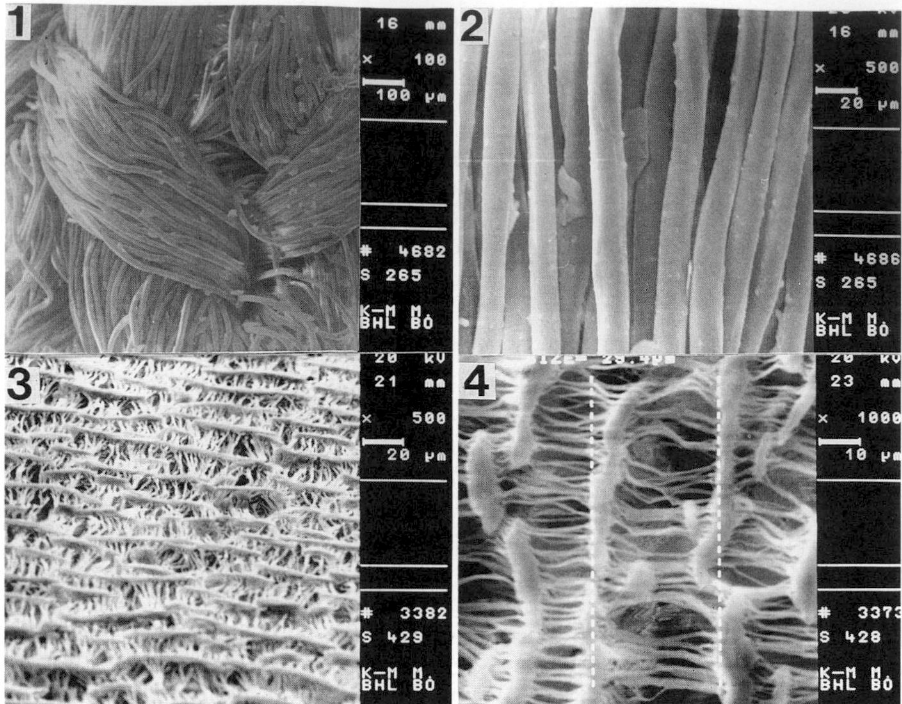

Fig. 3. Scanning electron micrographs 20 kV of: *1*, knitted Dacron prosthesis (native preparation), × 100; *2*, knitted Dacron prosthesis (native preparation), × 500; *3*, e-PTFE prosthesis (native preparation), × 500; *4*, e-PTFE prosthesis (native preparation), × 1000

4.2 Dacron Prostheses (Trevira / Diolen / Polyethylene terephthalate)

The synthetic material used for Dacron prostheses has been employed clinically since the beginning of the 1950s; the various types differ in shape, possible crimping, method of manufacture and degree of porosity. Compared with PTFE, Dacron prostheses with large pores have the advantage of better incorporation into prosthetic gaps (GUIDON et al. 1977). However, the histiocytic foreign-body reaction in the region of the outer coat is more pronounced at the beginning of the incorporation (see Figs. 2a and 3, parts 1 and 2).

5 Complications After Vascular Reconstruction

Apart from possible postoperative complications, occlusion from poor surgical technique can occur, as may formation of large perivascular haematomas in connection with coating of the transplant, or thrombus formation (VAN DONGEN

1980). A "peri-graft reaction" i.e. an aseptic, perivascular fluid accumulation, is rarely regarded as due to an excessive foreign-body reaction (KULENKAMPFF and SIMONIS 1976).

Further complications include aneurysms, haemorrhages, stenoses and detachment from the point of anchorage (cf. FORMICHI et al. 1988; TAKENAKA et al. 1985). The layer covering the inner prosthetic coat is subject to chronic recurrent degeneration resembling arterial sclerosis (SPERLING 1976; MARNACH 1988). Regressive alteration caused by a dissection of the inner layer may lead to distal embolism or recurring thrombus formation. As long ago as 1962, Wesolowski reported on fissuration or degeneration of the material of the prosthesis.

Apart from those complications described above, the use of alloplastic vascular transplants has limitations due to intrinsic "biological weaknesses": the loss of lumen due to the formation of the inner coat, loss of flexibility due to solidification, defective or completely deficient endothelial covering (especially after the age of 50) and degeneration of the inner capsule.

6 Microscopic Structure of Native Prostheses

We have found that the fibrous and porous synthetic tube, together with its free prosthetic gaps, serves as a fundamental frame for incorporation. The architectural arrangement of the organic tissue adapts to the interfibrous gaps. In cross-sections through native preparations of grid or arcade-like e-PTFE prostheses, interfibrous spaces become visible together with nodules in the shape of illuminated areas, which are typical of this type of prosthesis; delicately extended Teflon fibres can be seen in between. Using the same type of incision and thickness on Dacron prostheses, it becomes evident that the prosthetic gaps are situated adjacent to the fibrillar arrangement of the synthetic filamentous bundles. The fibres themselves can be seen as transversely and longitudinally arranged fibrils of homogeneous structure.

7 Morphological Changes After Implantation of Alloplastic Vascular Prostheses

The processes following implantation of synthetic vascular prostheses bring about fibrous tissue encapsulation of the transplant. Generally speaking, the endogenous tissue reactions to Teflon or Dacron are similar to the incorporation of inert, aseptic foreign bodies. There were only slight differences in the reaction patterns, and only the most obvious morphological deviations will be described in detail here. In order to gain a more detailed knowledge of the processes of incorporation, components of the extracellular matrix (collagen type I, collagen type III, laminin and fibronectin) were demonstrated by means of immunofluorescence microscopy and scanning electron microscopy during the various phases of incorpora-

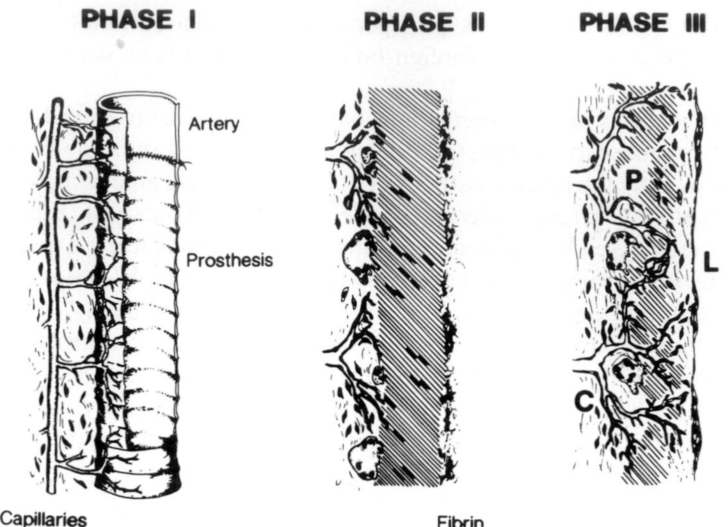

Fig. 4. Schema of the three phases of incorporation. Phase I: Longitudinally cut prosthesis with surrounding soft tissue coat; proliferation of capillaries toward prosthesis. Phase II: the *hatched area* represents intact prosthetic structures; in the lumen on the *right*, capillary buds are beginning to develop activation of the reticulo-endothelial system. Phase III: Sporadic transprosthetic capillarisation, degradation of the prosthesis, increased foreign body reaction and fibrosing connective tissue in the outer and inner prosthetic coats. *P*, prosthesis; *C*, capillary; *L*, lumen

tion. Immunohistochemical characterisation of cellular infiltration allowed complementary statements about typical reaction patterns and interactions between the extracellular matrix and the mesenchymal cellular components.

The incorporation of alloplastic vascular material follows a chronological pattern and can be subdivided into early, organisation and late (scarring) phases (Fig. 4). However, morphologically comprehensible alterations during the individual phases can overlap.

7.1 Early Phase (Phase I)

The early phase starts at the time of implantation and ends after approximately 2 weeks. Depending on the degree of porousness, the prostheses are either impregnated with the patients' blood before implantation or after implantation of a so-called primarily blood-dense prosthesis and release of blood flow. Some are impregnated with a fibrin-rich exudate and blood components. In the perivascular region, a small periprosthetic haematoma usually forms during this phase.

7.1.1 Morphology of the Early Phase

The inner surface of the vascular replacement is covered by a fibrinous film of varying thickness. In the region of the anastomoses, this type of coating can be particularly well developed and may lead to an early clinically relevant decrease in blood flow, which in turn can be enhanced by cell proliferation of an adjacent artery. All preparations with a blood flow duration of only 30 min show slight penetration by fibrin and protein, as well as an accretion of erythrocytes and white blood cells. All prostheses which have been exposed to blood flow for an hour show penetration of the gaps in the wall of the prostheses by fibrin, protein and erythrocytes. On the luminal side isolated round cells and granulocytes are found whose concentration is equivalent to that of the flowing blood. The perivascular haematoma initially formed is resorbed within the first few days after implantation. It is replaced by loose granulation tissue after approximately 1–2 weeks (see Fig. 10).

At this point a degree of attachment to the surrounding tissue is accomplished. During this phase the outer coat tends to grow towards the prostheses. While the organism is dealing with the synthetic implant, the inevitable chronic inflammation is weakly developed. Initially general postoperative inflammatory reactions predominate; however, typical features of granulation tissue can be recognised during the early phase and are preserved throughout the following phases. While the tissue components of the inner and outer coats arrange themselves concentrically, all tissue components in the intraprosthetic region react in exactly the opposite way: they have a radial arrangement. This observation applies to both cellular and extracellular components.

7.1.2 Examination of the Cellular Reaction Pattern

The intraluminal prosthetic fibrin accretions are of varying thickness and contain just a small number of neutrophil granulocytes, lymphocytes or plasma cells. Some lysozyme-positive macrophages can be seen here and there in the outer organisation tissue at the end of the first week. The morphological structure of the inner coat changes slightly during this phase. At the beginning of the early phase (30 min to 24 h) there is an accretion of erythrocytes and other blood cells in the prosthetic gaps. After the resorption of the haematoma which formed around the prosthesis, a continuous rearrangement starts in the perivascular region on approximately the second postoperative day. Granulocytes, which have predominated up to this point, are now degraded and are only sporadically found in the inner and outer coating. In addition to the activation of the reticulo-endothelial system, a perivascular increase in lymphocytes and plasma cells within the delicate fibrin framework is observed. There is also an increase in the number of monocytes, whose nuclei become enlarged and lysozyme-positive. Foreign-body giant cells have not yet appeared, and it is only from day 12 onwards that perivascular macrophages are seen. These fuse to become multinucleated giant cells and factor VIII-positive capillary precursors. In the peripheral region early fibroblasts become visible.

7.1.3 Characterisation of the Extracellular Matrix

In addition to those components located in the anastomotic tisssue of the extracellular matrix, only delicate, fibrous and sparse collagen type III can be found at the beginning of phase I. It is attached to the outer prosthetic structures of the anastomosis. Collagen type I, laminin and fibronectin cannot be identified during the first few days. From the fourth day onwards small amounts of collagen type I and type III are found. Collagen type I is seen in the form of a thin inner lining above the inner coat and as delicate, fibrous material between the synthetic structures. It is noteworthy that the Dacron fibrils arranged in bundles bear some deposition, mainly on the lengthwise fibrils. Collagen type III displays a different distribution pattern. It is only found in intraprosthetic and perivascular regions. Again, a pronounced arrangement around the longitudinally orientated, Dacron fibrils is found; however, the deposits have a rather focal cushion-like arrangement and a higher distribution density. At this point laminin is present in the same concentration as collagen type I and type III along the longitudinally arranged fibres. Laminin can even be demonstrated in the vicinity of the anastomoses. On the other hand, the distribution of fibronectin is similar to that of collagen type I and type III, but the accretions are more dense and are not yet demonstrable in the prosthetic part of the anastomosis.

As the duration of the implantation period increases, the amount of matrix components within the prosthetic gaps increases rapidly (between the 5th and 14th days).

7.2 Organisation Phase (Phase II)

The organisation phase starts approximately 2 weeks after implantation and lasts for up to 6 months.

7.2.1 Morphology of the Organisation Phase

After approximately 2–3 weeks the developing granulation tissue penetrates the prosthetic mesh (Fig. 5). The texture of the newly formed connective tissue framework adapts to the delicate reticulated prosthetic structures. The cell-rich granulation tissue develops, in a varying temporal sequence, a mesenchymal tissue which is rich in fibres but lacking in cells. Organisation of the extravascular part of the prosthesis is often complete after 3–4 weeks, leading to a firm connective

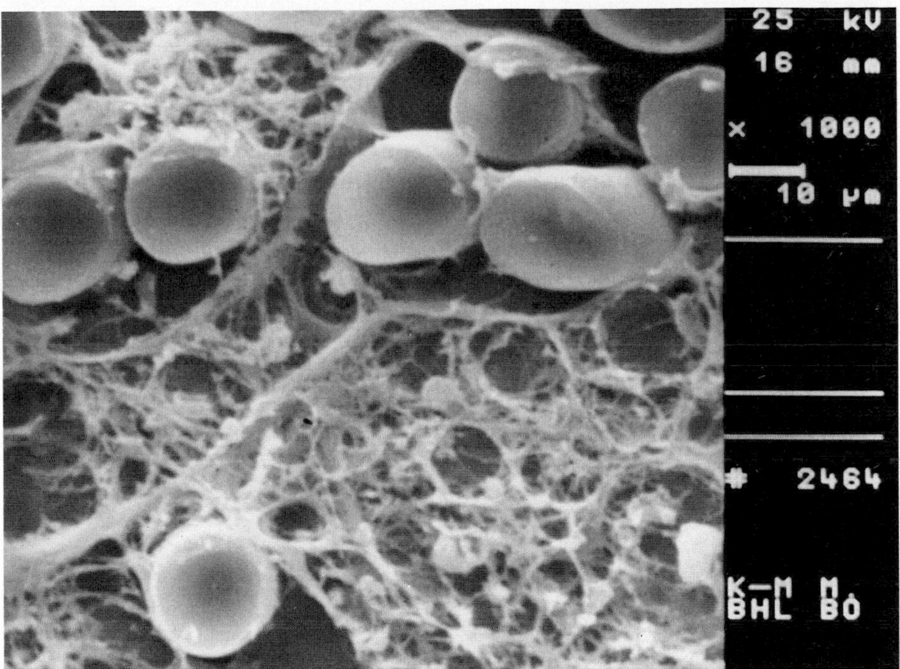

Fig. 5. Scanning electron micrograph. Cross-section showing delicate fibrous connective tissue between the fibres of a Dacron vascular prosthesis that had been implanted for 17 days × 1000

tissue attachment of the transplant. Mesenchymal proliferation of the tissue forming the outer coat into the prosthetic gaps continues. Intravascular fibrin accretions which were formed during the early phase detach and new accretions are laid down. The inner surface is now characterised by areas without any coating or by map-like deposits. These processes last for varying periods of time and show remarkable differences in intensity in different patients. In almost all implants, transformation processes in the outer and inner coats lead to the formation of loosely arranged fibrous tissue. There is an occasional excessive formation of inner prosthetic lining, with a progressive growth of thrombi which may require removal in case of obstruction without lysis or recanalisation. Deficiency of the endothelial lining is regarded as the main cause of possible thrombus formation in alloplastic prostheses. From phase II onwards endothelialisation is only seen near anastomoses, in the form of tongue-shaped proliferations derived from the original vascular endothelium and extending over the inner prosthetic lining. At the end of this phase of organisation a clear distinction can be made between the inner and outer limitations of the prosthesis and the lumen and the transplant bed. At this point the prosthesis is firmly anchored.

7.2.2 Examination of the Cellular Reaction Pattern

At the beginning of this phase an increased number of round cells, lymphocytes, plasma cells and smaller macrophages are found in the inner coat of the prosthesis (Fig. 6). Occasionally, small capillary precursors can be detected using factor VIII-associated antigen. A marked increase in the number of foreign body giant cells, which are quite rare up to this point, is seen after 4 weeks. The number of fibroblasts present is also increased, and these tissue changes occur in the inner coat in a much less evident form than in the outer coat. Endothelialisation can only be detected in areas near the anastomoses. The myoendothelial cells of endogenous arteries proliferate. Tongue-shaped or pannus-like areas form, possibly taking their origin from the changes in flow associated with localised currents or increased fibrin deposits, and may lead to occlusion of the vascular replacement. Delicate filamentous connective tissue can be seen in the interfibrillary prosthetic gaps,

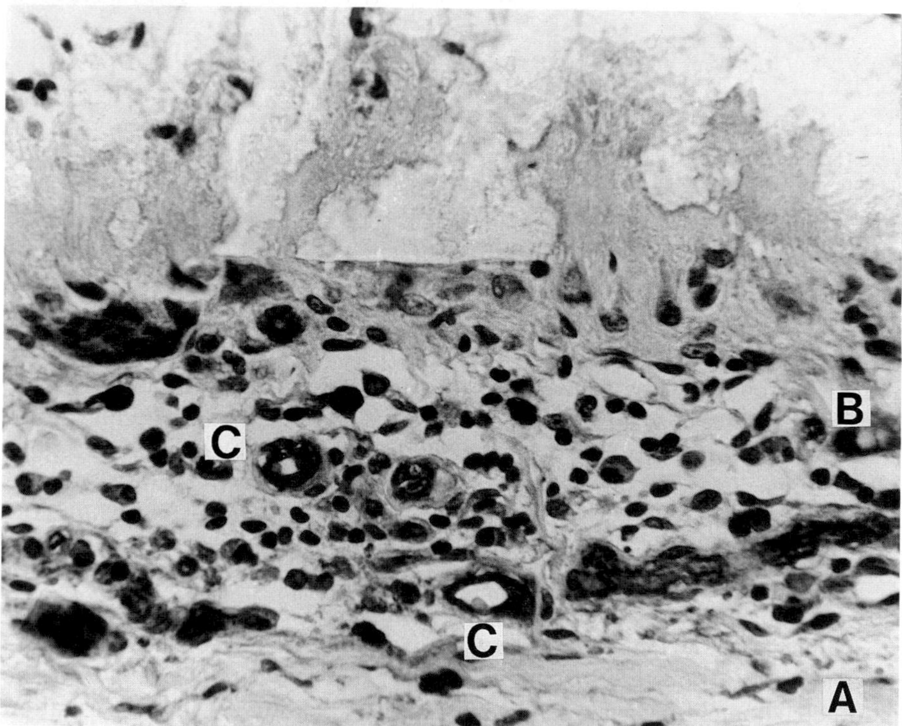

Fig. 6. Micrograph of the outer zone of a 3-month-old Teflon prosthesis in a 64-year-old woman with occlusive arterial disease. *A*, Outer prosthetic zone of organisation including the incorporation of fibrin, matrix structures, blood cells and fibroblasts between degraded synthetic fibres. *B*, Accumulation of monocytes, multinucleated giant cells and fibroblasts on the surface of the prosthesis between filamentous matrix structures. *C*, Demonstration of newly formed capillaries in the region of reactive inflammation by the use of factor VIII-associated antigen. Avidin-biotinbinding method with factor VIII-associated antigen. × 350

particularly in the outer third. Monocytes and macrophages from the inner and the outer connective tissue capsule have penetrated into the prosthesis. Neovascularisation continues. Capillaries and their precursors proliferate and show a general tendency towards confluency and dilatation. Initial vascular precursors penetrate as far as the outer prosthetic gaps. A marked accumulation of meganucleated macrophages, isolated monocytes, lymphocytes and plasma cells occurs in the transitional region near the outer third of the prosthesis. At the same time a steadily increasing number of foreign body giant cells are found.

Overall the cellular reaction within the outer fibrous tissue is much more pronounced than that within the inner prosthetic lining. Only a small number of cells can be detected here, predominantly lymphocytes and plasma cells, with scanty infiltration of fibroblasts and macrophages (Fig. 7). The periprosthetic tissue at this point shows a dense circle of lysozyme-positive reticulo-endothelial-cells very close to the synthetic structures of the outer third of the vascular prosthesis. Occasionally, foreign body giant cells which have phagocytosed small synthetic particles can be seen (Figs. 8–10).

The larger factor VIII-positive vessels derived from gap-like cavities and capillaries within the outer coat display a markedly close spatial relationship with

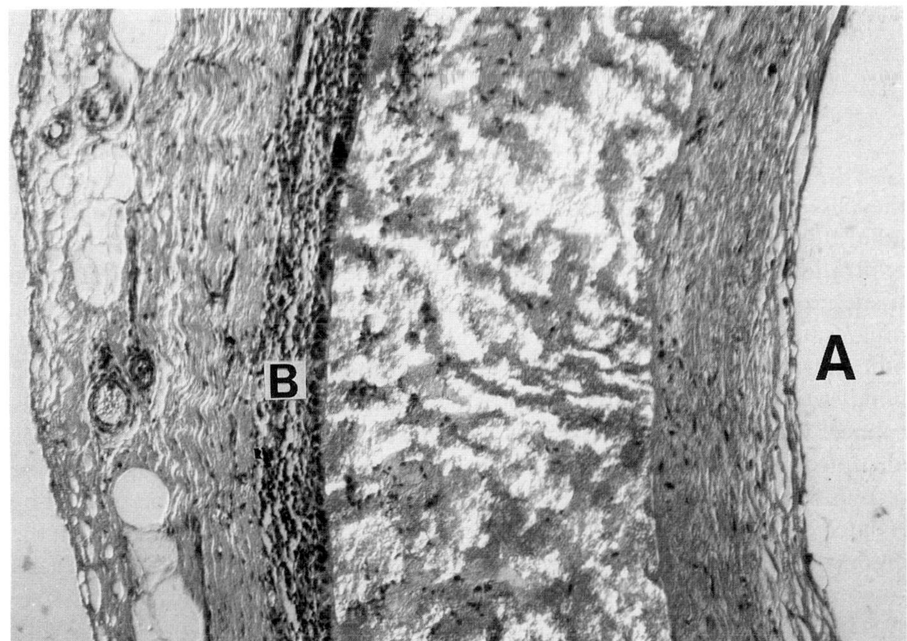

Fig. 7. Micrograph illustrating a cross-section of a Teflon prosthesis implanted for 12 months in a 52-year-old man with occlusive arterial disease. *A*, The inner coating with a mesenchymal proliferation. Between the birefringent prosthetic substances a fibrous connective tissue has formed. *B*, The macrophages and multinucleated foreign body giant cells are seen penetrating from the outer and inner capsule into the interspaces. Plane polarised light, H&E, × 220

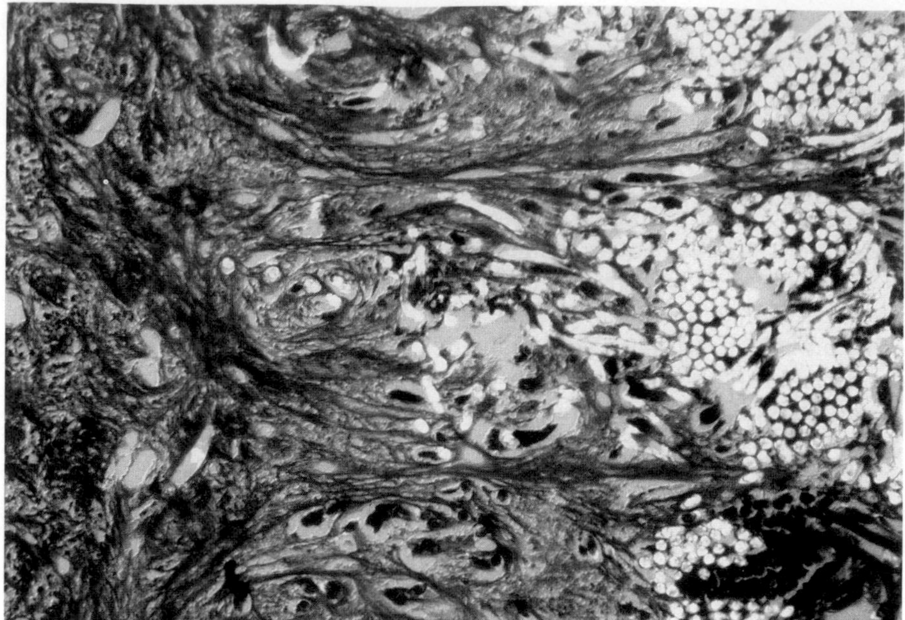

Fig. 8. Micrograph of a Dacron vascular prosthesis, implanted for 12 months in a 78-year-old man with occlusive arterial disease. There is advanced degradation and incorporation of fibres and fragments of fibres by multinucleated giant cells of the foreign body type. H&E, × 110

the cells of the reticulo-endothelial system. In some cases a moderate inflammatory infiltrate is seen in the granulation tissue and is accompanied by loose cellular infiltration of plasma cells and lymphocytes. Delicate filamentous connective tissue, cross-linked to the synthetic fibres, develops transprosthetically during the organisation phase. A distinctive arrangement can be identified between the cut outer fibrous coat and the outer third of the prosthesis, where delicate, fan-shaped bundles of fibres radiate into the prosthetic gaps (Fig. 11). They subsequently connect with the delicate, transprosthetically situated fibrous tissue and can be identified in the late phase. In the outer fibrous coat, macrophages can be recognised penetrating into the prosthetic gaps. The inner coat is permeated by isolated cells; however, this cellular reaction is much less pronounced than in the outer coat. On both sides a tendency towards migration into the prosthetic gaps can be seen. The thinning of the prosthetic structures is particularly impressive.

There is a gradual difference between Teflon and Dacron prostheses with respect to the foreign body giant cell reactions in the transitional zone between the inner capsule and the synthetic structures: Dacron prostheses show a marked accumulation during the organisation phase, whereas similar processes in Teflon prostheses are only rarely observed at this stage.

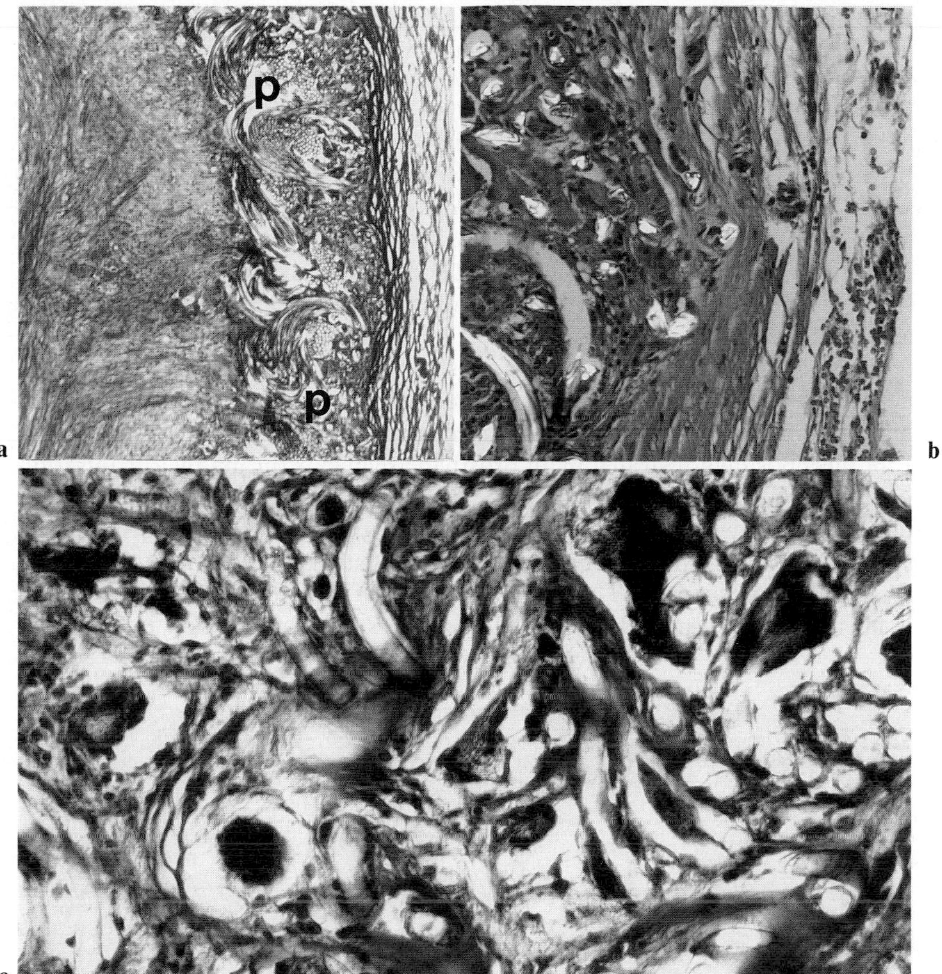

Fig. 9. a,b Overall view with outer capsule. **c** Detail: Multinucleated foreign body giant cells beside fibres and fragments of the Dacron vascular prosthesis

7.2.3 Characterisation of the Extracellular Matrix

In contrast to the relatively small amounts of matrix components synthesised during the early phase of incorporation, greater amounts of extracellular matrix are demonstrable during the organisation phase. Collagen type I can be seen as delicate filamentous or trabecular deposits found mainly in the outer third of the fibrous inner coat of the Teflon or Dacron prostheses. There is remarkably close spatial relationship with the heavy cellular infiltrate of monocytes and macrophages during this phase of incorporation. Collagen type I, synthesised by fibroblasts and macrophages, is deposited transprosthetically along longitudinally and transversely sectioned fibrils of Dacron prostheses, and in some circumscribed areas it assumes a cushion-like arrangement within the prosthetic gaps. In Teflon prostheses, however, collagen type I can be found as cushion-like deposits around isolated "cloud-like" Teflon structures. In the outer capsule the amount of collagen type I is comparable to that found in the inner coat and can be seen as trabecular deposits. Macrophages in the immediate vicinity of collagen are also seen. Collagen type III deposits display a distribution pattern comparable to that of collagen type I, as well as a similar distribution density. However, in the transitional region between the inner coat and the lumen a sickle-shaped arrangement can be seen whereas between synthetic structures a rather filamentous arrangement is common.

The synthesis and deposition of these matrix structures most often can be demonstrated near macrophages. In the periphery of multinucleated foreign body giant cells only very delicate filamentous collagen type III structures are identified. Fibronectin is demonstrated in all prosthetic segments during the organisation phase, becoming evident in the inner capsule as a trabeculated lining and as a delicate frame-work in the filamentous connective tissue. Less pronounced synthesis and deposition are found in the prosthetic gaps and in the connective tissue of the outer capsule. The distribution pattern is of interest in that fibronectin is always found near newly formed vessels. Neovascularisation is especially

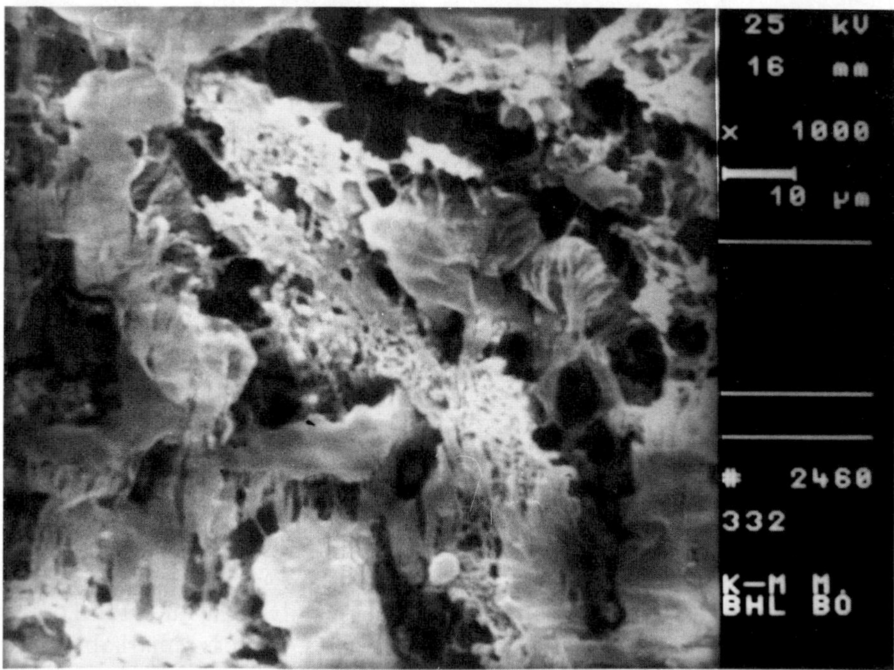

Fig. 10. Scanning electron micrograph of a Teflon vascular prosthesis implanted for 9 days. Delicate filamentous connective tissue with fibrin deposits and structures of the extracellular matrix extend between the interspaces of the Teflon particles. × 1000

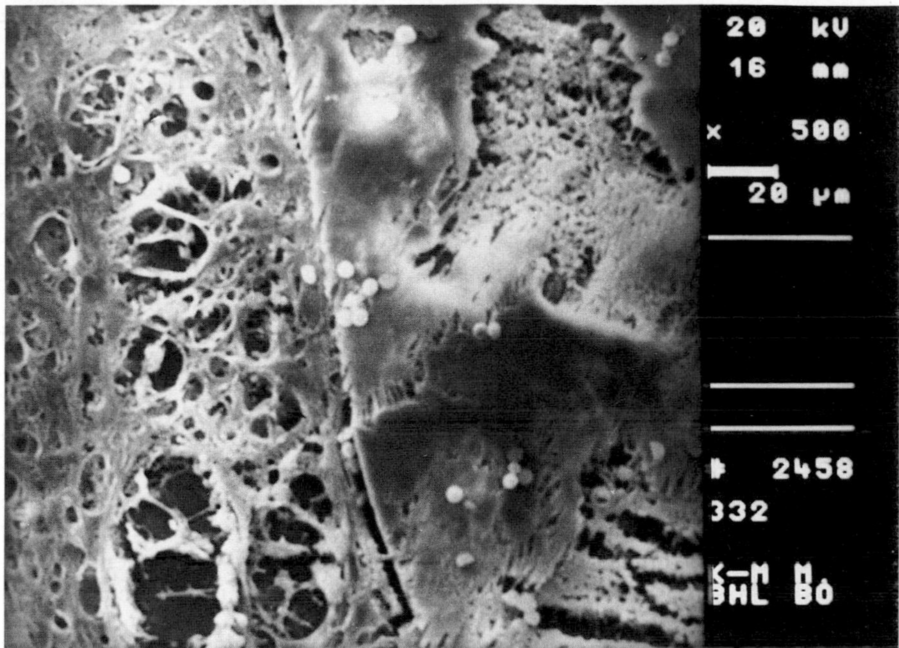

Fig. 11. Scanning electron micrograph of a Teflon vascular prosthesis implanted for 3 months. Fibrous and partly reticular structures are situated between the Teflon gaps and on the left side in the outer layer. × 500

pronounced during this phase. The glyco-protein laminin is deposited in the form of discrete, delicate lines on the synthetic structures and also on the basal membrane of the newly formed vessels. If a thrombus or connective tissue causes total or subtotal luminal occlusion, then a massive, focal accumulation of reticulated fibronectin or laminin is found in those parts of former thrombi where organisation is taking place. Organised thrombi are only slightly permeated by a cellular infiltration of neutrophil granulocytes, plasma cells, endothelial cells and isolated fibroblasts. The initial vascularisation of transprosthetic gaps, which can often be observed at this point during the incorporation, is clearly indicative of laminin accumulation. It is also worth mentioning that in the spiral reinforcements of Teflon vascular prostheses laminin and fibronectin are identified in the form of highly delicate fringes, and collagen type I as a delicate reticular structure around the spiral reinforcement.

7.3 Late (Scarring) Phase (Phase III)

7.3.1 Morphology of the Late Phase

After incorporation without complications the late phase is reached 6 months after implantation. It is characterised by decreasing mesenchymal activity on the outside of the prosthesis. Mesenchymal tissue which is rich in fibres and poor in cells can be seen here and is best demonstrated by scanning electron microscopy (Figs. 12–14). An occasional loosening of the prosthetic structure can be observed. Active mesenchymal proliferation of a less obvious extent can now be observed only within the inner coating.

7.3.2 Examination of the Cellular Reaction Pattern

The inner coating of the vascular prosthesis displays mesenchymal proliferation, including macrophages, monocytes, confluent capillaries and blood vessels. Occasionally multinucleated foreign body giant cells can be seen in this area, and in some cases also within the area of a monocyte/macrophage border at the point of transition to the synthetic structures. Those areas within the lumen which are not covered by cells can be coated with myoendothelial cells or fibroblasts. In addition, fine, transitory fibrinous membranes or thrombi are still formed at this point. Sporadically, the overall loosely structured mesenchymal tissue is permeated by lymphocytes and plasma cells. In those segments with longer existing cellular coats, collagen fibres are formed, and at the points of prosthetic attachment elastic fibres are also developed. Capillarisation continues discretely within

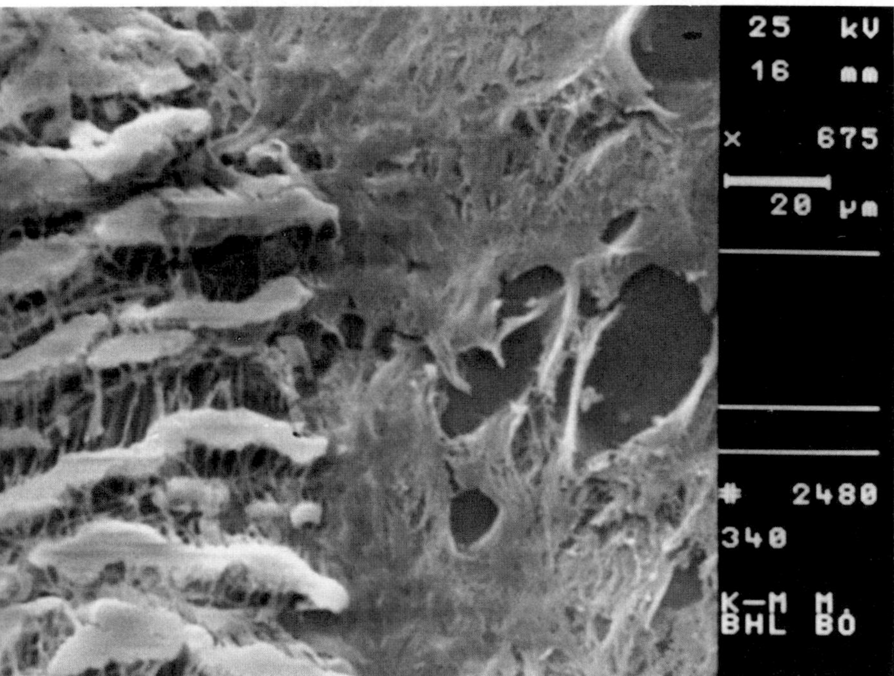

Fig. 12. Scanning electron micrograph. Cross-section of a Teflon vascular prosthesis implanted for 10 years demonstrating reticular dense connective tissue (*right*) in the outer capsule. × 675

the prosthetic gaps. A demonstration of birefringent material within the cytoplasm of cells of the reticulo-endothelial system is not as frequent on the luminal side as in the outer fibrous coat. Delicate fibrous connective tissue has formed within the prosthesis (see Fig. 5). Macrophages and multinucleated foreign body giant cells penetrating from the outer and inner capsule are directly attached to the synthetic particles. During increasing periods of incorporation, further degradation of synthetic particles continues to take place. Sometimes varying distances between fibres and fibrils are seen due to phagocytosis and clearance.

In several Teflon vascular prosthesis implantations of long duration, gap-like voids filled with Teflon particles were found within the outer coat. In the peripheral region of these spaces, massive accumulations of macrophages and foreign body giant cells are found. However, the synthetic particles are rarely situated intracellularly. Apart from these "streets", which are often perpendicularly orientated to the ring-like Teflon structures, a concentric border can be demonstrated around the prosthesis, this border being composed of detached Teflon fragments. An accumulation of cells of the reticulo-endothelial system is particularly evident in the vicinity of detached Teflon fragments. These reaction patterns are always found in connection with degradation and thus thinning of the prosthetic frame. If there is a greater distance between the pores, capillaries push forward into the

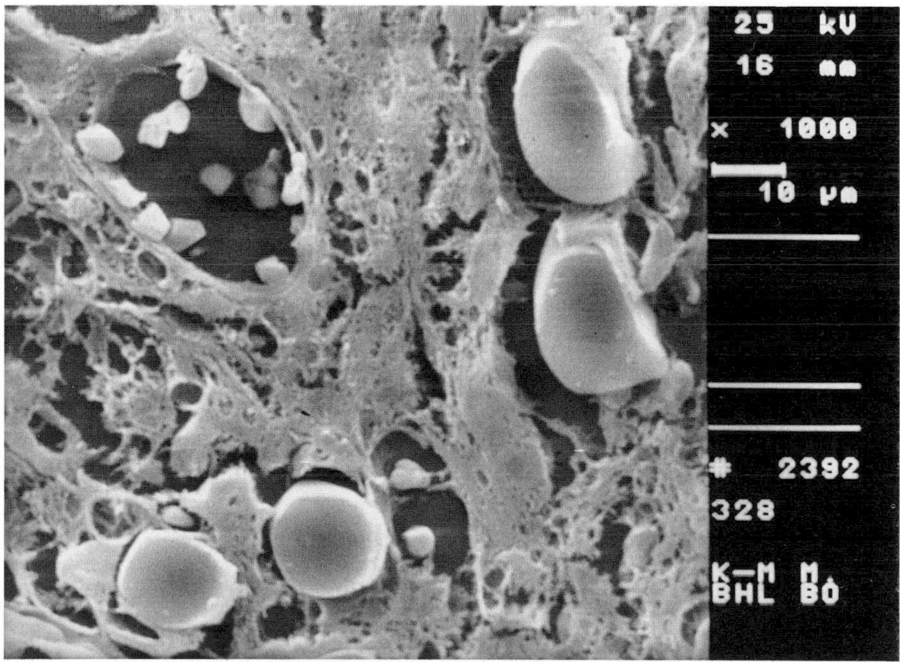

Fig. 13. Scanning electron micrograph. Cross-section of a Dacron vascular prosthesis implanted for 2 years. Dense connective tissue and small capillaries are seen between the Dacron fibres. × 1000

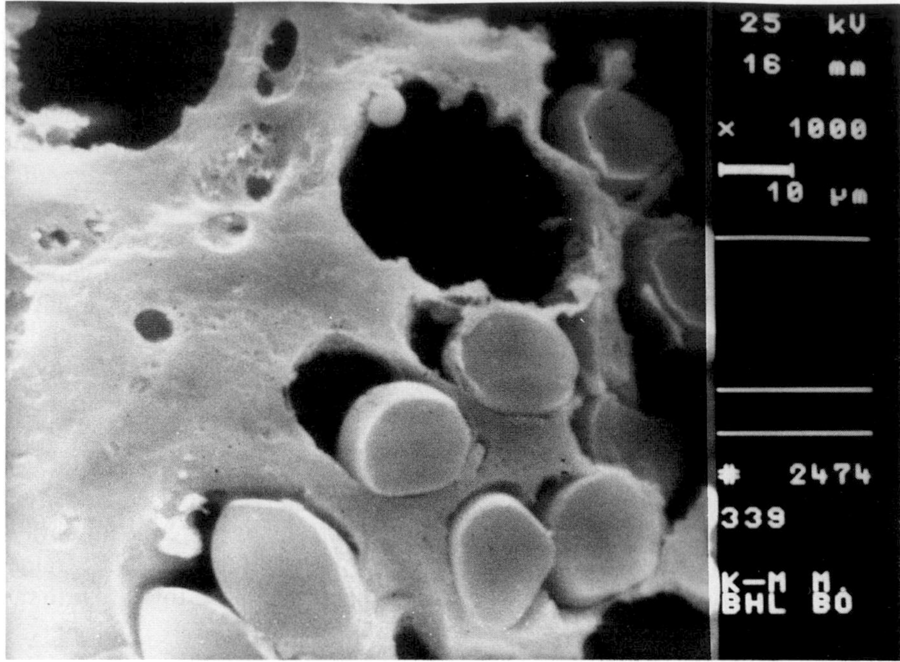

Fig. 14. Scanning electron micrograph. Cross-section after implantation for 6 years. Between the Dacron fibres there is very dense fibrous tissue with occasional capillarisation. × 1000

inner layer of the prosthesis and partly anastomose with small blood vessels growing inwards from the inner capsule. Thus an occasional capillarisation is brought about, which leads to the formation of isolated endothelial islets on the luminal side. A continuous coating with endothelial cells, however, cannot be demonstrated within the inner capsule. In the dense, fibril-rich connective tissue of the outer coat, an almost regular circle of monocytes, macrophages and foreign body giant cells is formed only in the transitional region of the prosthesis (Fig. 12). Vascular proliferation has largely reached a standstill. Vessels of a large relative calibre derived from capillaries and capillary precursors are demonstrable (Fig. 13). At the end of the scarring phase the prosthesis is firmly connected to the surrounding tissue by cell-poor but fibre-rich connective tissue and lined by fibrous tissue; it can function well for years (Fig. 14). In addition to findings of chronic inflammation, however, an increased tendency to proliferation of the inner capsule or recurring thrombotic complications is found.

7.3.3 Characterisation of the Extracellular Matrix

During the late phase, which is characterised by decreasing proliferation, collagen type I can only be recognised as fine, delicate, fibrous and trabeculated accretions within the inner and outer coat and reticular structures near the synthetic fibrils.

Again, greater deposits are seen near the cells of the reticulo-endothelial system. Comparable amounts of type I and type III collagen are found in the tissue of the inner and outer capsule. Intraprosthetically only tongue-shaped or maculate deposits are identifiable; longitudinally cut Dacron fibrils are occasionally surrounded by a broad border of type III collagen. Some of the foreign body giant cells are recognised by the surrounding fibrillated type III collagen. Laminin is only detected in vessels in the inner and outer tissue coats; here, however, an intensive accumulation of finely structured material can be seen. In prostheses with older thrombi undergoing organisation, a delicately trabeculated and diffuse arrangement of laminin is found, and like thrombi which have reached an equivalent level of organisation, an extensive accumulation of fibronectin can be seen. Fibroblasts and endothelial cell accumulations can be identified in these thrombi. Fibronectin itself shows a non-uniform distribution pattern. It is mostly evident as a thin, filamentous, inner luminal lining and as a delicate fibrous network between the synthetic particles. However, the intensity of its accumulation varies. In some Teflon and Dacron prostheses almost all gaps are filled; in others, however, only isolated and sparse deposits can be seen. If fibronectin is found in the mesenchymal tissue surrounding the prosthesis, its arrangement is always predominantly perivascular.

8 Discussion

Although there is extensive documentation in respect of alloplastic arterial prostheses, the processes involved in their incorporation still raise questions. The tissue reactions seen, including phagocytosis of foreign body material, have been examined with respect to degradation of prosthetic material and its possible removal, raising questions about the various possibilities for cell transformation and activation of the reticulo-endothelial monocyte-macrophage system. The interactions between organism and implanted synthetic vascular prosthesis represent an exceptional state. There is, initially, neither an elaborate tissue architecture resembling that in the surrounding stroma, nor a localised cellular response in the prosthetic gaps. Nevertheless, it seems justified to compare the fibrous infiltration of the implant with the processes leading to the formation of granulation tissue – which means to compare it with the general pathology of inflammation. From a modern point of view there are basically two possible ways to bring about tissue formation, a regular arrangement of the extracellular matrix and a corresponding arrangement of two binding sites for the cellular components.

Tissue can be derived from cells of neighbouring tissue. The proliferation of local cells at the implantation site with a continuous building-up of extracellular cells allows the ingrowth of cells into the prosthetic spaces. After primary migration of individual blood-borne cells over short distances, a secondary connection to cells and matrix of the local tissue follows. Subsequently various cell types can be transformed and contribute to the formation of extra-cellular matrix. Migration, however, requires the presence of mechanisms which specifically attract cells, for instance chemotaxis or thigmotaxis within the structures of the matrix. The extracellular matrix constitutes a loose network of large, extracellulary located organic molecules, which consist predominantly of protein fibres and polysaccharide molecules. They are secreted locally, mostly by fibroblasts. These structures used to be regarded as a relatively inert frame whose function was to stabilise the tissue; nowadays its much more active function, and complex influence on the behaviour of cells which are in contact with it, has been recognised. The matrix is said to have the ability to influence development, migration, multiplication and morphological and metabolic functions of cells. Knowledge of the complex interactions, molecular composition and structure is still fragmentary. In our investigations the laminin identified was only evident in the basal membranes of newly formed vessels. Its main biological characteristic is the ability to attach to fibroblasts and epithelial cells (AUMAILLEY et al. 1983; FOIDART et al. 1982), and VAHERI et al. (1983) observed inhibition of fibroblastic growth by laminin.

8.1 Interactions Between Matrix and Cells

Fibronectin is demonstrable during the various phases of prosthetic incorporation. In its capacity as a binding protein it can either inhibit or promote fibroblastic growth, can cause formation of an endothelial single layer, and can initiate capillary budding (POTT et al. 1982, 1983; VAHERI et al. 1983). It appears that fibronectin plays an important part as a connecting link between the cells and connective tissue matrix. It promotes cell adhesion, and it can be detected in high concentrations in regions of increased cellular migration. Its chemotactic influence on connective tissue cells explains its particular importance in wound healing (VOSS et al. 1980; VOSS and RAUTERBERG 1985).

In connection with the synthetic structures of the prostheses which we have examined, it is worth mentioning that fibronectin can complex with these filamentous structures, and can opsonise synthetic particles to bring about later phagocytosis. SIMONIS and KOCH (1980) also found intracellular uptake of birefringent substances as a result of their experiments with Dacron prostheses which were opsonised. The demonstrated synthesis and distribution pattern of fibronectin, laminin and collagen types I and III, in addition to the arrangement of the cellular infiltration during the various phases of incorporation of vascular prostheses, show that a strong interaction exists between cells and extracellular matrix at a very early stage (from day 4 on), reaching a peak on day 14. In our investigations, however, no identifiable structures were found within the prosthetic gaps during the early organisation phase. It is generally presumed that the cytoskeleton of the cell and the secreted matrix molecules possess the ability to organise each other. If, however, those cells which produce the extracellular matrix come into contact with synthetic surfaces like Teflon or Dacron, they start producing less glycogen and proteoglycans (TERRANOVA et al. 1983). The basal cell surface becomes irregular, the intracellular order is disturbed, and the cytoskeleton is deformed (compare also YAMADA 1982, 1983). Our findings seem to support these observations since the fibrous organisation of the vascular prosthesis was delayed in comparison with the formation of regular granulation tissue. While cells attach themselves to basal membranes or other extracellular macromolecules which are present at a later stage, no alteration of the intracellular arrangement was observed. It must be noted, however, that fibronectin is known to be connected to intracellularly located fibroblastic actin filaments. In regularly structured connective tissue, an identical, longitudinal alignment of cells is found, and similar observations were made with respect to the distribution of collagen among fibroblasts.

It can be concluded that a high degree of order within the cell can be transferred to the extracellular matrix, constituting the centre of formation and preservation of cellular patterns. Matrix molecules bound to the cell surface have both binding and adaptational functions in the interaction between cells and matrix during these processes of organisation. Under the assumption that the matrix components are interconnected in forms of different three-dimensional structures and that their arrangement is partly governed by matrix synthesising cells, it can be concluded that the developing cellular organisation is passed on from cell to cell by means of the matrix, leading to typical morphological reaction patterns. Possible proof of such order within new tissues was found in the form of "cell locks" on the outer surface of our vascular prostheses. This structural arrangement found in the extracellular matrix was almost always demonstrable after infiltration of fibroblasts into the prosthetic spaces.

8.2 Matrix Structures During the Various Phases of Implantation

8.2.1 Early Phase (Phase I)

The events occurring during the initial phase after implantation can be compared with the exudative-inflammatory reactions of acute inflammation. In contrast to wound healing, the infiltrating granulocytes and macrophages within the innermost part of the prosthesis are not involved in degradation and removal of necrobiotic tissue, since only fibrin and proteins were found on the luminal aspect and intraprosthetically. A different situation occurred in the outer prosthetic layer. Here the perivascular haematoma and the subordinate wound area were contiguous. Cells migrating from the wound area reached the perivascular haematoma and soon became responsible for the production of collagen and non-collagenous glycoproteins. A subsequent narrowing of the wound gap was observed. During these changes, platelet-derived growth factor which is stored in thrombocytes, displays a chemotactic effect on fibroblasts and neutrophilic granulocytes and plays an important role in the cellular reaction pattern. Our findings show differences in time with respect to the identification of fibroblasts and capillary precursors; these are explained by the different conditions prevailing in the lumen and on the outside of the vascular prosthesis. All subsequent morphological changes taking place in the inner coat which were observed in our investigations became obvious much later and at a modest intensity. From the 12th day of the early phase on, fibroblasts and capillary precursors and foreign body giant cells were identified in periprosthetic regions; they obviously permeated from the surrounding tissue, and grew in.

It is noteworthy that during the early phase there is no cellular infiltration in the prosthetic gaps, but rather an initial focal permeation of proteinaceous material, fibrin and erythrocytes. Cottier et al. (1980) pointed out that neutrophilic granulocytes possess a great locomotive ability, but their energy requirements depend mostly on anaerobic glycolysis and thus disturbances of the extracellular and subsequent cellular metabolism can lead to a decrease in the number of cells (compare also Bremm and König 1988) and blood-borne neutrophilic granulocytes do not penetrate the prosthetic gaps despite the absence of normal vascular membrane in artificial vascular replacements. Different metabolic conditions are found in the prosthetic gaps and in the transplant bed, compared with surrounding tissue, since neither vessels nor capillaries exist at the beginning of the early phase to provide a natural nutritional environment. Initial capillary precursors were identified in the outer coat even before the end of the first week. Gabbiani et al. (1976) found capillary precursors penetrating granulation tissue after the third day, and from the sixth day on fully developed capillaries could be seen. Polverini et al. (1977) showed that macrophages appeared to participate in the induction of vascular budding. Between the fifth and 14th day, extracellular matrix structures (fibronectin, collagen types I and III), including their sites of attachment for fibroblasts, basal membrane structures and collagen fibres, are identifiable in the form of deposits along synthetic particles; larger amounts, however, can only be demonstrated intraprosthetically at the end of the early phase. Up to this point of time only synthetic surface structures are available as attachment sites for phagocytic cells. According to Helpap (1987) neutrophilic granulocytes, macrophages and stimulated fibroblasts secrete collagenases, so that the collagen content that can now be found results from a balance between collagen synthesis and its degradation. The quantitatively higher content of collagen type III found in our experiments resembled the findings of Gabbiani et al. (1976) that collagen type III synthesis predominated during the early phase. Kang (1978) and Gauss-Müller et al. (1980) emphasised the importance of collagen type III in attracting other inflammatory cells and as a matrix structure for cell migration.

8.2.2 Organisation Phase (Phase II)

The organisation phase is comparable to the reparative proliferative phase of normal inflammatory processes and its picture in our preparations is dominated by monocytes and by cells which have been transformed into macrophages; in addition fibroblasts, foreign body giant cells, capillaries and isolated plasma cells are present. Strictly speaking, however, no repair of injured tissue follows since the organisation of the prosthesis is the main objective. In contrast with the initially predominant neutrophil response, the monocytes produced are much more capable of intercellular contact formation (COTTIER et al. 1980). The increased cellular permeation into prosthetic gaps may be dependent on this. The phagocytic processes observed are carried out by macrophages, which play a central part during the reparative-proliferative phase. Macrophages are found in the outer coat and are assumed to originate from ingrowing capillary buds and local connective tissue cells of the periprosthetic tissue. The ones found in the inner coat originate from flowing blood. These blood-borne macrophages have retained the ability to proliferate (cf. BRIELER 1981). According to COTTIER et al. (1980), blood monocytes transform into macrophages in granulation tissue, with a strong hydrolytic and oxidative potential. Small fibrin deposits can sometimes be seen intraluminally during phase II and III and can be phagocytosed by macrophages (see HELPAP 1987). In addition to enzymatic degradation by phagocytosis (FREYRIA et al. 1991) and mechanical destruction (GEIGER and KREMPIEN 1988), clearance of exudate by the lymphatic system is of great importance to the functioning of the prosthesis. Since this clearance is secured only to a limited extent, there is no perivascular lymphatic sheath to minimise the fluid accumulation which has been observed by various authors (KULENKAMPFF and SIMONIS 1976; VOLLMAR et al. 1982; KAUPP et al. 1979; BLUMENBERG et al. 1985). The lack of flexibility and rigidity of the synthetic tube after increased retention time may be explained by a sporadic periprosthetic fibrosis readily induced in persistently oedematous tissue (SPERLING 1976; VOLLMAR et al. 1982). As a result of activation of the reticulo-endothelial system, lysozyme-positive macrophages can be demonstrated by immunohistochemical methods, particularly in the vicinity of newly formed vessels.

After persistent inflammatory irritation, they showed a tendency towards phagocytosis and formation of foreign body giant cells. They were always located in close proximity to the synthetic particles, which could also be demonstrated intracellularly. KULENKAMPFF and SIMONIS (1976) also described birefringent synthetic particles as vacuolar inclusions within the macrophages, and assumed they represented the biological degradation of the prosthetic structures. The foreign body giant cells thus corresponded to syncytial macrophages brought about by fusion (COTTIER et al. 1980; KRAUS 1980).

The fact that macrophages can only incompletely eliminate the prosthetic foreign body by phagocytosis suggests that the formation of foreign body giant cells is due to failure of degradation of prosthetic material, which must be regarded as a possible cause of periprosthetic granuloma formation. Loosening of the prosthetic structures together with a persistent histiocytic-monocytic foreign body reaction can be observed from the start of the organisation phase, and the loss of stability produced is minimised by the endogenous connective tissue vessel wall which has developed. Geiger and co-workers conducted a study of Teflon prostheses which had been implanted for a long time, using light and scanning electron microscopy as well as structural analysis after treatment with sodium hypochloride; following the foreign body reaction, inhomogeneous surface structure was identified (GEIGER et al. 1980; GEIGER and KREMPIEN 1988). The Teflon vascular prostheses used in our investigations were all wrapped in a thin band made of Teflon fibres in order to prevent aneurysmal pouch formation, and these small fibres seem very subject to phagocytosis. We also found distorsion and stenosis of the synthetic tube in addition to the alterations caused by foreign body reactions. Since the developing connective tissue adapts to the prosthetic architecture, strong connective tissue strands may cause such changes in shape. For example, wedge-shaped fibrous connective tissue proliferation within an older puncture channel was found on one Teflon prosthesis which had been implanted to function as an arteriovenous shunt. Subsequently the prosthetic lumen became obliterated by fibrous connective tissue and therefore removal was required.

Little is documented on the mechanism of activation of fibroblasts; however, it is assumed that fibrin and the products of fibrinogen degradation have a stimulating effect. At the beginning fibrin accretions were found in the perivascular region and on the luminal surface, where isolated patches could even be found after weeks and months. "Macrophage-dependent stimulating activity" is said to play an important part in the activation of fibroblasts (COTTIER et al. 1980). POSTLETHWAIT and KANG (1983) and KANG (1978) demonstrated that this factor, synthesised by macrophages, was effective in fibroblasts. According to MILLIKAN (1981) and LINDNER (1982), infiltrated fibroblasts are capable of synthesising ground substance and collagens and furthermore they can secrete hydrolytic enzymes. When fibro-blasts have penetrated into the prosthetic tissue, components of the extracellular matrix such as collagen fibres, fibronectin and fibrin from the exudate serve as guidance tracks (GAUSS-MÜLLER et al. 1980) and are also responsible for the chemotactic attraction of fibroblasts (HELPAP 1980). The increasing number of fibroblasts in the cellular infiltrate during a reparative-proliferative phase is probably caused by local fibroblasts proliferation and permeation from the flowing blood according to the autoradiographic studies of HELPAP (1980), HELPAP and GROULS (1981) and STEWART et al. (1981). HELPAP (1981) found greater increase in the number of cells than was evident from the autoradiographic marking index and interpreted this as proof of local fibroblastic proliferation. Mucopolysaccharide synthesis occurs prior to collagen synthesis (LINDNER 1982).

These results agree with our present findings. We found an increase in the cellular infiltration and in the amount of extracellular matrix components in the inner and outer capsule as well as in the prosthetic gaps as early as the 5th–14th days. In a recent tissue lesion collagen synthesis starts approximately between the third and sixth day and reaches a peak around the 10th–12th days (LINDNER 1982). According to our observations, confirmed by the findings of CLORE et al. (1979), the quantitative ratio changes with time in favour of collagen type I, which mainly serves to provide stability. They also found a comparable quantitative ratio of collagen type I and type III in granulation tissue. Generally speaking, collagen type III serves as a track for growth and guidance of the cellular infiltrate, particularly during the early phase and organisation phase. With the emergence of cellular infiltrates (monocytes and fibroblasts) and the beginning of the synthesis of collagen type I and type III, the transprosthetic cellular penetration also commences. This process is supported by the "macrophage growth factor" produced by activated macrophages and fibroblasts. The distinct neovascularisation seems to be of crucial importance for the accumulation of cells of the reticulo-endothelial system, since cellular infiltration is frequently found in close spatial relation to the vessels. Fibronectin, which is deposited along newly formed vessels and prosthetic structures, is also thought to possess catalytic functions for the cellular permeation of the prosthesis. It is interesting to find fan-shaped arrangements of fibronectin in the transitional zone of the outer connective tissue capsule and the synthetic structures from the second phase onwards. This arrangement can be seen as a "cell-sluice", since fibronectin possesses sites of attachment for numerous cells, which are then intraprosthetically demonstrable during later phases, and which in turn produce components of the extracellular matrix. Collagen type I, which was already present in abundance at the beginning of the organisation phase, made possible the firm attachment of the vascular prosthesis to the soft tissue coat.

8.2.3 Late Phase (Phase III) and "Chronic Final Stage"

Since the tissue reactions of the organism caused by Teflon and Dacron are basically comparable to the incorporation of inert, aseptic foreign bodies, a chronic inflammatory tissue reaction persists during phase III. In agreement with the results of examinations of granulation tissues (Helpap 1980), an increased transformation of macrophages can be regarded as a reaction to Teflon and Dacron, which is very difficult to eliminate. Macrophages are able to prolong and possibly increase the inflammation due to the secretion of inflammation mediators (Bitter-Suermann 1980) and proliferation of fibrous elements can continue as a result of increased macrophage activation. Usually a fibre-rich, cell-poor granulation tissue is found during the late phase, but different individual reaction patterns are also present during the late phase. If the chronic inflammatory reaction persists in the organism, vascular prostheses may fail as a result of uncontrolled proliferation of mesenchymal cells and excessive synthesis of extracellular matrix components. Lack of stromal architecture can be regarded as the main reason for excessive growth of the inner prosthetic capsule, but if the surrounding tissue is intact – as is the case with a prosthetic bed – proliferation standstill seems to be guaranteed by the attachment of newly formed granulation tissue to the pre-existing connective tissue areas. Such tissue contact is not possible within the lumen, and this may lead to progressive obliteration of the vessel due to continuously proliferating tissue. The degeneration of the inner coat observed during late phases (Wesolowski 1962) together with atherosclerotic changes (lipid accumulation, necrosis, calcification, tissue ruptures, collagen exposure and subsequent platelet aggregation) may be regarded as a consequence of underlying arterial sclerosis inducing generalised mesenchymal activation.

In addition to the obliteration and degeneration of alloplastic vascular prostheses described by numerous authors (DeBakey et al. 1965; Borchard et al. 1975; Bürger et al. 1978; Echave et al. 1979; Hamann and Vollmar 1979; Bisler et al. 1980; Johnson and Baker 1980; Schejbal and Könn 1980; Silver and Wilson 1991; How et al. 1992), a further essential disadvantage of alloplastic vascular prostheses compared to autologous venous transplants has become obvious. In contrast to the findings obtained from animal experiments which led to the concept of a fibrous permeation of the synthetic framework and subsequent intima-like lining (Anders et al. 1983), it has not yet been convincingly demonstrated that the prosthesis becomes lined with a functioning endothelium comparable to the proper anatomical endothelium. Factor VIII-positive endothelial cells in our preparations were only found in the form of small islets of luminal lining, together with transprosthetic capillary permeation. They were seen in the vicinity of anastomoses, arising from continuous division and growth in length of preexisting endothelial cells situated in the neighbouring arterial segment (cf. also Illig 1961). In animal experiments, Stump et al. (1967) and Zacharias et al. (1987) also found capillaries growing basally into Dacron prostheses. Loose et al. (1976) demonstrated transprosthetic endothelial cell proliferation in a Dacron prosthesis which had remained in a patient for 5 years; however, only a delicate endothelial extension was visible in the lumen. In a 10-year experimental study with dogs, it was found that venous prostheses with a large calibre and high porosity were completely endothelialised (Kogel et al. 1989a,b). Additionally, factor VIII-positive endothelial cells could be demonstrated in some cases were thrombus formation together with a partial recanalisation had occurred.

As long ago as 1963 it was pointed out that the inner surface lining of synthetic prostheses lacks fibrinolytic characteristics (Poche 1963) and so in addition to the frequent complications of luminal narrowing through the formation of a broad fibrous inner coat, the accretion of thrombi is also favoured because the inner coat does not possess antithrombogenic potential, in contrast to regular endothelium. Over the past years numerous experiments have been carried out in order to replace the deficient lining by breeding endothelial cells which originate from autologous veins and seeding them onto an alloplastic prosthesis before implantation. In 1976 Loose et al. tried to line arterial prostheses with vital endothelial cells with the help of cryopreservation of endothelial cells; however, only discontinuously distributed and regressively altered endothelial cells persisted. In the endothelial cell seeding procedure published by Herring in 1979 (Herring et al. 1984, 1987a,b) and in procedures developed thereafter, endothelial cells were enzymatically "harvested" in vital venous segments and transferred to Dacron or Teflon prostheses at the time of implantation. It is thus assumed that the fibrous invasion of the prosthesis is not a prerequisite for the attachment of endothelial cells. After numerous studies based on animal experiments (Allen et al. 1984; Callow 1987; Pasquinelli et al. 1987; Zilla and Reichart 1989), with results suggesting improved permeability rates and decreased thrombogenicity, this procedure was applied in human medicine for the first time in 1984 by HERRING. When it was recognised that the degree of endothelialisation is dependent upon the initial cellular surface adherence, the number of adherent cells per unit area, the shear-strength resistant growth and the surface tension of the material to be endothelialised, further tests with differently pre-lined prosthetic surfaces were carried out. The prelinings include fibronectin, laminin, collagen types I, III and V, ε-aminocaproic acid and fibrin adhesives. A high cell density was seen in the groups lined with fibronectin and collagen types I and IV (cf. VOHRA et al. 1991a,b) whereas an increased resistance to shear strength was observed in the groups with pre-linings of ε-aminocaproic acid and fibrin adhesives (DEUTSCH et al. 1988). KADLETZ et al. (1987, 1989) confirmed these findings through their own test results. Although endothelial cell seeding can be regarded as a step forward in the search for a less thrombogenic prosthesis, due to the prevention of direct contact between thrombocytes and subsequently formed endothelial collagenous structures, there are still numerous questions which remain to be answered.

Overall it is not clear whether the cells following the endothelial cell seeding remain capable of performing their original functions with respect to synthesis and control within the scope of vascular haemostasis. HOLLIER et al. (1986) even raised the question of whether the inner prosthetic lining following endothelial cell seeding was composed of the originally applied cells. In animal experiments with male and female endothelial cell donors it was shown by chromosome analysis that the covering cell layer was not derived from the originally applied cells, but from the cells of the male host animal. A question that remains open is whether the endothelial cells whose molecular structure is altered by culture are responsible for the frequently observed transformation of haematogenous monocytes into activated macrophages leading to phagocytosis or induction of cell division (cf. VOSS 1985). After seeding, the cultured endothelial cells frequently show detachment of their intercellular connections. There are no data available on the moment of maximum cellular attachment following the application to the synthetic material. Comparable test results with respect to the antithrombogenic characteristics of arterial, venous and seeded endothelial cells are not available.

9 Summary

In order to analyse the incorporation pattern of synthetic prostheses made of Teflon and Dacron in the arterial system, 21 prostheses removed surgically and seven prostheses obtained from autopsies were examined; the duration of the implantation periods ranged from 30 min up to 10 years.

Essentially the early phase of prosthetic incorporation (phase I) includes exudative inflammatory reactions as part of acute inflammatory processes. The degree of order within the tissue architecture and the mutual influence of matrix and cells in the reaction appeared to be slight. The cellular infiltrate found on the outer prosthetic surface is of local origin whereas the inner prosthetic lining contains cells of haematogenous origin. The organisation phase (phase II), which is comparable to the reparative-proliferative phase of an inflammatory reaction, showed activation of the reticulo-endothelial system together with the start of phagocytosis and a thinning of the prosthetic structures. Collagen type I and type III and fibronectin served both as a guidance and a growth tract for the cells during the cellular permeation of the prosthesis. Fibronectin and collagen type III have a special "catalytic" function. Collagen type I causes the firm anchoring of the vascular prosthesis in the periprosthetic tissue. The loss of stability of the prosthesis due to phagocytosis of fibres is balanced by the newly formed connective tissue within the wall of the vessel. The fibroblasts involved in the organisation must be derived from the flowing blood and from local mesenchymal cells. A chronic inflammatory reaction persisted during the late phase. In some cases increased proliferation of the inner mesenchymal lining of the prosthesis was observed together with regressive changes. The lack of a continuous surrounding stromal architecture on the luminal side of the vessel can be regarded as the main reason for this proliferation. Transformation of haematogenous cells into angioblasts or endothelial cells was not seen. Small endothelialised areas were only seen in the vicinity of anastomoses and following transprosthetic permeation by capillaries.

Acknowledgements. I would like to express my special thanks to Dr. rer. nat. Voss, Berufsgenossenschaftliches Forschungsinstitut für Arbeitsmedizin (BGFA), for technical advice concerning the immunohistochemical examinations, Frau Dr. rer. nat. Schmitz, Institut für Pathologie an den Krankenanstalten Bergmannsheil, Universitätsklinik, Bochum, for electron microscopic investi-gations, and Frau Elisabeth Harrer and Frau Sandra Ketzler for the translation of the manuscript.

References

Alberts B, Dennis B, Lewis J, Raff M, Roberts K, Watson JD (1986) Molekularbiologie der Zelle. VCH, Weinheim

Allen BT, Long JA, Clark RE, Sicard GA, Hopkins KT, Welch MJ (1984) Influence of endothelial cell seeding on platelet deposition and patency in small-diameter Dacron arterial grafts. J Vasc Surg 1: 224–232

Anders A, Poutot M, Böse-Andgraf J, Apitzsch D (1983) Der Einbau kleinkalibriger PTFE-Prothesen im Tierexperiment – Mikroangiographische, elektronen-und lichtoptische Befunde. In: Müller-Wiefel H (ed) Gefäßersatiz. 2. Gemeinsame Jahrestagung der Angiologischen Gesellschaften Deutschlands, Österreichs und der Schweiz, Düsseldorf, 26–29.9.1979, Tagungsbericht (part II). Gerhard Witzstrock, Baden-Baden, pp 116–121

Aumailley M, Nowack H, Timpl R (1983) Laminin: structure and cell-binding activity. In: Popper H (ed) Structural carbohydrates in the liver. proceedings of an international conference held during Basel Liver Week, 12-18 October 1982. MTP Press, Lancaster, England, pp 375–384

Bisler H, Alemany J, Kurt R (1980) Verwendung verschiedener Kunststoffimplantate in der Gefäßchirurgie-Zehn-Jahresergebnisse. In: Muller-Wiefel H (ed) Gefäßersatz. 2. Gemeinsame Jahrestagung der Angiologischen Gesellschaften Deutschlands, Österreichs und der Schweiz, Düsseldorf, 26–29.9.1979, Tagungsbericht (part II). Gerhard Witzstrock, Baden-Baden, pp 157–160

Bitter-Suermann D (1980) Die Funktionseinheit Makrophage-Komplement. Verh Dtsch Ges Pathol 64: 63–76

Blumenberg RM, Gelfand ML, Dale WA (1985) Perigraft seromas complicating arterial grafts. Surgery 97: 194–203

Borchard F, Loose DA (1980) Die Morphologie des Arterienersatzes. In: Müller-Wiefel H (ed) Gefäßersatz. 2. Gemeinsame Jahrestagung der Angiologischen Gesellschaften Deutschlands, Österreichs und der Schweiz, Düsseldorf, 26–29.9.1979, Tagungsbericht (part II). Gerhard Witzstrock, Baden-Baden, pp 6–24

Borchard F, Kremer K, Loose DA (1975) Licht- und elektronenmikroskopische Befunde bei neun autoalloplastischen Arterienprothesen nach Sparks. Thoraxchirurgie 23: 83–97

Borchard F, Kemkes BM, Loose DA (1980) Arterienersatz durch biologische Gefäßprothesen: Morphologie und klinische Erfahrungen. Gefäß-Patient-Therapie. 6. Internationales angiographisches und angiologisches Seminar. 15–17.3.1979, Baden-Baden. Gerhard Witzstrock, Baden-Baden, pp 191–203

Boyce B (1982) Physical characteristics of expanded polytetrafluoroethylene grafts. In: Stanley JC (ed) Biologic and synthetic vascular prostheses. Grune & Stratton, New York, pp 553–561

Bremm KD, König E (1988) Die Rolle der neutrophilen Granulozyten bei der mikrobiellen Infektabwehr – Signalübertragung und Freisetzung proinflammatorischer Mediatoren. Dtsch Med Wochenschr 113: 392–402

Brieler HS (1981) Autoalloplastischer Gefäßersatz bei Ratten. Mikrochirurgie und autoradiographische Untersuchungen zur Herkunft der Prothesenendothelzellen. Ergebnisse der Angiologie, vol 24. F.K. Schattauer, Stuttgart

Bürger K, Schröder G, Preis R (1978) Spätkomplikationen nach alloplastischem Gefäßersatz. Zentralbl Chir 103: 197–205

Callow AD (1987) Endothelial cell seeding: problems and expectations. J Vasc Surg 6: 318–319

Clore JN, Cohen IK, Diegelmann RF (1979) Quantitation of collagen types I and III during wound healing. Proc Soc Exp Biol Med 161: 337–340

Cottier H, Hess MW, Keller HU, Schaffner T (1980) Chemokinese, Chemotaxis und Funktionen von Phagozyten, mit besonderer Berücksichtigung der Makrophagen. Verh Dtsch Ges Pathol 64: 24–44

Dasbach G (1989) Inkorporationsphasen arterieller Kunststoffprothesen: Immunhistochemische Charakterisierung von Matrixstrukturen. Inaugural-Dissertation zur Erlangung des Doktorgrades der Medizin einer Hohen Medizinischen Fakultät der Ruhr-Universität Bochum

Dasbach G, Voss B, Tiemann H, Müller K-M (1990) Charakterisierung des zellulären Reaktionsmusters und der Bestandteile der Extrazellularmatrix nach Implantation von allopolastischem Gefässersatz. Z Herz Thorax Gefäßchir 4: 21–24

De Bakey ME, Jordan GL, Beall AC, O'Neal RM, Abbott JP, Halpert B (1965) Basic biologic reactions to vascular grafts and prostheses. Surg Clin North Am 43: 477–497

Deutsch M, Fasol R, Zilla P, Fischlein T (1988) In vitro Endothelialisierung von PTF-Kunststoffprothesen. Angio 10 (4): 159–168

Echave V, Koornick AR, Haimov MJ, Jacobsen JH II (1979) Intimal hyperplasia as a complication of the use of the polytetrafluoroethylene graft for femoro-popliteal bypass. Surgery 86 (6): 791–798

Feigl W, Susani M, Ulrich W, Matejka M, Losert U, Sinzinger H (1985) Organisation of experimental thrombosis by blood cells. Virchows Arch [A] 406: 133–148

Foidart J-M, Timpl R, Furthmayer H, Martin GR (1982) Laminin, a glycoprotein from basement membranes. In: Furthmayr H (ed) Immunochemistry of the extracellular matrix, vol I. Methods. CRC Press, Boca Raton, Fl., pp 125–134

Formichi MJ, Guidoin RG, Jausseran J-M, et al. (1988) Expanded PTFE prostheses as arterial substitutes in humans: late pathological findings in 73 excised grafts. Ann Vasc Surg 1: 14–27 (1988)

Freyria AM, Chignier E, Guidollet J, Louisot P (1991) Peritoneal macrophage response: an in vivo model for the study of synthetic materials. Biomaterials 12(2): 111–118

Gabbiani G, Lelons M, Bailey AJ, Bazin S, Delaunay A (1976) Collagen and myofibroblasts of granulation tissue. A chemical, ultrastructural and immunological study.; Virchows Arch [B] 21: 133–145

Gauss-Müller V, Kleinman HK, Martin GR, Schiffmann E (1980) Role of attachment factors and attractants in fibroblast chemotaxis. J Lab Clin Med 96: 1071–1080

Geiger G, Krempien B (1988) Strukturanalyse von expanded Polytetrafluoräthylen-Prothesen nach Langzeitimplantation beim Menschen. Angio 10 (4): 169–178

Geiger G, Rückert U, Krempien B (1980) Histologische und rasterelektronenmikroskopische Untersuchungen an expanded PTFE-Prothesen an mechanisch belasteten Stellen im chronischen Tierversuch. In: Müller-Wiefel H (ed) Gefäßersatz 2. Gemeinsame Jahrestagung der Angiologischen Gesellschaften Deutschlands, Österreichs und der Schweiz, Düsseldorf, 26–29.9.1979, Tagungsbericht (part II). Gerhard Witzstrock, Baden-Baden, pp 118–120

Giessler R (1987) Gefäßrekonstruktionen. In: Heberer G, Pichlmayer R (eds) Kirschnersche allgemeine

und spezielle Operationslehre, vol XI, Gefäßchirurgie. Springer, Berlin Heidelberg New York, pp 73–88
Guidon RC Gosselin C, Domurado D et al. (1977) Dacron as arterial prosthetic material: nature, properties, brands, fate and perspectives. Biomater Med Dev Artif Organs 5: 177–203
Guidon RC, Snyder RW, Awad JA, King MW (1992) Biostability of vascular prostheses. In: Hastings GW (ed) Cardiovascular biomaterials. Springer, London Berlin Heidelberg New York, pp 143-172
Hamann H, Vollmar J (1979) Expanded-PTFE-Gefäßprothesen – ein neuer Weg des Arterien- und Venenersatzes? Chirurg 50: 249–256
Helpap B (1980) Der kryochirurgische Eingriff und seine Folgen. Morphologische und zellkinetische Analyse. In: Doerr W, Leonhardt H (eds) Normale und pathologische Anatomine, vol 40. Thieme, Stuttgart
Helpap B (1987) Leitfaden der Allgemeinen Entzündungslehre. Springer, Berlin Heidelberg New York
Helpap B, Cremer H (1972) Zellkinetische Untersuchungen zur Wundheilung der Mäuseleber. Virchows Arch [B] 10: 134–144
Helpap B, Grouls V (1981) The cellular reaction of the kidney after different physical injuries. Urol Res 9: 115–121
Herring MB, Baughman S, Glover J et al. (1984) Endothelial seeding of Dacron and polytetrafluoroethylene grafts: the cellular events of healing. Surgery 96: 745–755
Herring MB, Compton RS, LE Grand DR, Gardner AL, Madison DL, Glover, JL (1987a) Endothelial seeding of polytetrafluoroethylene popliteal bypass. A preliminary report. J Vasc Surg 6: 114–118
Herring MB, Gardner A, Glover JL (1987b) Seeding human arterial prostheses with mechanically derived endothelium. The detrimental effect of smoking. J Vasc Surg 1: 279–287
Hollier LH, Fowl RJ, Pennell RC, Heck CF, Winter KAH, Fass DN, Kaye MP (1986) Are seeded endothelial cells the origin of neointima on prosthetic vascular grafts? J Vasc Surg 1: 65–73
How TV (1992) Mechanical properties and arterial grafts In: Hastings GW (ed) Cardiovascular biomaterials. Springer, London Berlin Heidelberg New York, pp 1–35
Hsu S-M, Raine L, Fanger H (1981) Use of avidin-biotin-peroxidase complex (ABC) in immunoperoxidase techniques: a comparison between ABC and unlabeled antibody (PAP) procedures. J Histochem Cytochem 29: 577–580
Illig L (1961) Die terminale Strombahn. Capillarbett und Mikrozirkulation. In: Hegglin R, Leuthardt F, Schoen R, Schwiegk H, Zollinger HU (eds) Pathologie und Klinik in Einzeldarstellungen vol XI. Springer, Berlin Göttingen Heidelberg, pp 210–232
Johnson JM, Baker LD Jr (1980) Experience with IMPRA-graft as a vascular substitute In: Müller-Wiefel H (ed) Gefäßersatz. 2. Gemeinsame Tagung der Angiologischen Gesellschaften Deutschlands, Österreichs und der Schweiz, Düsseldorf, 26–29.9.1979, Tagungsbericht (part II). Gerhard Witzstrock, Baden-Baden, pp 94–101
Kadletz M, Moser R, Preiss P, Deutsch M, Zilla P, Fasol R (1987) In vitro lining of fibronectin coated PTFE grafts with cryopreserved saphenous vein endothelial cells. Thorac Cardiovasc Surg 35: 143–147
Kang AH (1978) Editorial: fibroblast activation. J Lab Clin Med 92: 1–4
Kaupp HA, Matulewicz TJ, Lattimer GL, Kremen JE, CelaniVJ (1979) Graft infection of graft reaction? Arch Surg 114: 1419–1422
Kogel A, Amselgruber W, Froesch D, Mohr W, Cyba-Altunbay S (1989a) New techniques of analyzing healing process of artificial vascular grafts, transmural vascularization, and endothelialization. Res Exp Med 189: 61–68
Kraus B (1980) Mehrkernige Riesenzellen in Granulomen. Verh Dtsch Ges Pathol 64: 103–124
Kulenkampff H, Simonis G (1976) Zur Frage der biologischen Verträglichkeit von Gefäßprothesen aus Dacron und synthetischem Fadenmaterial. Chirurg 47: 189–192
Lindner J (1982) Morphologie und Biochemie der Wundheilung. Langenbecks Arch Chir 358: 153–160
Loose DA, Borchardt F, Lenz W (1976) Zur Frage der Endothelialisierung von Gefäßprothesen. In: Walter F, Schmitz H (eds) Der heterologe Gefäßersatz. Editio Aulendorf, Aulendorf 115–124
Marnach H (1988) Einheilungsphasen arterieller Gefäßprothesen - Histomorphologische Befunde und Komplikationen. Inaugural-Dissertation zur Erlangung des Doktorgrades der Medizin einer Hohen Medizinischen Fakultät der Ruhr-Universität Bochum
Millikan LE (1981) Skin anatomy in wound healing. Ear Nose Throat J 60: 10–22
Müller-Wiefel H (1986) Gefäßprothesen. Chirurg 57: 64–71
Pasquinelli G, Preda P, Curti T, D'Addato M, Laschi R (1987) Endothelialization of new Dacron graft in an experimental model: light microscopy, electron microscopy and immunocytochemistry. Scanning Microsc 1: 1327–1338

Poche R (1963) Über das Schicksal alloplastischer Teflonprothesen im Gefäßsystem. Langenbecks Arch Klin Chir 304: 972–981

Polverini PJ, Cotran RS, Gimbrone MA, Unanue ER (1977) Activated macrophages induce vascular proliferation. Nature 269: 804–806

Postlethwait AE, Kang AH (1983) Induction of fibroblast proliferation by human mononuclear leukocyte-derived proteins. Arthritis Rheum 26: 22–27

Pott G, Zündorf P, Gerlach U, Voss B, Rauterberg J (1982) Die Bedeutung struktureller Glykoproteine, dargestellt am Beispiel der Fibronectine. Z Gastroenterol 20: 649–658

Pott G, Voss B, Rauterberg J, Gerlach U (1983) Fibronectin and induction of fibroplasia in the liver. In: Popper H (ed) Structural carbohydrates in the liver: proceedings of an international conference held during Basel Liver Week, 12–18 October 1982. MTP Press, Lancaster, England, pp 385–398

Sandmann W, Kremer K (1987) Materialprobleme in der Gefäßchirurgie. Chirurg 54: 433–443

Schejbal V, Könn G (1980) Über morphologische Befunde bei der Einheilung synthetischer arterieller Prothesen. In: Tiemann H (ed) Gefäßchirurgie aktuell. TM, Bad Oeynhausen, pp 127–130

Silver MD, Wilson JW (1991) Pathology of mechanical heart valve prostheses and vascular grafts made of artificial materials In: Silver MD (ed) Cardiovascular pathology, vol 2, 2nd edn. Churchill Livingstone, New York, pp 1429–1464

Simonis G, Koch B (1980) Polarisationsmikroskopische Untersuchungen an Dacron-Prothesen mit Innenvelours. In: Müller-Wiefel H (ed) Gefäßersatz. 2. Gemeinsame Jahrestagung der Angiologischen Gesellschaften Deutschlands, Österreichs und der Schweiz, Düsseldorf, 26–29.9.1979, Tagungsbericht (part II). Gerhard Witzstrock, Baden-Baden, pp 49–52

Sperling M (1976) Die Problematik des arteriellen Gefäßersatzes. Med Klin 71: 1587–1593

Stewart RJ, Duley JA, Dewdney J, Allardyce RA, Beard MEJ, Fitzgerald PH (1981) The wound fibroblast and macrophage II. Their origin studied in a human after bone marrow transplantation. Br J Surg 68: 129–131

Stump MM, Jordan GL, De Bakey ME, Halpert B (1967) Endothelium grown from circulating blood on isolated intravascular Dacron hub. Am J Pathol 43: 361

Takenaka K, Kholoussy AM, Yang Y, Kodellas L, Matsumoto T (1985) The healing of thin walled, expanded polytetrafluoroethylene vascular graft. Vasc Surg 19: 383–389

Terranova VA, Kleinman HK, Martin GR (1983) Regulation of cellular activity by extracellular matrix molecules. In: Popper H (ed) Structural carbohydrates in the liver: proceedings of an international conference held during Basel Liver Week, 12–18 October 1982. MTP Press, Lancaster, England, pp 399–406

Vaheri A, Alitalo K, Hedman K, Keski-Oja J, Vartio T (1983) Fibronectin and epithelial cells. In: Popper H (ed) Structural carbohydrates in the liver: proceedings of an international conference held during Basel Liver Week, 12–18 October 1982. MTP Press, Lancaster, England, 385–398

Van Dongen RJAM (1980) Die Bedeutung der Vena saphena magna in der rekonstruktiven Arterienchirurgie. In: Müller-Wiefel H (ed) Gefäßersatz. 2. Gemeinsame Jahrestagung der Angiologischen Gesellschaften Deutschlands, Österreichs and der Schweiz, Düsseldorf, 26–29.9.1979, Tagungsbericht (part II). Gerhard Witzstrock, Baden-Baden, pp 93–94

Vohra R, Thomson GJ, Carr HM, Sharma H, Walker MG (1991a) Comparison of different vascular prostheses and matrices in relation to endothelial seeding. Br J Surg 78: 417–420

Vohra R, Thomson GJ, Carr HM, Sharma H, Welch M, Walker MG (1991b) In vitro adherence and kinetics studies of adult human endothelial cell seeded polytetrafluoroethylene and gelatin impregnated Dacron grafts. Eur J Vasc Surg 5: 93–103

Vollmar J (1980) Gefäßersatz – Trends und Handikaps. In: Müller-Wiefel H (ed) Gefäßersatz. 2. Gemeinsame Jahrestagung der Angiologischen Gasellschaften Deutschlands, Österreichs und der Schweiz, Düsseldorf, 26–29.9.1979, Tagungsbericht (part II). Gerhard Witzstrock, Baden-Baden, pp 1–5

Vollmar J (1982) Rekonstruktive Chirurgie der Arterien. Thieme, Stuttgart, pp 15–71, 566–574

Vollmar J, Hesse G, Mohr W (1982) Infektion oder Unverträglichkeit von Kunststoffprothesen? Aktuel Chir 17: 19–24

Von Falkai (1984) Synthesefasern. Verlag Chemie, Weinheim, pp 172–179, 218–219

Voss B (1985) Makrophagen beeinflussen das Wachstum von Nabelschnurendothelzellen des Menschen. Medwelt 36: 938–941

Voss B, Rauterberg J (1985) Bindegewebsproteine der Arterienwand und ihre mögliche Bedeutung für die Aktivierung von Monozyten. Medwelt 36: 826–829

Voss B, Kereny T, Herrenpoth B, Klein C (1980) Macrophages and endothelial cells in atherosclerosis. In: Revollard JP (ed) Local immunity, Imprimerie Marcolle, Suresnes Cédex, France pp 1–16

Wesolowski SA (1962) Etat actuel des connaissances concernant des protheses vasculaires. Mater Med Pol 2: 190–205

Yamada KM (1982) Isolation of fibronectin from plasma and cells. In: Furthmayer H (ed) Immunochemistry of the extracellular matrix, vol I. Methods CRC Press, Boca Raton, Fl., pp 111–124

Yamada KM (1983) Cell surface interactions with extracellular materials. Annu Rev Biochem 52: 761–799

Zacharias RK, Kirkman TR, Clowes AW, Clowes BA (1987) Mechanisms of healing in synthetic grafts. J Vasc Surg 6: 429–436

The Pathology of Intra-Uterine Contraceptive Devices

C.H. BUCKLEY

1 Introduction

The composition and structure of intra-uterine contraceptive devices (IUCDs) has changed over the years and thus data relating to women in the 1970s or early 1980s is almost certainly inapplicable to current users. Further, large-scale population studies of users, which are assumed to be objective, may be affected by bias because not all women are viewed as being equally suitable candidates for the device. Thus a degree of preselection has occurred even before we begin to examine the consequences, to the individual, of wearing an IUCD.

The early modern IUCDs were made of silk (RICHTER 1909), silver (GRAFENBERG 1929), human hair or rubber (OHTA 1974) but were used by only a small number of women. It was not until the 1960s, with the development of plastic devices, that they came into common use.

Currently IUCDs are made of plastic partly covered by coils of closely wound copper wire or are made of plastic impregnated by progestagen. Although inert, non-medicated plastic devices are no longer inserted, women who have worn them for many years still have them in situ and it is appropriate, when considering the pathology of IUCDs, to include data relating to these devices.

Two monofilamentous threads, forming a tail, are attached to the device to facilitate removal. The Dalkon shield, which was an inert plastic device and is no longer inserted, had a multifilamentous tail and certain difficulties were attributed to its presence.

Current Topics in Pathology
Volume 86. Ed. C. Berry

Problems associated with the wearing of an IUCD may occur at the time of insertion or later and may be minor or may compromise fertility and produce life-endangering disease.

2 Problems Associated with Insertion of an IUCD

Perforation of the uterus occurs in between 0.012% and 0.29% of insertions (Key and Kreutner 1980; Van Os and Edelman 1989), the variation being due to differences in operative skill and training (Craig 1975). It is said to be a particular hazard in the postpartum or postabortive state when the tissues are soft (Kiilholma et al. 1990) but this has not always been substantiated (Mishell and Roy 1982) unless the patient is lactating (Heartwell and Schlesselman 1983).

The perforation may be partial or complete and indeed, evidence from the study of forces required to perforate the uterus in vivo and in vitro suggests that the majority of perforations may, initially, be partial (Goldstuck 1987). Perforation may occur in the corpus uteri or in the cervix (Rienprayura et al. 1973). When the perforation is partial, the tail of the IUCD may still be palpable at the external cervical os and, unless the patient complains of abnormal bleeding (Tadesse and Wamsteker 1985), the problem may remain undetected until the time comes to remove the device, when great difficulties may be encountered. The IUCD is usually found lying malaligned, partly within the uterine cavity and partly embedded in the myometrium.

When a complete perforation has occurred, or a partial perforation has become complete due to migration of the IUCD through the uterine wall, a complication perhaps more likely to occur if the patient is breast feeding (Mittal et al. 1986), the device may be found in the broad ligament, in the peritoneal cavity (Gorsline and Osborne 1985), in the bladder (Hefnawi et al. 1975; Thomalla 1986; Kiilholma et al. 1989; Khan and Wilkinson 1990), adjacent to the ureter (Timonen and Kurppa 1987), in the large bowel (Key and Kreutner 1980; Hays et al. 1986; Browning and Bigrigg 1988) or in the rectum (Sepulveda 1990). A vesico-uterine fistula has also been reported in association with an ectopic IUCD (Schwartzwald et al. 1986). A misplaced copper-covered device presents a particular hazard as the copper may elicit a brisk inflammatory response (Fig. 1) and when this is in the peritoneal cavity it may cause adhesions leading to intestinal obstruction (Mittal et al. 1986; Osborne and Bennett 1978; Adoni and Ben Chetrit 1991).

Cervical laceration is a rare complication of IUCD insertion, having been reported, in a multicentre review of the years 1977–1987, in 1.8% of insertions. The incidence is higher in nulliparous women and with copper and multiload devices than with loops (Chi et al. 1989).

Sampling the blood within a few minutes of replacing an IUCD is reported to detect a transient bacteraemia in 13% of women (Murray et al. 1987). This clearly has implications for the patient at risk of developing endocarditis.

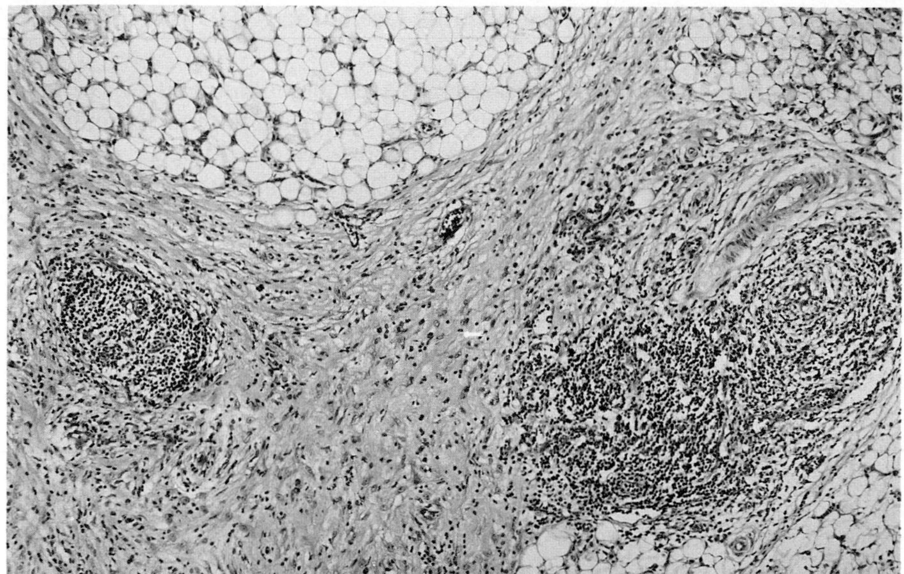

Fig. 1. Fibrosis and non-specific chronic inflammation in the omentum of a woman in whom a copper-containing IUCD had perforated the uterus. × 90

Multiple device insertion has been described when a woman believes, erroneously, that her previous device has been expelled (PORGES 1973) and a complaint of infertility may be made when the presence of a device has been forgotten (OLSON and JONES 1967; ABRAMOVICI et al. 1987).

3 Spontaneous Expulsion of the Device

The proportion of devices expelled depends on the type of device, on the duration of the study and on the patient; the reported incidence therefore varies considerably. Spontaneous expulsion rates for copper devices range from approximately 5.0% (19 821 treatment cycles) within 36 months of use (FYLLING 1987) to 1.8% (1038 women, 66% of whom were in the postpartum or post-abortive state) within 2 years (TSALIKIS et al. 1986). Expulsion rates are not affected by the timing of insertion in relation to the menstrual cycle (OTOLORIN and LADIPO 1985). There is, however, an increased rate of explusion if the device is fitted immediately following delivery of the placenta (THIERY et al. 1985) and this risk can be reduced if insertion is delayed for between 2 and 72 h (CHI et al. 1985).

4 General Problems Associated with the Use of the IUCD

Women commonly experience increased menstrual blood loss whilst wearing an IUCD (Christiaens et al. 1981) and this may be sufficient to require removal of the device. Rarely does haemorrhage, in the presence of an IUCD, reach life-threatening proportions (Glew and Singh 1989). In contrast, amenorrhoea or scanty menstrual loss occurs with the progestagen-impregnated devices and this may also be grounds for removal (Sivin et al. 1990) as it may be associated with intermenstrual spotting (Sivin 1985a; Scholten et al. 1987). Whilst prolonged menstrual bleeding may lead to depletion of body iron stores, the scanty menstrual loss caused by most progestagen-releasing devices enhances the body's iron stores (Haukkamaa et al. 1985; Andrade and Pizarro-Orchard 1987; Luukkainen et al. 1987; Faundes et al. 1988). This does not, however, apply to devices delivering only 2 µg levonorgestrel, which are less effective in reducing bleeding (WHO 1987).

Discontinuation rates for pain and bleeding with non-medicated IUCDs range from 11.0 to 19.6 per 100 women per year and for copper devices from 4.4 to 6.8 per 100 women in the first year of use (Andrade and Pizarro-Orchard 1987). Requests for removal, for oligomenorrhoea or amenorrhoea, of a device releasing 20 µg progestagen per day lie between 8.4 per 100 women (net rate) (Sivin et al. 1987) and 1.4% in the first year of use (Luukkainen et al. 1987).

On rare occasions the device may fracture in utero and this may hinder removal (Custo et al. 1986; Blaauwhof and Goldstuck 1988). Fragmentation of the copper on the device increases with duration of use but in only 0.1% of cases is this of sufficient degree as to impair future fertility (Edelman and Van Os 1990).

Uterine malignancy has developed in association with long-term use of an IUCD but no causal relationship has been demonstrated (Hsu et al. 1989). On the contrary, Pike (1990) has suggested that a progestagen-containing IUCD could reduce the incidence of endometrial carcinoma.

There is no evidence that copper absorbed from the device results in increased serum copper levels even after 12 months of continuous use (Arowojolu et al. 1989).

5 Local Effects of the IUCD on the Endometrium

In most IUCD wearers, the changes seen in the endometrium are the result of irritation (Davis 1972) and pressure, are relatively minor and are, to ordinary histological examination, limited to the contact sites of the IUCD and the immediately adjacent tissue. In the majority of cases, the changes are superficial and on removal of the device, the modified tissue is shed in the next menstrual cycle (Badrawi et al. 1988).

There is, almost invariably, a local inflammatory cell response at the contact sites. In the period immediately following insertion this is entirely a polymorphonuclear leucocyte infiltrate but with time, in the absence of infection, polymorphs

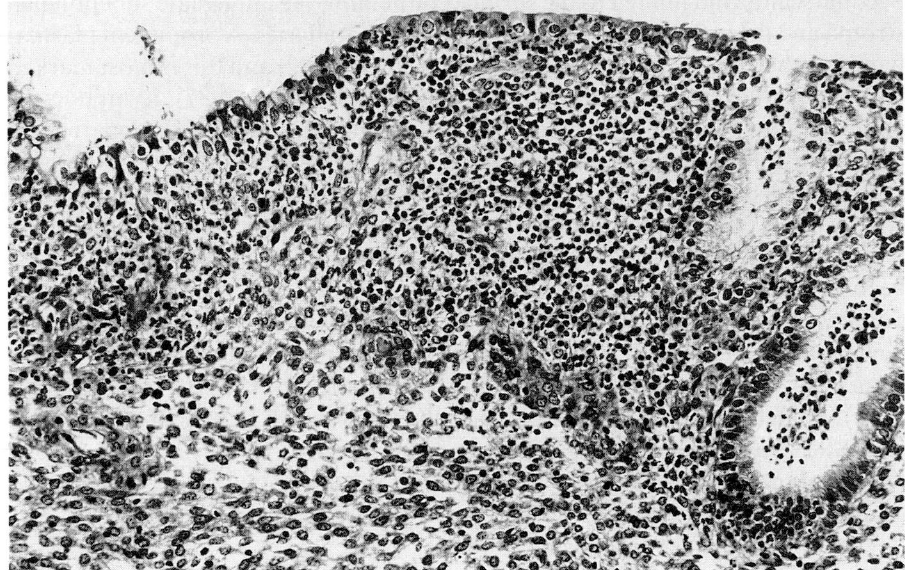

Fig. 2. A well-demarcated, discrete plasma-lymphocytic infiltrate marks the contact site of an IUCD in the endometrium. (From Buckley and Fox 1989) × 185

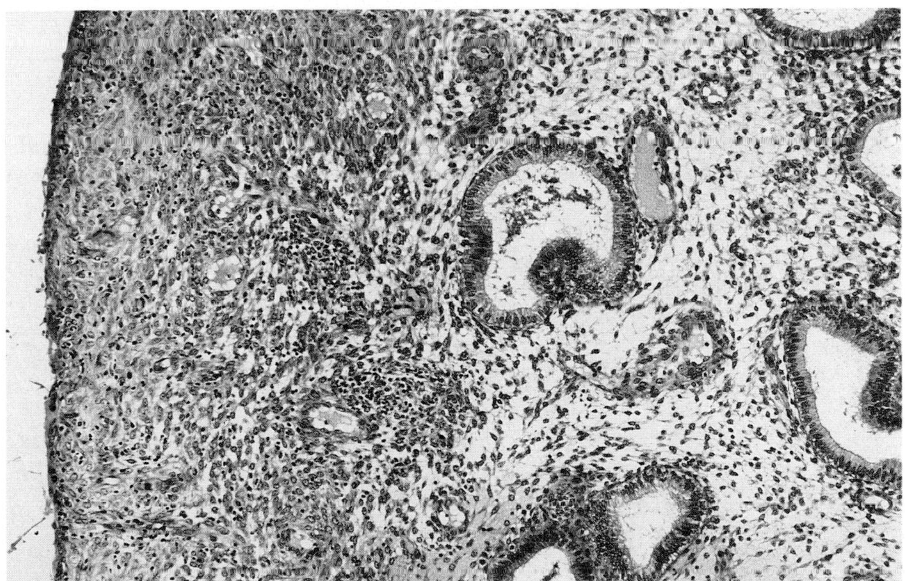

Fig. 3. Pseudodecidualisation of the superficial part of the endometrial stroma beneath the contact site of an IUCD (*left*). A focal inflammatory cell infiltrate is also present. (From Buckley and Fox 1989) × 120

become scanty and limited to the surface epithelium, the immediate subepithelial stroma and the lumina of the superficial stromal capillaries. A prominent plasma-lymphocytic infiltrate persists at the contact sites (Fig. 2) and this is most marked with copper-covered devices (Moyer et al. 1970; Sheppard 1987). Lymphocytes are generally increased throughout the tissue but this may not be apparent on routine histological examination (Mishell and Moyer 1969).

There is also, typically, at the contact sites, stromal pseudodecidualisation (Fig. 3) and compression artefact or atrophy of the functionalis, which may accurately reflect the surface contours of the device (Fig. 4). The surface epithelium becomes flattened or there may be reactive cellular atypia with some loss of nuclear polarity, mild nuclear pleomorphism, increased nucleo-cytoplasmic ratios, the development of nucleoli and cytoplasmic vacuolation (Buckley 1987). Less commonly there is ulceration of the surface epithelium (Moyer and Mishell 1971), sometimes with preservation of the underlying basement membrane, stromal fibrosis (Fig. 5) (Bonney et al. 1966; Shaw et al. 1979a) and, rarely, squamous metaplasia (Tamada et al. 1967) or the development of foreign body granulomata (Ragni et al. 1977).

With progestagen-impregnated devices there are, in addition to the local irritative effects, changes which are attributable to the progestagen and are dose dependent. Initially, in the tissue immediately adjacent to the device (Dallenbach-Hellweg 1981; Ermini et al. 1989), there is pseudodecidualisation of the stroma with progressive regression of glandular and surface epithelium, the epithelial cells becoming cuboidal. The glands become fewer, smaller in calibre and inactive

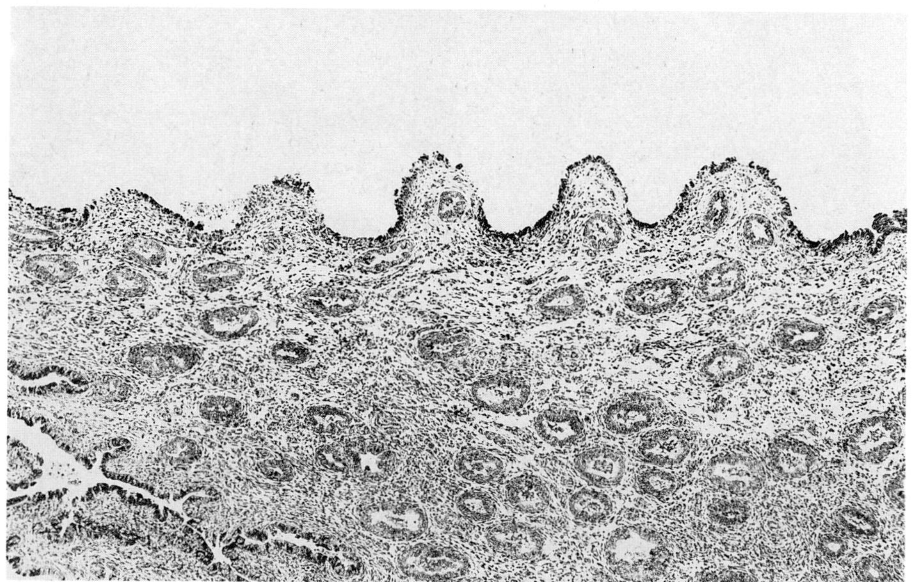

Fig. 4. The contact site of a copper-covered IUCD. The coils of copper on the stem of the device create a series of regular indentations on the endometrial surface. (From Buckley and Fox 1989) × 50

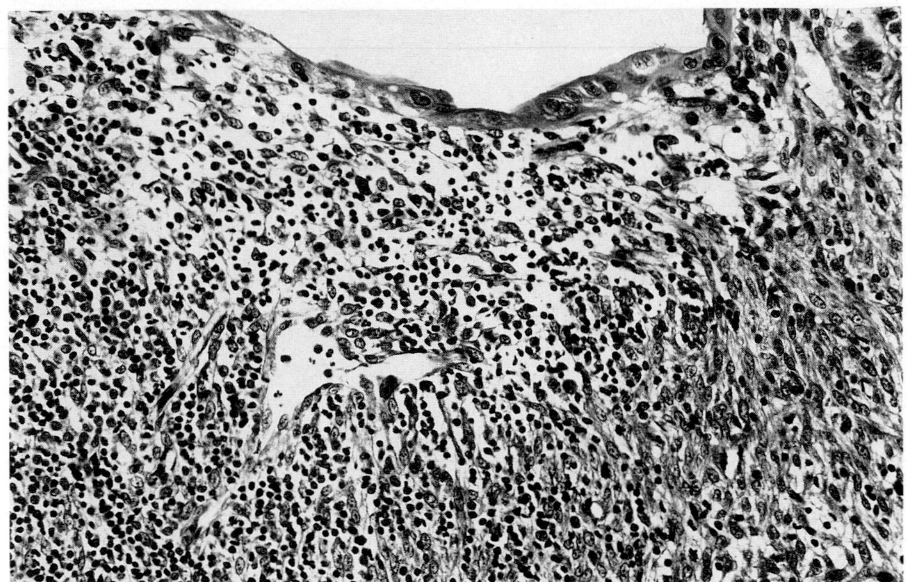

Fig. 5. IUCD contact site. A flattened epithelium covers an endometrium in which there are no glands and the stroma is replaced by maturing, non-specific granulation tissue. (From Buckley and Fox 1989) × 185

whilst the stroma becomes less mature, losing its decidualised appearance and appearing spindle celled. Over a period which may be as long as 6–12 months, if the amount of progestagen liberated is sufficient, these appearances may spread to the whole of the endometrium. The functionalis thus becomes thin, there are no cyclical changes and the appearances are similar throughout the cycle (El-Mahgoub 1980; Silverberg et al. 1986). They closely resemble those seen in systemic progestagen users (Buckley and Fox 1989). With devices delivering only a small dose, the changes may remain limited to the tissue adjacent to the contact site and the stroma may remain focally pseudodecidualised (Shaw 1985). With devices delivering 20–30 μg progestagen (Sheppard 1987) profound atrophy develops within a month of insertion of the device. Stromal calcification, microscopic polyps and thick-walled fibrotic blood vessels similar to those seen in endometrial polyps may develop after several years of use. Ulceration of the surface epithelium is less common with progestagen-impregnated devices than with either inert or copper-covered devices (Sheppard and Bonnar 1985).

Between the contact sites, particularly of inert devices, there is oedema (Fig. 6) and vascular congestion whilst immediately below the device there is vascular blanching (Shaw 1985). Both beneath and adjacent to the device there are microvascular defects with endothelial damage. With progestagen-impregnated devices, vascular damage also occurs, but there is a reduction in the vascularity of the tissues commensurate with the reduction in bleeding experienced by these women (Shaw et al. 1979b, 1981).

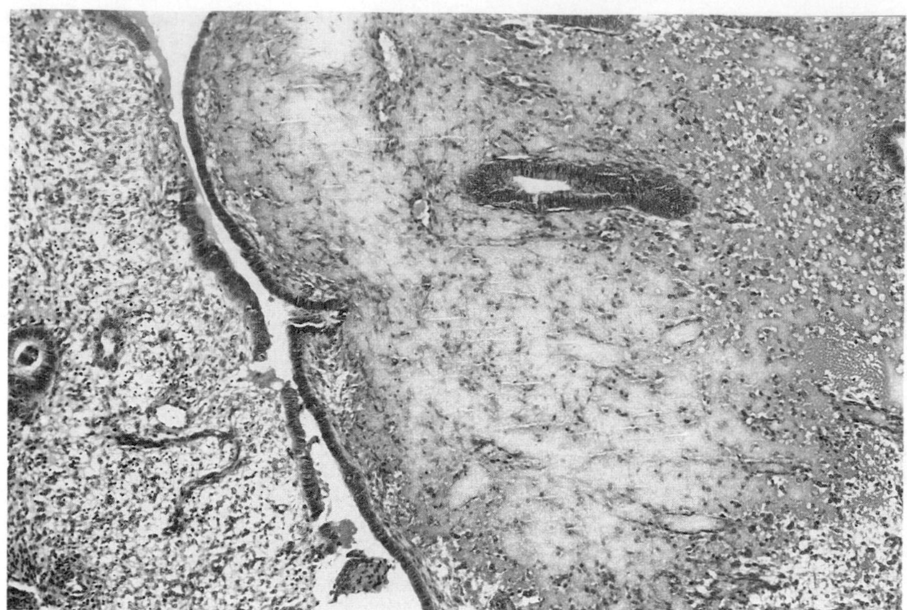

Fig. 6. The endometrium between the contact sites of an IUCD, to the *right*, is oedematous. It contrasts with the more normal endometrium, to the *left*. (From Buckley and Fox 1989) × 90

At a functional level, oestrogen and progesterone receptors are decreased in proportion to the amount of copper in the device (De Castro et al. 1986). As copper concentration becomes lower towards the end of the first year, the endometrium more consistently shows secretory changes indicating a return of steroid receptors, but with devices having a surface area of 375 mm^2, and hence delivering a larger concentration of copper, the endometrium remains shallow.

On occasions, the glands immediately deep to the contact site have a pattern of maturation which differs slightly from that in the adjacent areas; there may be delayed maturation or premature secretory maturation or, rarely, the glands may be inactive (Buckley and Fox 1989). Even when the endometrium is of apparently normal morphology, and ovarian function is normal, there is a reduction in expression of D9B1, a monoclonal antibody binding to a polypeptide-associated oligosaccharide epitope that is secreted by endometrial epithelium in the luteal phase (Seif et al. 1989).

Infection, which is less common with modern copper-covered than with earlier inert devices, causes widespread inflammation which may extend into the myometrium and persist after removal of the device. It is characterised by intraglandular polymorphs and a stromal infiltrate of plasma cells and lymphocytes (Fig. 7). The plasma cells are often predominantly periglandular whilst the lymphocytes may be diffuse or form aggregates or lymphoid follicles. The irritative cytological atypia in the epithelial cells (Fig. 8) may be so exaggerated that the detection of these cells in a cervical smear gives rise to a suspicion of malignancy (Gupta. et al. 1978a). Low-grade infection does not significantly

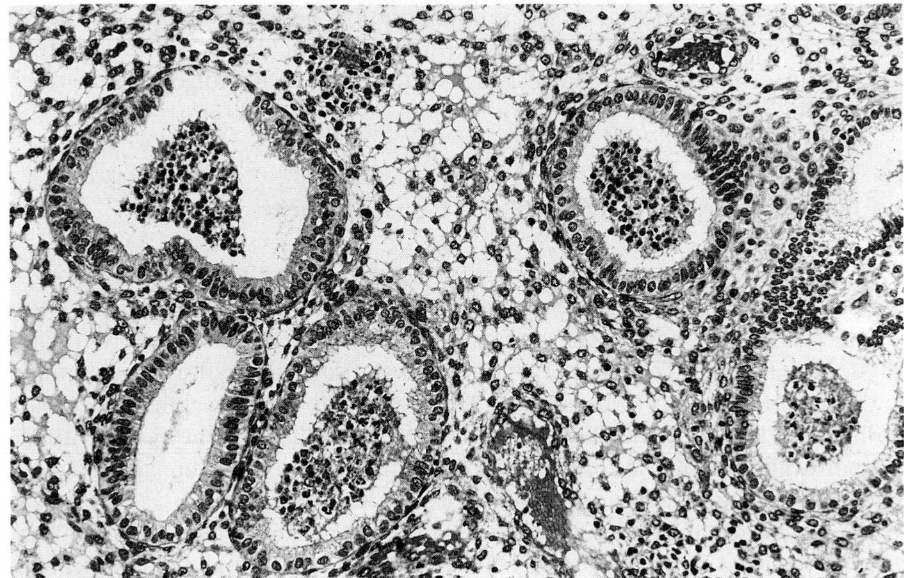

Fig. 7. A low-grade infection of the endometrium in an IUCD wearer. It is characterised by the presence of intraglandular polymorphonuclear leucocytes and a scanty stromal lymphocytic infiltrate. × 185

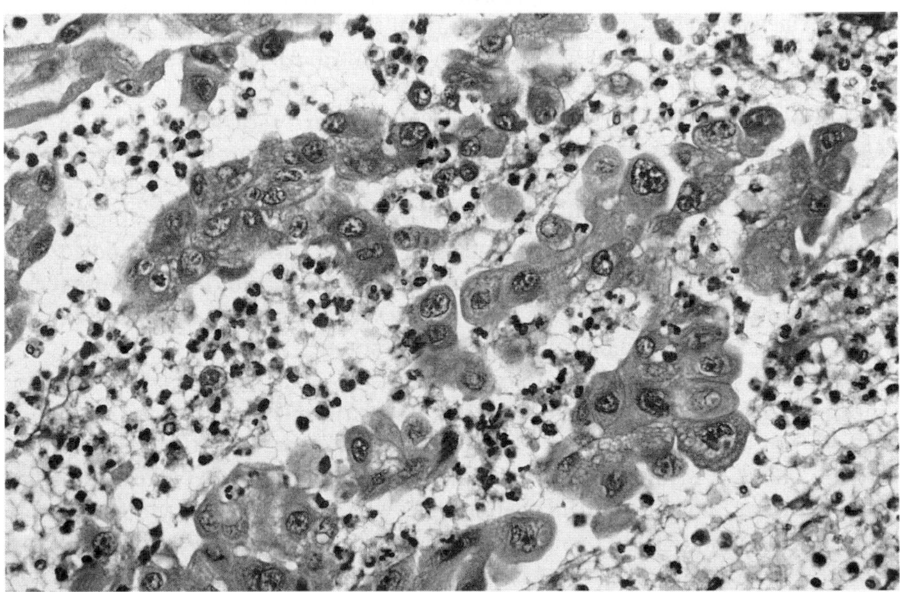

Fig. 8. Severe reactive cytological atypia in the epithelial cells from a woman with severe IUCD-associated endometritis. × 370

disturb the cyclical maturation; severe inflammation, however, interferes with the development or function of hormone receptors and cyclical changes are impaired.

On rare occasions endometritis may be the result of infection by *Actinomyces* (see below).

6 Changes in the Vagina, Cervix and Cervical Smear

A non-specific, non-infectious cervicitis occurs more often in both copper-containing and progestagen-releasing IUCD wearers (Winkler and Richart 1985; Fahmy et al. 1990) than in women using other forms of contraception. This is associated with cytological atypia in both the squamous and the columnar epithelium of the cervix (Gupta et al. 1978a) and is more severe with copper than inert devices (Misra et al. 1977). In the squamous epithelium the nuclear atypia is usually mild, but in the columnar epithelium it may be so severe as to suggest the presence of an adenocarcinoma or adenocarcinoma in situ.

The presence of organisms in the smear, in the absence of an inflammatory response, should be treated warily. In asymptomatic, sexually active healthy women using an IUCD or steroid contraceptives, the vaginal flora is more likely to contain anaerobes than is the cervix from a barrier contraceptive user (Haukkamaa et al. 1986). There are, however, no significant differences between users of copper-containing devices and progestagen-containing devices (Ulstein et al. 1987).

Candida strains are present in the vagina in 20% of IUCD wearers in whom there are no factors predisposing to infection, as compared with 6% of controls. In some the fungus is also found on the tail of the device (Parewijck et al. 1988)

The prevalence of *Actinomyces*-like organisms in cervical smears is reported as being between 11.6% (n = 973) and 2.8% (Nayar et al. 1985; Mali et al. 1986; Cleghorn and Wilkinson 1989) and the majority of these women are asymptomatic. Indeed, many of these organisms have neither the immunological nor the cultural characteristics of *Actinomyces* (Gupta et al. 1978b; Valicenti et al. 1982). Proven *Actinomyces israelii* may be found in women using copper-covered or inert plastic devices and tend to be more common when the device has been in place for several years Cleghorn and Wilkinson 1989). In the absence of inflammation *Actinomyces* can be regarded as saprophytic but in the presence of inflammation an aetiological role should be assumed.

So-called pseudo-sulphur granules (O'Brien et al. 1981, 1985) may be confused with bacterial colonies (Fig. 9). This is material that forms on the surface of IUCDs of all types and is amorphous or filamentous, eosinophilic and often partly calcified. It is composed of a mixture of leucocytes, erythrocytes, epithelial cells, sperm and bacteria, fibrillary material, which is mainly fibrin, and amorphous acellular material consisting of calcite, calcium phosphate (Khan and Wilkinson 1985) and magnesium (Rizk et al. 1990). It forms over a period of time on the surface of the device and resembles dental plaque. In a histological or cytological preparation it may be mistaken, by the unwary, for colonies of micro-

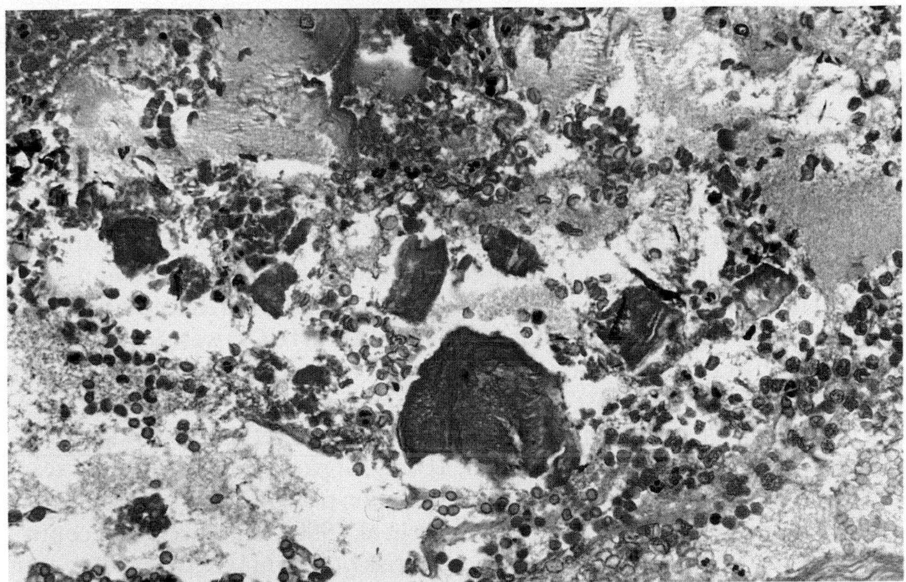

Fig. 9. The debris from the surface of an IUCD forming so-called pseudo-sulphur granules. × 370

organisms. Such deposits are found on the surface of all IUCDs, and in patients who have had heavy bleeding there is often a very thick layer of amorphous deposits (RIZK et al. 1990).

In women wearing copper-covered devices, immunoglobulin levels (IgG, IgA and IgM) in the serum and in the mucus on the tail of the device are significantly higher than in women using steroid contraception or no contraceptive (EISSA et al. 1985). It is uncertain whether this represents a response to the bacteria that are present in these patients or is a form of foreign body response to the device.

Changes in the fatty acid composition of mid-cycle lecithin in the cervical mucus, which is similar to that detected in women with unexplained primary infertility, suggests that part of the contraceptive effect of copper IUCDs may be due to changes in the cervical mucus (PSCHERA et al. 1988).

In a comparison between IUCD users and combined steroid contraceptive users, FIORE (1986) found that mild dyskaryosis was more likely to be found in the cervical smears from IUCD users (17.6%) than in those from steroid contraceptive users (10.53%).

7 Infection and the IUCD

Early reports indicated that IUCD wearers had a 1.6–3 times increased risk of developing pelvic inflammatory disease (PID), that is, infection centred on the fallopian tube and adjacent tissues, when compared with an otherwise similar group of non-users (FLESH et al. 1979; BURKMAN 1981). More recent reports (LEE et al. 1988; Kessel 1989; Kronmal et al 1991) have questioned the interpretation of the original data and have evaluated the more modern copper-covered and progestagen-releasing devices.

Case control studies which have been widely used to evaluate the risk of PID are vulnerable to bias even when carefully conducted (Edelman and Porter 1986b). Firstly, most series are hospital based and as women with acute PID who use an IUCD are more likely to be admitted to hospital than are women with PID who are not wearing an IUCD, the risk of acute PID in IUCD wearers appears higher than it really is. Secondly, case control studies only provide a comparison between the two chosen groups of women so that if there is a reduced risk of PID in women forming the control group, the risk of PID in IUCD wearers will appear relatively higher though the rate of infection may actually be similar to that of the general population. Most case-control studies have not considered the contraceptive methods of their control patients (Edelman 1985) yet there is evidence that methods of contraception other than the IUCD, in particular steroid contraceptives and barrier methods, provide some protection from PID (Keith and Berger 1985; Wolner-Hanssen et al. 1985; Buchan et al. 1990). Moreover, case control studies almost invariably reveal an increased risk of PID in IUCD wearers whilst cohort studies usually reveal an increase in only certain groups of IUCD wearers (Edelman and Porter 1986b).

In certain circumstances there is undoubtedly an increased risk of developing PID (Daling et al. 1985). There is a transient increased risk in the first few months after insertion (Mishell et al. 1966; Vessey et al. 1981; Wright and Aisien 1989; Lovset 1990), but the incidence declines the longer the device remains in place (Vessey et al. 1981). Cautious interpretation of these data is, however, required as while in asymptomatic women the device is left in place, in women with PID the device is often removed.

The risk of PID is computed to be greater for women with multiple sexual partners who are at risk of contracting sexually transmitted disease (Burkman 1981; Cramer et al. 1985; Huggins and Cullins 1990). Many believe that there is little risk for women in a monogamous relationship who are not at risk of sexually transmitted disease and who are parous at the time of insertion (Cramer et al. 1985; Lee et al. 1988; Burkman 1990; Lovset 1990).

In the Oxford Family Planning study (Buchan et al. 1990) an increased overall risk of PID was identified for non-medicated IUCD users (with 95% CI) of 3.3 (2.3–5.0); these devices are, however, no longer used. For those with medicated devices the relative risk is 1.8 (0.8–4.0) and for ex-users 1.3 (0.7–2.3). Toivonen and colleagues (1991) found that PID is less likely to develop with a device releasing 20 μg levonorgestrel per day than with a standard copper device.

The presence of an IUCD of any type may compromise the sterility of the uterine cavity (Hill et al. 1986) and small numbers of bacteria are present in the cavity of both mono- and multifilamentous tailed device wearers (Sparks et al. 1977, 1981). In contrast, devices which are tailless or ones in which the tail no longer lies in the endocervical canal will be sterile in 50% of cases (Wolf and Kriegler 1986).

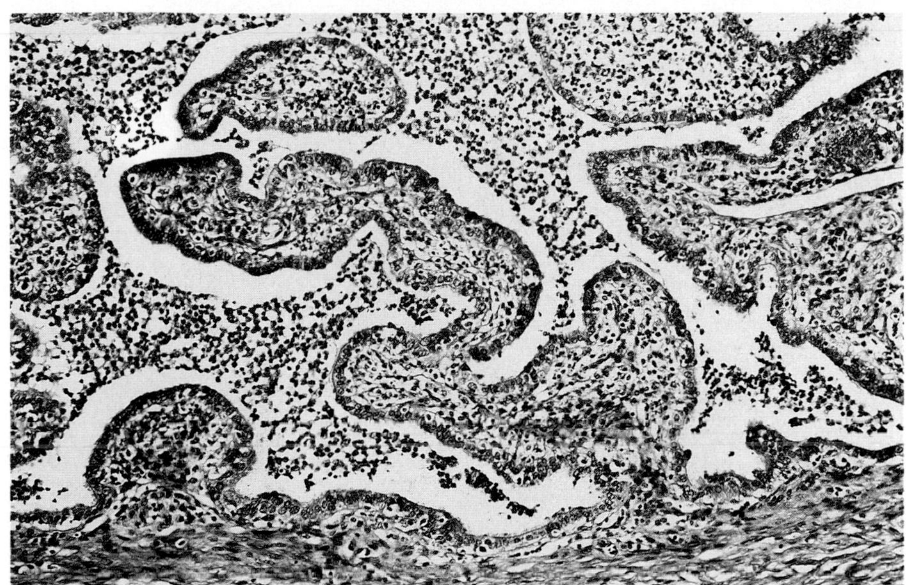

Fig. 10. A non-specific, active, chronic endosalpingitis in a patient wearing an IUCD who underwent hysterectomy for uterine leiomyomata. The mucosal folds are infiltrated by lymphocytes and the lumen contains neutrophil polymorphs, histiocytes and lymphocytes. × 120

It is important to recognise that inflammation sufficient to cause structural or functional damage to the fallopian tubes may occur in the absence of symptoms. Asymptomatic sterile, histologically proven endosalpingitis may also be detected more often in IUCD wearers than "never wearers" or former wearers during hysterectomy for non-IUCD-associated disease (Fig. 10) (Kajanoja et al. 1987; Vanlancker et al. 1987; Ghosh et al. 1989) and is more frequent in copper-device users (Vanlancker et al. 1987). At an ultrastructural level, in a small series, Wollen et al. (1990) have described a reduction in tubal epithelial cilial length, less well-orientated cilia and a reduction in the proportion of cilia with a ciliary crown.

Pelvic inflammatory disease in IUCD users may be caused by a variety of organisms, including pneumococci (Goldman et al. 1986), but is frequently polymicrobiol with a preponderance of anaerobic organisms (Landers and Sweet 1985). PID can range from minor, asymptomatic episodes of endosalpingitis to major pelvic sepsis with tubo-ovarian abscess, which may be unilateral or bilateral (Landers and Sweet 1985), local or generalised peritonitis (Brinson et al. 1986), hepatic phlebitis and intrahepatic or subphrenic abscess formation. Such complications are, however, rare and reports frequently predate the introduction of copper-containing devices.

Exceptionally, infection may be due to *Actinomyces* (Fig. 11) and may result in the development of endometritis, endocervicitis, salpingitis (Hansen 1989), ovarian abscess (Maroni and Genton 1986; de Clercq et al. 1987), tubo-ovarian abscess (Schmidt et al. 1980) abdominopelvic abscess (Yoonessi et al. 1985;

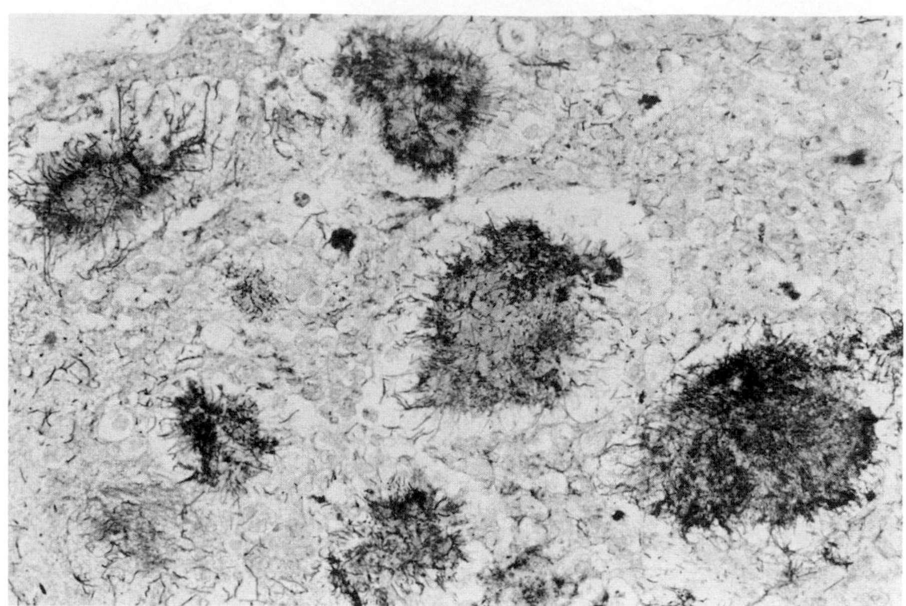

Fig. 11. Colonies of *Actinomyces* in the uterine curettings from a woman with severe endometritis. Grocott stain, × 370

MAENPAA et al. 1988) or an abdominal wall abscess (ADACHI et al. 1985). On rare occasions disseminated infection (FISHER 1980) or hepatic abscess has occurred secondary to the pelvic infection (SHURBAJI et al. 1987). Actinomycosis of the cervix may result in the formation of a cervical mass which may mimic a cervical carcinoma (SNOWMAN et al. 1989). A case in which the both *Actinomyces* and amoebae were identified in the cervical smear has also been reported in an IUCD wearer (ARROYO and QUINN 1989).

8 Pregnancy and the IUCD

Pregnancy may occur in an intra–uterine or ectopic site in IUCD users and occasionally in both simultaneously (CLAUSEN et al. 1990).

8.1 Intra-uterine Pregnancy

Unintended pregnancy occurs in less than 1 woman per 100 wearing a copper-impregnated device in the first year of use (SIVIN 1985a). The risk is similar with inert and low-dose copper devices but is lower with both modern high-dose copper devices and those delivering 20 μg levonorgestrel daily (SIVIN and SCHMIDT 1987; LOVSETT 1990; TOIVONEN et al. 1991). The cumulative gross pregnancy rate at 5 years of use is 1.1 ± 0.5 with levonorgestrel-releasing devices and 1.4 ± 0.4 for copper device users (SIVIN et al. 1990). The reason for the lower rate with progestagen-releasing devices is that they act not only locally: there is evidence that the amount of progestagen absorbed, although small, may be sufficient to disturb the pituitary ovarian axis and impair ovarian follicular development (BARBOSA et al. 1990).

Of women who conceive with an IUCD in situ ($n = 154$) (TEWS et al. 1988) up to three-quarters will request a termination of pregnancy, and of those who become pregnant when their device has been removed because of complications, 29% will request a termination (SKJELDESTAD and BRATT 1988).

With regard to the outcome of pregnancies in patients who were reported to the University of Exeter, Family Planning Research Unit, and in whom the outcome of the pregnancy was known, 27% were live births, 1% were stillbirths, 41% were terminated, 26% aborted spontaneously and 5% were ectopic (SNOWDEN et al. 1977).

Overall, approximately 50% of pregnancies that occur in IUCD wearers end in spontaneous abortion (DOMMISSE 1977). Early removal of the device can reduce this to approximately 25% (ALVIOR 1973), although abortion may occur during removal if the device lies lateral or cephalad to the foetus (SERR and SHALEV 1985). A comparison of women with and without IUCDs who presented for termination of pregnancy in Trondheim, Norway ($n = 962$) (SKJELDESTAD et al. 1988), revealed that, despite removal of the device in the first trimester, women who had an IUCD in place when they became pregnant were more likely to experience a spontaneous abortion (15.6% compared with 7.0%, $P = 0.05$). In the 1970s, mid trimester abortion accompanied by pyrexia was frequently reported (KIM-FARLEY et al. 1978). This seems to have been a hazard with a particular inert device and is no longer a problem. The adverse publicity associated with this was largely responsible for the withdrawal of the IUCD from the American market.

In pregnancies going to term, there is no evidence of an increased risk of fetal abnormalities and the device is usually found embedded in the placenta, where, if copper covered, it elicits a minor degree of focal inflammation. Occasionally, intra-uterine monilial infection of the foetus and placenta have occurred (SPAUN and KLUNDER 1986; SMITH et al. 1988; MICHAUD et al. 1989).

There is a statistically significant negative relationship between the IUCD and complete molar pregnancies (HONORÉ 1986) and a reduced risk of having a spontaneous abortion with morphological evidence suggestive of heteroploidy (HONORÉ 1985), suggesting that the IUCD may selectively inhibit chromosomally abnormal conceptuses.

The fact that some women with an IUCD become pregnant whilst others do not has led to speculation as to the reason, but few data are available. It is known, however, that in women who become pregnant there is a lower percentage of CD3+ mature T lymphocytes among the cells adherent to the device than in non-pregnant women. CD4+ cells are increased and CD8+ cells are decreased. This raises the possibility that immunological factors play a part. The percentage of B lymphocytes is similar in pregnant and non-pregnant IUCD wearers (Randic et al. 1990).

8.2 Ectopic Pregnancy

The proportion of ectopic pregnancies occurring in the fallopian tube and ovary is greater in IUCD wearers than in women using other forms of contraception (Paavonen et al. 1985). A statistically insignificant number also occur in other sites (Muzsnai et al. 1980; Goldman et al. 1988). Between 5% and 7.8% of accidental pregnancies in IUCD wearers are ectopic compared with 0.5%–1.3% in non-users (Dommisse 1977; Tatum and Schmidt 1977: Skjeldestad et al. 1988). The significance of these figures is, however, difficult to evaluate and conflicting opinions are reported.

A multinational case control study (WHO 1985) describes an increased relative risk of ectopic pregnancy of 6.4 for IUCD wearers compared with pregnant non-users matched for parity and marital status whilst Edelman and Porter (1986a), analysing published data, reached the conclusion that there is no increased risk of ectopic pregnancy in current and past users of the IUCD. The risk is, however, different for different types of device and the various series may not have compared like with like.

The lowest rate of ectopic pregnancy is found in copper device users and the highest rate in those using low-dose (2 μg/24 h) progestagen-releasing devices (WHO 1987; Sivin 1991). There is also some evidence of an increased risk of ectopic pregnancy for users of progestagen-impregnated devices delivering high doses of up to 65 μg per day (Fylling and Fagerhol 1979; Larsen et al. 1981) but the risk for those using devices delivering between 20 and 30 μg progestagen daily (Sivin 1985b) is similar to that found in wearers of copper-covered or inert devices.

Sivin (1991) analysed randomised trials of copper IUCDs and confirmed that the ectopic pregnancy rate varied, not only according to the dose of progestagen, but also inversely with the surface area of the copper on the device.

The incidence of ectopic pregnancy doubled between the eighth and ninth decades of this century and there is a consensus that the increase is related to the increased incidence of tubal damage secondary to sexually transmitted disease (Sivin 1985b). This increase has coincided with a time when the IUCD has been more widely used (Tuomivaara et al. 1986; Thorburn et al. 1987). It is important, therefore, to distinguish between an increased incidence of ectopic pregnancy in the population as a whole and that which might be attributable to the use of IUCD. Evaluation of the role of IUCD in the increased reporting of ectopic gestation is complex although multivariate analysis (Makinen et al. 1989) indicates that it does play an aetiological role.

Tubal damage is a potent and well-recognised cause of tubal ectopic pregnancy and this may be a factor in the development of ectopic pregnancy in IUCD wearers. This presupposes, however, that conception regularly occurs in IUCD users, that there is sufficient tubal damage in IUCD users to account for the increased incidence and that it is the tubal damage, together with the greater protection against intra-uterine compared with extra-uterine pregnancy afforded to IUCD wearers, which determines the tubal implantation site. This is not, however, supported by the evidence.

Firstly, in women wearing the newer, high-dose copper and progestagen-releasing IUCDs, monitoring of human chorionic gonadotropin in the latter part of the menstrual cycle indicates that covert pregnancies do not routinely occur (SEGAL et al. 1985; WILCOX et al. 1987; SIVIN 1989). Indeed, recovery of ova flushed from the fallopian tubes also shows that conception rates are lower than would be expected in normally ovulating women having unprotected coitus (ALVAREZ et al. 1988). It may be that in the past, frequent conception did play an important part in the development of ectopic pregnancies because, in women wearing an inert IUCD, conception occurs in about 20% of cycles (VIDELA-RIVERO et al. 1987).

Secondly, the ratio of ovarian to all ectopic pregnancies in IUCD wearers lies between 1:10 and 1:13 compared with 1:78 to 1:111 in a group of non-IUCD wearers (HERBERTSSON et al. 1987; SANDVEI et al. 1987) and it seems unlikely that tubal damage alone would cause this.

Thirdly, it is only in women who are at risk of developing sexually transmitted PID that the tubes are likely to be damaged, and they constitute a small proportion of wearers (see above).

The single most important clinical correlate remains the history of PID, which increases the risk of subsequent ectopic pregnancy in both pregnant and non-pregnant controls (2.8 and 2.0 relative risk respectively), and the risk may be further increased with multiple episodes of PID (HERBERTSSON et al. 1987). It may be that the reported incidence of ectopic gestation in IUCD wearers represents simply a combination of an increased risk, in certain users, of tubal damage secondary to PID, the device's somewhat reduced efficiency in preventing tubal implantation and its inefficiency in preventing ovarian implantation.

9 Long-Term Consequences of IUCD Use and Fertility

In the absence of significant PID, removal of the device, in asymptomatic women, is accompanied by the return of normal fertility as measured by the pregnancy rate; this is true independent of the type of device (RIOUX et al. 1986). RANDIC et al. (1985) found that 55.9% of women wishing to conceive became pregnant within 3 months of IUCD removal, and in longer term follow-up 94.3% conceived. In India, GUPTA et al. (1989) reported a pregnancy rate of 96.7% in the 18 months after the removal of an IUCD. The duration of use, the type of IUCD, and the timing of insertion have no influence on the return to fertility. Older age at removal is, however, associated with a reduced conception rate, which is almost certainly a consequence of the natural decline in fertility with age.

The relative risk of primary tubal infertility in nulligravid women who have ever used an IUCD lies between 2.0 and 2.6 times that in women who have never used one (Cramer et al. 1985; Daling et al. 1985). The risk has been found to be greatest for those using the Dalkon shield (3.3–6.8) and lower for those using the Lippes Loop and Saf-T-coil (2.9–3.2). The smallest risk is for those using copper-covered devices (1.6–1.9), and if they have used only a copper-covered device it is 1.3.

When insertion of an IUCD is postponed until after the first live birth, if the device is copper covered tubal infertility is not significantly increased (Cramer et al. 1985), but when inert devices were used there is a significant risk.

10 Summary

The IUCD is a simple and effective way of producing contraception without the need for patient compliance. It is not rendered ineffective by other drugs, as may be steroid contraceptives, and its side-effects, for carefully selected patients, are considered by most practitioners to be acceptably low (Van Kets et al. 1989).

References

Abramovici H, Faktor JH, Bornstein J, Sorokin Y (1987) The "forgotten" intrauterine device. Fertil Steril 47: 519–521

Adachi A, Kleiner GJ, Bezahler GH, Greston WM, Friedland GH (1985) Abdominal wall actinomycosis with an IUD. A case report. J Reprod Med 30: 145–148

Adoni A, Ben Chetrit A (1991) The management of intrauterine devices following uterine perforation. Contraception 43: 77–81

Alvarez F, Brache V, Fernandez E et al. (1988) New insights on the mode of action of intrauterine contraceptive devices in women. Fertil Steril 49: 768–773

Alvior GT Jr (1973) Pregnancy outcome with removal of intrauterine device. Obstet Gynecol 41: 894–896

Andrade AT, Pizarro-Orchard E (1987) Quantitative studies on menstrual blood loss in IUD users. Contraception 36: 129–144

Arowojolu AO, Otolorin EO, Ladipo OA (1989) Serum copper levels in users of multiload intra-uterine contraceptive devices. Afr J Med Sci 18: 295–299

Arroyo G, Quinn JA Jr (1989) Association of amoebae and actinomyces in an intrauterine contraceptive device user. Acta Cytol 33: 298–300

Badrawi HH, Van Os WA, Edelman DA, Rhemrev PE (1988) Effects of intrauterine devices on the surface ultrastructure of human endometrium before and after removal. Adv Contracept 4: 295–305

Barbosa I, Bakos O, Olsson SE, Odlind V, Johansson ED (1990) Ovarian function during use of a levonorgestrel-releasing IUD. Contraception 42: 51–66

Blaauwhof PC, Goldstuck ND (1988) Intrauterine breakage of a Multiload Cu250 intrauterine device: report of a case. Adv Contracept 4: 217–220

Bonney WA, Glasser SR, Clewe TH, Noyes RW, Cooper CL (1966) Endometrial response to the intrauterine device. Am J Obstet Gynecol 96: 101–113

Brinson RR, Kolts BE, Monif GR (1986) Spontaneous bacterial peritonitis associated with an intrauterine device. J Clin Gastroenterol 8: 82–84

Browning JJ, Bigrigg MA (1988) Recovery of the intrauterine contraceptive device from the sigmoid colon. Three case reports. Br J Obstet Gynaecol 95: 530–532

Buchan H, Villard-Mackintosh L, Vessey M, Yeates D, McPherson K (1990) Epidemiology of pelvic inflammatory disease in parous women with special reference to intrauterine device use. Br J Obstet Gynaecol 97: 780–788

Buckley CH (1987) Pathology of contraception and hormonal therapy. In: Fox H (ed) Haines and Taylor: obstetrical and gynaecological pathology. Churchill Livingstone, Edinburgh, pp 839–873

Buckley CH, Fox H (1989) Biopsy pathology of the endometrium. Chapman and Hall, London, pp 72–79

Burkman R (1981) Women's Health Study: association between intrauterine contraceptive devices and pelvic inflammatory disease. Obstet Gynecol 57: 269–276

Burkman RT (1990) Modern trends in contraception. Obstet Gynecol Clin North Am 17: 759–774

Chi IC, Wilkens L, Rogers S (1985) Expulsions in immediate postpartum insertions of Lippes loop D and Copper T IUDs and their counterpart Delta devices – an epidemiological analysis. Contraception 32: 119–134

Chi IC, Wilkens LR, Robinson N, Dominik R (1989) Cervical laceration at IUCD insertion – incidence and risk factors. Contraception 39: 507–518

Christiaens GCML, Sixma JJ, Haspels AA (1981) Haemostasis in menstrual endometrium in the presence of an intrauterine device. Br J Obstet Gynaecol 88: 825–837

Clausen I, Borium KG, Frost L (1990) Heterotopic pregnancy. The first case with an IUD in situ. Zentralbl Gynakol 112: 45–47

Cleghorn AG, Wilkinson RG (1989) The IUCD-associated incidence of *Actinomyces israelii* in the female genital tract. Aust NZ J Obstet Gynaecol 29: 445–449

Craig JM (1975) The pathology of birth control. Arch Pathol 99: 233–236

Cramer DW, Schiff I, Schoenbaum SC, et al. (1985) Tubal infertility and the intrauterine contraceptive device. N Engl J Med 312: 941 947

Custo G, Saitto C, Cerza S, Cosmi EV (1986) Intrauterine rupture of the intrauterine device "ML Cu 250": an uncommon complication: presentation of a case. Fertil Steril 45: 130–131

Daling JR, Weiss NS, Metch BJ, Chow WH, Soderstrom RM, Moore DE (1985) Primary tubal infertility in relation to the use of an intrauterine device. N Engl J Med 312: 937–941

Dallenbach-Hellweg G (1981) Histopathology of the endometrium, 3rd edn. Springer, Heidelberg Berlin New York, pp 126–256

Davis HJ (1972) Intrauterine contraceptive devices. Present status and future prospects. Am J Obstet Gynecol 114: 134–151

de Castro A, Gonzalez-Gancedo P, Contreras F, Lapena G (1986) The effect of copper ions in vivo on specific hormonal endometrial receptors. Adv Contracept 2: 399–404

de Clercq AG, Bogaerts J, Thiery M, Claeys G (1987) Ovarian actinomycosis during first trimester pregnancy. Adv Contracept 3: 167–171

Dommisse J (1977) Intra-uterine contraceptive devices. S Afr Med J 52: 495–496

Edelman DA (1985) Selection of appropriate comparison groups to evaluate PID risk in IUD users. In: Zatuchni GI, Goldsmith A, Sciarra JJ (eds) Intrauterine contraception. Advances and future prospects. Harper & Row, Philadelphia, pp 412–419

Edelman DA, Porter CW (1986a) The intrauterine device and ectopic pregnancy. Adv Contracept 2: 55–63

Edelman DA, Porter CW Jr (1986b) Pelvic inflammatory disease and the IUD. Adv Contracept 2: 313–325

Edelman DA, van Os WA (1990) Duration of use of copper releasing IUDs and the incidence of copper wire breakage. Eur J Obstet Gynecol Reprod Biol 34: 267–272

Eissa MK, Sparks RA, Newton JR (1985) Immunoglobulin levels in the serum and cervical mucus of tailed copper IUD users. Contraception 32: 87–95

El-Mahgoub BS (1980) The Norgestrel-T IUD. Contraception 22: 271–286

Ermini M, Carpino F, Petrozza V, Benagiano G (1989) Distribution and effect on the endometrium of progesterone released from a Progestasert device. Hum Reprod 4: 221–228

Fahmy K, Ismail H, Sammour M, el-Tawil A, Ibrahim M (1990) Cervical pathology with intrauterine contraceptive devices – a cyto-colpo-pathological study. Contraception 41: 317–322

Faundes A, Alvarez F, Brache V, Tejada AS (1988) The role of the levonorgestrel intrauterine device in the prevention and treatment of iron deficiency anemia during fertility regulation. Int J Gynaecol Obstet 26: 429–433

Fiore N (1986) Epidemiological data, cytology and colposcopy in IUD (intrauterine device), E-P (estro-progestogens) and diaphragm users. Study of cytological changes of endometrium IUD related. Clin Exp Obstet Gynecol 13: 34–42

Fisher MS (1980) "Miliary" actinomycosis. J Can Assoc Radiol 31: 149–150

Flesh G, Weiner J, Corlett R, et al. (1979) The intrauterine contraceptive device and acute salpingitis: a multifactor analysis. Am J Obstet Gynecol 135: 402–408

Fylling P (1987) Clinical performance of Copper T 200, Multiload 250 and Nova-T: a comparative multicentre study. Contraception 35: 439–446

Fylling P, Fagerhol M (1979) Experience with two different medicated intrauterine devices: a comparative study of the Progestasert and Nova T. Fertil Steril 31: 138–141

Ghosh K, Gupta I, Gupta SK (1989) Asymptomatic salpingitis in intrauterine contraceptive device users. Asia Oceania J Obstet Gynaecol 15: 37–40

Glew S, Singh A (1989) Uterine bleeding with an IUD requiring emergency hysterectomy. Adv Contracept 5: 51–53

Goldman GA, Dicker D, Ovadia J (1988) Primary abdominal pregnancy: can artificial abortion, endometriosis and IUD be etiological factors. Eur J Obstet Gynecol Reprod Biol 27: 139–143

Goldman JA, Yeshaya A, Peleg D, Dekel A, Dicker D (1986) Severe pneumococcal peritonitis complicating IUD: case report and review of the literature. Obstet Gynecol 41: 672–674

Goldstuck ND (1987) Insertion forces with intrauterine devices: implications for uterine perforation. Eur J Obstet Gynecol Reprod Biol 25: 315–323

Gorsline JC, Osborne NG (1985) Management of the missing intrauterine contraceptive device: report of a case. Am J Obstet Gynecol 153: 228–229

Grafenberg E (1929) cited by Zatuchni GI, Goldsmith A, Sciarra JJ (eds) (1985) Intrauterine contraception. Advances and future prospects. Harper & Row, Philadelphia, p xvii

Gupta BK, Gupta AN, Lyall S (1989) Return of fertility in various types of IUCD users. Int J Fertil 34: 123–125

Gupta PK, Burroughs F, Luff RD, Frost JK, Erozan YS (1978a) Epithelial atypias associated with intrauterine contraceptive devices (IUD). Acta Cytol 22: 286–291

Gupta PK, Erozan YS, Frost JK (1978b) Actinomycetes and the IUD: an update. Acta Cytol 22: 281–282

Hansen LK (1989) Bilateral female pelvic actinomycosis. Acta Obstet Gynecol Scand 68: 189–190

Haukkamaa M, Allonen H, Heikkila, Luukkainen T, Lahteenmaki P, Nilsson CG, Toivonen J (1985) Long-term clinical experience with levonorgestrel-releasing IUD. In: Zatuchni GI, Goldsmith A, Sciarra JJ (eds) Intrauterine contraception. Advances and future prospects. Harper & Row, Philadelphia, pp 232–237

Haukkamaa M, Stranden P, Jousimies-Somer H, Siitonen A (1986) Bacterial flora of the cervix in women using different methods of contraception. Am J Obstet Gynecol 154: 520–524

Hays D, Edelstein JA, Ahmad MM (1986) Perforation of the sigmoid colon by an intrauterine contraceptive device. Contraception 34: 413–416

Heartwell SF, Schlesselman S (1983) Risk of uterine perforation among users of intrauterine devices. Obstet Gynecol 61: 31–36

Hefnawi F, Hosni M, El-Shiekha Z, Serour GI, Hasseeb F (1975) Perforation of the uterine wall by Lippes loop in postpartum women. In: Hefnawi F, Segal SJ (eds) Analysis of intrauterine contraception. North-Holland, Amsterdam, pp 469–476

Herbertsson G, Magnusson SS, Benediktsdottir K (1987) Ovarian pregnancy and IUCD use in a defined complete population. Acta Obstet Gynecol Scand 66: 607–610

Hill JA, Talledo E, Steele J (1986) Quantitative transcervical uterine cultures in asymptomatic women using an intrauterine contraceptive device. Obstet Gynecol 68: 700–704

Honoré LH (1985) The negative effect of the IUCD on the occurrence of heteroploidy-correlated abnormalities in spontaneous abortions: an update. Contraception 31: 253–260

Honoré LH (1986) The intrauterine contraceptive device and hydatidiform mole: a negative association. Contraception 34: 213–219

Hsu CT, Hsu ML, Hsieh TM, Lin CT, Wang TT, Lin YN (1989) Uterine malignancy developing after long-term use of IUCD additional report. Asia Oceania J Obstet Gynaecol 15: 237–243

Huggins GR, Cullins VE (1990) Fertility after contraception or abortion. Fertil Steril 54: 559–573

Kajanoja P, Lang B, Wahlstrom T (1987) Intra-uterine contraceptive devices (IUDs) in relation to uterine histology and microbiology. Acta Obstet Gynecol Scand 66: 445–449

Keith LG, Berger GS (1985) The pathogenic mechanisms of pelvic infection. In: Zatuchni GI, Goldsmith A, Sciarra JJ (eds) Intrauterine contraception. Advances and future prospects. Harper & Row, Philadelphia, pp 232–237

Kessel E (1989) Pelvic inflammatory disease with intrauterine device use: a reassessment. Fertil Steril 51: 1–11

Key TC, Kreutner AK (1980) Gastrointestinal complications of modern intrauterine devices. Obstet Gynecol 55: 239–244

Khan SR, Wilkinson EJ (1985) Scanning electron microscopy, X-ray diffraction, and electron microprobe analysis of calcific deposits on intrauterine contraceptive devices. Hum Pathol 16: 732–738

Khan SR, Wilkinson EJ (1990) Bladder stone in a human female: the case of an abnormally located intrauterine contraceptive device. Scanning Microsc 4: 395–398

Kiilholma P, Makinen J, Vuori J (1989) Bladder perforation: uncommon complication with a misplaced IUD. Adv Contracept 5: 47–49

Kiilholma P, Makinen J, Maenpaa J (1990) Perforation of the uterus following IUD insertion in the puerperium. Adv Contracept 6: 57–61

Kim-Farley RJ, Cates W, Ory HW, Hatcher RA (1978) Febrile spontaneous abortion and the IUD. Contraception 18: 561–569

Kronmal RA, Whitney CW, Mumford SD (1991) The intrauterine device and pelvic inflammatory disease: the Women's Health Study reanalysed. J Clin Epidemiol 44: 109–122

Landers DV, Sweet RL (1985) Current trends in the diagnosis and treatment of tuboovarian abscess. Am J Obstet Gynecol 151: 1098–1110

Larsen S, Hansen MK, Jacobsen JC, Ladehoff P, Sorensen T, Westergaard JG (1981) Comparison between two IUDs: Progestasert and CuT 200. Contracept Deliv Syst 2: 281–286

Lee NC, Rubin GL, Borucki R (1988) The intrauterine device and pelvic inflammatory disease revisited: new results from the Women's Health Study. Obstet Gynecol 72: 1–6

Lovest T (1990) A comparative evaluation of the Multiload 250 and Multiload 375 intra-uterine contraceptive devices. Acta Obstet Gynecol Scand 69: 521–526

Luukkainen T, Allonen H, Haukkamaa M, et al. (1987) Effective contraception with the levonorgestrel-releasing intrauterine device: 12-month report of a European multicenter study. Contraception 36: 169–179

Maenpaa J, Taina E, Gronroos M, Soderstrom KO, Ristmaki T, Narhinen L (1988) Abdominopelvic actinomycosis associated with intrauterine devices. Two case reports. Arch Gynecol Obstet 243: 237–241

Makinen JI, Erkkola RU, Laippala PJ (1989) Causes of the increase in the incidence of ectopic pregnancy. A study on 1017 patients from 1966 to 1985 in Turku, Finland. Am J Obstet Gynecol 160: 642–646

Mali B, Joshi JV, Wagle U, et al. (1986) Actinomyces in cervical smears of women using intrauterine contraceptive devices. Acta Cytol 30: 367–371

Maroni ES, Genton CY (1986) IUD-associated ovarian actinomycosis causing bowel obstruction. Arch Gynecol 239: 59–62

Michaud P, Lemaire B, Tescher M (1989) Avortement spontane d'une grossesse sur DIU par chorioamniotite a *Candida*. Rev Fr Gynecol Obstet 84: 45–46

Mishell DR Jr, Moyer DL (1969) Association of pelvic inflammatory disease with the intrauterine device. Clin Obstet Gynecol 12: 179–197

Mishell DR Jr, Roy S (1982) Copper intrauterine contraceptive device event rates following insertion 4 to 8 weeks post partum. Obstet Gynecol 143: 29–35

Mishell DR Jr, Bell JH, Good RG, Moyer DL (1966) The intrauterine device: a bacteriological study of the endometrial cavity. Am J Obstet Gynecol 96: 119–126

Misra JS, Engineer AD, Tandon P (1977) Cytological studies in women using copper intrauterine devices. Acta Cytol 21: 514–518

Mittal S, Gupta I, Lata P, Mahajan U, Gupta AN (1986) Management of translocated and incarcerated intrauterine contraceptive devices. Aust NZ J Obstet Gynaecol 26: 232–234

Moyer DL, Mishell DR Jr (1971) Reactions of human endometrium to the intrauterine foreign body. 2. Long-term effects on the endometrial histology and cytology. Am J Obstet Gynecol 111: 66–80

Moyer DL, Mishell DR Jr, Bell J (1970) Reactions of the human endometrium to the intrauterine device. I. Correlation of the endometrial histology with the bacterial environment of the uterus following short-term insertion of the IUD. Am J Obstet Gynecol 106: 799–809

Murray S, Hickey JB, Houang E (1987) Significant bacteremia associated with replacement of intrauterine contraceptive device. Am J Obstet Gynecol 156: 698–700

Muzsnai D, Hughes T, Price M, Bruksch L (1980) Primary abdominal pregnancy with the IUD (2 case reports). Eur J Obstet Gynecol Reprod Biol 10: 275–278

Nayar M, Chandra M, Chitraratha K, Kumari-Das S, Rai-Chowdhary G (1985) Incidence of actinomycetes infection in women using intrauterine contraceptive devices. Acta Cytol 29: 111–116

O'Brien PK, Roth-Moyo LA, Davis BA (1981) Pseudo-sulfur granules associated with intrauterine contraceptive devices. Am J Clin Pathol 75: 822–825

O'Brien PK, Lea PJ, Roth-Moyo LA (1985) Structure of a radiate pseudocolony associated with an intrauterine contraceptive device. Hum Pathol 16: 1153–1156

Ohta T (1974) Record of Ohta ring. Ohta Ring Research Institute, 2-1, Kanda, Ogawa-machi, Chiyoda, Tokyo

Olson RO, Jones S (1967) The forgotten IUD as a cause of infertility. Review of the world literature and report of a case. Obstet Gynecol 29: 579–580

Osborne JL, Bennett MJ (1978) Removal of intra-abdominal intrauterine contraceptive devices. Br J Obstet Gynaecol 85: 868–871

Otolorin EO, Ladipo OA (1985) Comparison of intramenstrual IUD insertion with insertion following menstrual regulation. Adv Contracept 1: 45–49

Paavonen J, Varjonen-Toivonen M, Komulainen M, Heinonen PK (1985) Diagnosis and management of tubal pregnancy: effect on fertility. Int J Gynaecol Obstet 23: 129–133

Parewijck W, Claeys G, Thiery M, van Kets H (1988) Candidiasis in women fitted with an intrauterine contraceptive device. Br J Obstet Gynaecol 95: 408–410

Pike MC (1990) Reducing cancer risk in women through lifestyle-mediated changes in hormone levels. Cancer Detect Prev 14: 595–607

Porges RF (1973) Complications associated with the unsuspected presence of intrauterine contraceptive devices. Am J Obstet Gynecol 116: 579–580

Pschera H, Larsson B, Lindhe BA, Kjaeldgaard A (1988) The influence of copper intrauterine device on fatty acid composition of cervical mucus lecithin. Contraception 38: 341–348

Ragni N, Rugiati S, Rossato P, Venturini PL, Foglia G, Capitanio GL (1977) Histological and ultrastructural changes of the endometrium in women using inert and copper coiled IUDs. Acta Eur Fertil 18: 193–210

Randic L, Vlasic S, Matrljan I, Waszak CS (1985) Return to fertility after IUCD removal for planned pregnancy. Contraception 32: 253–259

Randic L, Haller H, Susa M, Rukavina D (1990) Cells adherent to copper-bearing intrauterine contraceptive devices determined by monoclonal antibodies. Contraception 42: 35–42

Richter R (1909) cited by Zatuchni GI, Goldsmith A, Sciarra JJ (eds) (1985) Intrauterine contraception. Advances and future prospects. Harper & Row, Philadelphia, p xvii

Rienprayura D, Phaosavasdi S, Semboonsuk S (1973) Cervical perforation by the copper-T intrauterine device. Contraception 7: 515–521

Rioux JE, Cloutier D, Dupont P, Lamonde D (1986) Pregnancy after IUD use. Adv Contracept 2: 185–192

Rizk M, Shaban N, Medhat I, Moby el Dien Y, Ollo MA (1990) Electron microscopic and chemical study of the deposits formed on the copper and inert IUCDs. Contraception 42: 643–653

Sandvei R, Sandstad E, Steier JA, Ulstein M (1987) Ovarian pregnancy associated with the intra-uterine contraceptive device. A survey of two decades. Acta Obstet Gynecol Scand 66: 137–141

Schmidt WA, Bedrossian CW, Ali V, Webb JA, Bastian FO (1980) Actinomycosis and intrauterine contraceptive devices – the clinicopathologic entity. Diagn Gynecol Obstet 2: 165–177

Scholten PC, Christaens GC, Haspels AA (1987) Intrauterine steroid contraceptives. Wien Med Wochenschr 137: 479–483

Schwartzwald D, Moopan UM, Tancer ML, Gomez-Leon G, Kim H (1986) Vesicouterine fistula with menouria: a complication from an intrauterine contraceptive device. J Urol 136: 1066–1067

Segal SJ, Alvarez-Sanchez F, Adejuwon CA, Brache-de-Mejia V, Leon P, Faundes A (1985) Absence of chorionic gonadotropin in sera of women who use intrauterine devices. Fertil Steril 44: 214–218

Seif MW, Aplin JD, Awad H, Wells D (1989) The effect of the intrauterine contraceptive device on endometrial secretory function: a possible mode of action. Contraception 40: 81–89

Sepulveda WH (1990) Perforation of the rectum by a Copper-T intra-uterine contraceptive device. Eur J Obstet Gynecol Reprod Biol 35: 275–278

Serr DM, Shalev J (1985) Ultrasound guidance for IUD removal in pregnancy. In: Zatuchni GI, Goldsmith A, Sciarra JJ (eds) Intrauterine contraception. Advances and future prospects. Harper & Row, Philadelphia, pp 194–197

Shaw ST (1985) Endometrial histopathology and ultrastructural changes with IUD use. In: Zatuchni GI, Goldsmith A, Sciarra JJ (eds) Intrauterine contraception. Advances and future prospects. Harper & Row, Philadelphia, pp 276–296

Shaw ST Jr, Macaulay LK, Hohman WR (1979a) Vessel density in endometrium of women with and without intrauterine contraceptive devices: a morphometric evaluation. Am J Obstet Gynecol 135: 202–206

Shaw ST Jr, Macaulay LK, Hohman WR (1979b) Morphologic studies on IUD-induced metrorrhagia. I. Endometrial changes and clinical correlations. Contraception 19: 47–61

Shaw ST Jr, Macaulay LK, Aznar R, Gonzalez-Angulo A, Roy S (1981) Effects of a progesterone-releasing intrauterine contraceptive device on the endometrial blood vessels: a morphometric study. Am J Obstet Gynecol 141: 821–827

Sheppard BL (1987) Endometrial morphological changes in IUD users: a review. Contraception 36: 1–10
Sheppard BL, Bonnar J (1985) Endometrial morphology and IUD-induced bleeding. In: Zatuchni GI, Goldsmith A, Sciarra JJ (eds) Intrauterine contraception. Advances and future prospects. Harper & Row, Philadelphia, pp 297–306
Shurbaji MS, Gupta PK, Newman MM (1987) Hepatic actinomycosis diagnosed by fine needle aspiration. A case report. Acta Cytol 31: 751–755
Silverberg SG, Haukkamaa M, Arko H, Nilsson CG, Luukkainen T (1986) Endometrial morphology during long-term use of levonorgestrel-releasing intrauterine devices. Int J Gynecol Pathol 5: 235–241
Sivin I (1985a) Intrauterine contraception. In: Zatuchni GI, Goldsmith A, Sciarra JJ (eds) Intrauterine contraception. Advances and future prospects. Harper & Row, Philadelphia, pp 70–78
Sivin I (1985b) IUD-associated ectopic pregnancies, 1974 to 1984. In: Zatuchni GI, Goldsmith A, Sciarra JJ (eds) Intrauterine contraception. Advances and future prospects. Harper & Row, Philadelphia, pp 340–353
Sivin I (1989) IUDs are contraceptives, not abortifacients: a comment on research and belief. Stud Fam Plann 20: 355–359
Sivin I (1991) Dose-and age-dependent ectopic pregnancy risks with intrauterine contraception. Obstet Gynecol 78: 291–298
Sivin I, Schmidt F (1987) Effectiveness of IUDs: a review. Contraception 36: 55–84
Sivin I, Stern J, Diaz MM, et al. (1987) Two years of intrauterine contraception with levonorgestrel and with copper: a randomized comparison of the TCu 380Ag and levonorgestrel 20 mcg/day devices. Contraception 35: 245–255
Sivin I, el Mahgoub S, McCarthy T, Mishell DR Jr, Shoupe D, Alvarez F (1990) Long-term contraception with the levonorgestrel 20mcg/day (LNg 20) and the copper T 380Ag intrauterine devices: a five-year randomized study. Contraception 42: 361–378
Skjeldestad F, Bratt H (1988) Fertility after complicated and non-complicated use of IUDs: a controlled prospective study. Adv Contracept 4: 179–184
Skjeldestad FE, Hammervold R, Peterson DR (1988) Outcomes of pregnancy with an IUD in situ – a population based case-control study. Adv Contracept 4: 265–270
Smith CV, Horenstein J, Platt LD (1988) Intraamnoiotic infection with *Candida albicans* associated with a retained intrauterine contraceptive device: a case report. Am J Obstet Gynecol 159: 123–124
Snowden R, Williams M, Hawkins D (1977) The IUD: a practical guide. Croom Helm, London, p 38
Snowman BA, Malviya VK, Brown W, Malone JM Jr, Deppe G (1989) Actinomycosis mimicking pelvic malignancy. Int J Gynaecol Obstet 30: 283–286
Sparks RA, Purrier BGA, Watt PJ, Elstein M (1977) The bacteriology of the cervix and uterus. Br J Obstet Gynaecol 84: 701–704
Sparks RA, Purrier BGA, Watt PJ, Elstein M (1981) Bacteriological colonisation of the uterine cavity: role of tailed intrauterine contraceptive device. Br Med J 282: 1189–1191
Spaun E, Klunder K (1986) Candida chorioamnionitis and intrauterine contraceptive device. Acta Obstet Gynecol Scand 65: 183–184
Tadesse E, Wamstcker K (1985) Evaluation of 24 patients with IUD-related problems: hysteroscopic findings. Eur J Obstet Gynecol Reprod Biol 19: 37–41
Tamada T, Okagaki T, Maruyama M, Matsumoto S (1967) Endometrial histology associated with an intrauterine contraceptive device. Am J Obstet Gynecol 98: 811–817
Tatum HJ, Schmidt FH (1977) Contraceptive and sterilization practices and extrauterine pregnancy: a realistic perspective. Fertil Steril 28: 407–421
Tews G, Arzi W, Stoger H (1988) 74 Schwangerschaften trotz liegendem IUD. Geburtshilfe Frauenheilkd 48: 349–351
Thiery M, Van Kets H, Van der Pass H (1985) Immediate post-placental IUD insertion: the expulsion problem. Contraception 31: 331–349
Thomalla JV (1986) Perforation of urinary bladder by intrauterine device. Urology 27: 260–264
Thorburn J, Friberg B, Schubert W, Wassen AC, Lindblom B (1987) Background factors and management of ectopic pregnancy in Sweden. Changes over a decade. Acta Obstet Gynecol Scand 66: 597–602
Timonen H, Kurppa K (1987) IUD perforation leading to obstructive nephropathy necessitating nephrectomy: a rare complication. Adv Contracept 3: 71–75
Toivonen J, Luukkainen T, Allonen H (1991) Protective effect of intrauterine release of levonorgestrel on pelvic infection: three years' comparative experience of levonorgestrel- and copper-releasing intrauterine devices. Obstet Gynecol 77: 261–264

Tsalikis T, Stamatopoulos P, Kalachanis J, Mantalenakis S (1986) Experience with the MLCu250 IUD. Adv Contracept 2: 393–398

Tuomivaara L, Kauppila A, Puolakka J (1986) Ectopic pregnancy – an analysis of the etiology, diagnosis and treatment in 552 cases. Arch Gynecol 237: 135–147

Ulstein M, Steier AJ, Hofstad T, Digranes A, Sandvei R (1987) Microflora of cervical and vaginal secretion in women using copper- and norgestrel-releasing IUCDs. Acta Obstet Gynecol Scand 66: 321–322

Valicenti JF, Pappas AA, Graber CD, Williamson HO, Willis NF (1982) Detection and prevalence of IUD-associated *Actinomyces* colonization and related morbidity – a prospective study of 69 925 cervical smears. JAMA 247: 1149–1152

Vanlancker M, Dierick AM, Thiery M, Claeys G (1987) Histologic and microbiologic findings in the fallopian tubes of IUD users. Adv Contracept 3: 147–157

van Kets HE, Thiery M, van der Pas H, Dieben TO (1989) Long-term experience with Multiload intrauterine devices. Adv Contracept 5: 179–188

Van Os WA, Edelman DA (1989) Uterine perforation and use of the Multiload IUD. Adv Contracept 5: 121–126

Vessey MP, Yeates D, Flavel R, McPherson K (1981) Pelvic inflammatory disease and the intrauterine device: findings in a large cohort study. Br Med J 282: 855–857

Videla-Rivero L, Etchepareborda JJ, Kesseru E (1987) Early chorionic activity in women bearing inert IUD, copper IUD and levonorgestrel-releasing IUD. Contraception 36: 217–226

Wilcox AJ, Weinberg CR, Armstrong EG, Canfield RE (1987) Urinary human chorionic gonadotropin among intrauterine device users: detection with a highly specific and sensitive assay. Fertil Steril 47: 265–269

Winkler B, Richart RM (1985) Cervical/uterine pathologic considerations in pelvic infection. In: Zatuchni GI, Goldsmith A, Sciarra JJ (eds) Intrauterine contraception. Advances and future prospects. Harper & Row, Philadelphia, pp 438–449

Wolf AS, Kriegler D (1986) Bacterial colonization of intrauterine devices (IUDs). Arch Gynecol 239: 31–37

Wollen AL, Flood PR, Sanvei R (1990) Altered ciliary substructure in the endosalpinx in women using an IUCD. Acta Obstet Gynecol Scand 69: 307–312

Wolner-Hanssen P, Svensson L, Mardh PA, Westrom L (1985) Laparoscopic findings and contraceptive use in women with signs and symptoms suggestive of acute salpingitis. Obstet Gynecol 66: 233–238

World Health Organization's Special Programme of Research, Development and Research Training in Human Reproduction (1985) Task Force on Intrauterine Devices for Fertility Regulation. A multinational case-control study of ectopic pregnancy. Clin Reprod Fertil 3: 131–143

World Health Organization's Special Programme of Research, Development and Research Training in Human Reproduction (1987) Task Force on Intrauterine Devices for Fertility Regulation. Microdose intrauterine levonorgestrel for contraception. Contraception 35: 363–379

Wright EA, Aisien AO (1989) Pelvic inflammatory disease and the intrauterine contraceptive device. Int J Gynaecol Obstet 28: 133–136

Yoonessi M, Crickard K, Cellino IS, Satchidanand SK, Fett W (1985) Association of actinomyces and intrauterine contraceptive devices. J Reprod Med 30: 48–52

Subject Index

Index of Volumes 83–85 Current Topics in Pathology

Volume 83: Cell Receptors. Edited by G. Seifert

P. Karlson, Historical Development of the Receptor Concept
R. D. Hesch, Classification of Cell Receptors
H. Jüppner, R. D. Hesch, Biochemical Characterization of Cellular Hormone Receptors
M. Dietel, Morphological Characterization of Cell Receptors
D. Richter, W. Meyerhof, F. Buck, S. D. Morley, Molecular Biology of Receptors for Neuropeptide Hormones
J. Lloyd, R. Tibolt, G. V. Childs, Peptide Hormone Receptors
I. Damjanov, Growth Factor Receptors
A. Niendorf, U. Beisiegel, Low Density Lipoprotein Receptors
A. Probst, G. Mengod, J. M. Palacios, Neurotransmitter Receptors in Human Brain Diseases
M. Vierbuchen, Lectin Receptors
E. V. Jensen, Steroid Hormone Receptors
H. Höfler, Oncogene and Receptor Expression
H.-E. Stegner, W. Jonat, Breast Carcinoma
N. Wernert, G. Seitz, Prostatic Cancer – Immunohistochemistry of Steroid Hormone Receptors
M. R. Parwaresch, H. Kreipe, H. J. Radzun, G. Griesser, Malignant Lymphomas – Lineage Specific Receptors in the Diagnosis of Malignant Lymphomas and Myelomonocytic Neoplasias

Volume 84/1: Reaction Patterns of the Lymph Node.
Edited by E. Grundmann, E. Vollmer

A. Castenholz, Architecture of the Lymph Node with Regard to Its Function
G. Sainte-Marie, C. Bélisle, F. S. Peng, The Deep Cortex of the Lymph Node: Morphological Variations and Functional Aspects
S. Fossum, Differences Between Lymph Node Structure and Function in Normal and Athymic Rats
P. P. H. de Bruyn, Y. Cho, Structure and Function of High Endothelial Postcapillary Venules in Lymphocyte Circulation
F. G. M. Kroese, W. Timens, P. Nieuwenhuis, Germinal Center Reaction and B Lymphocytes: Morphology and Function
J. J. van den Oord, F. Facchetti, J. Delabie, C. de Wolf-Peeters, T. Lymphocytes in Non-neoplastic Lymph Nodes

B. Brado, P. Möller, The Plasmacytoid T Cell or Plasmacytoid Monocyte – A Sessile Lymphoid Cell with Unique Immunophenotype and Unknown Function, Still Awaiting Lineage Affiliation
H.-H. Wacker, H. J. Radzun, M. R. Parwaresch, Accessory Cells in Normal Human and Rodent Lymph Nodes: Morphology, Phenotype, and Functional Implications
E. W. A. Kamperdijk, E. B. J. van Nieuwkerk, M. A. M. Verdaasdonk, E. C. M. Hoefsmit, Macrophages in Different Compartments on the Non-neoplastic Lymph Node
S. Bödewadt-Radzun, H.-H. Wacker, H. J. Radzun, M. R. Parwaresh, Phenotypic Characterization of Macrophages in Non-neoplastic Lymph Nodes
M.-L. Hansmann, H.-H. Wacker, Immunoelectron-microscopic Investigations of Lymph Nodes

Volume 84/2: Reaction Patterns of the Lymph Node.
Edited by E. Grundmann, E. Vollmer

E. Vollmer, V. Krieg, F. Shimamoto, E. Grundmann, Reaction Patterns of Lymph Nodes in the Development and Spread of Cancer
N. Beck, D. Lorke, P. Möller, Patterns of Fibronection Induction in Lymph Nodes Affected by Metastatic Growth of Adenocarcinomas
E. Vollmer, F. Shimamoto, V. Krieg, E. Grundmann, Macrophages/ Reticulum Cells in Early and Late Phases of Lymphogenous Matastasis
H. Cottier, R. Kraft, F. Meister, Primary Immunodeficiency Syndromes and Their Manifestations in Lymph Nodes
G. R. F. Krueger, D. V. Ablashi, P. Lusso, S. F. Josephs, Immunological Dysregulation of Lymph Nodes in AIDS Patients
J. Diebold, J. Audouin, A. Le Tourneau, S. Prevot, G. Szekeres, Lymph Node Reaction Patterns in Patients with AIDS or AIDS-Related Complex

Volume 85: Gynecological Tumors. Edited by N. Sasano

G. Dallenbach-Hellweg, Endometrial Carcinomas
S. G. Silverberg, Mixed Müllerian Tumors
K. Noda, Cervical Intraepithelial Neoplasia and Microinvasive Carcinoma of the Cervix
R. Kudo, Cervical Adenocarcinoma
R. H. Young, R. E. Scully, Endocrine Tumors of the Ovary
A. Talerman, Germ Cell Tumors
Y. Tomoda, T. Ishizuka, S. Goto, Y. Furuhashi, Trophoblastic Disease
M. K. Sidawy, Cytology in Gynecological Disorders
T. Okagaki, Impact of Human Papillomavirus Research on the Histopathologic Concepts of Genital Neoplasms
G. Ueda, M. Yamasaki, Neuroendocrine Carcinoma of the Uterus
D. A. Bell, Flow Cytometry of Ovarian Neoplasms
H. Sasano, C. T. Garrett, Oncogenes in Gynecological Tumors

Springer-Verlag and the Environment

We at Springer-Verlag firmly believe that an international science publisher has a special obligation to the environment, and our corporate policies consistently reflect this conviction.

We also expect our business partners – paper mills, printers, packaging manufacturers, etc. – to commit themselves to using environmentally friendly materials and production processes.

The paper in this book is made from low- or no-chlorine pulp and is acid free, in conformance with international standards for paper permanency.